THE **BEAUTY** BIBLE

From acne to
wrinkles and
everything in
between

Every woman's skin-care
and makeup application guide

By
Paula Begoun

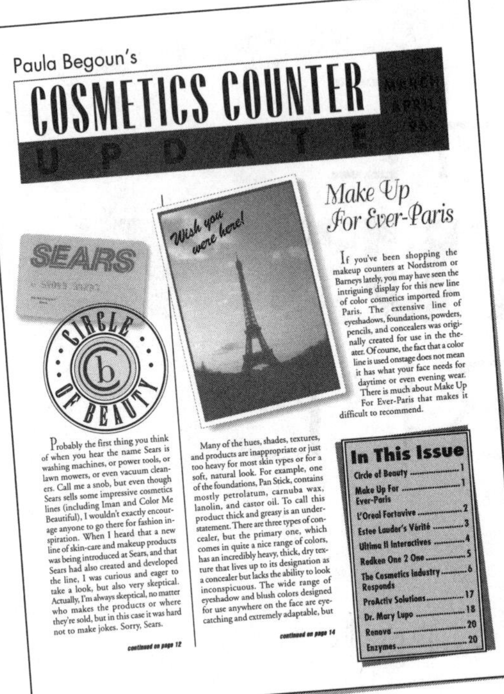

Paula Begoun's

COSMETICS COUNTER UPDATE

SEARS

CIRCLE OF BEAUTY

Wish you were here!

Make Up For Ever-Paris

If you've been shopping the makeup counters at Nordstrom or Barneys lately, you may have seen the intriguing display for this new line of color cosmetics imported from Paris. The extensive line of eyeshadows, foundations, powders, pencils, and concealers was originally created for use in the theater. Of course, the fact that a color line is used onstage does not mean it has what your face needs for daytime or even evening wear. There is much about Make Up For Ever-Paris that makes it difficult to recommend.

Probably the first thing you think of when you hear the name Sears is washing machines, or power tools, or lawn mowers, or even vacuum cleaners. Call me a snob, but even though Sears sells some impressive cosmetics lines (including Iman and Color Me Beautiful), I wouldn't exactly encourage anyone to go there for fashion inspiration. When I heard that a new line of skin-care and makeup products was being introduced at Sears, and that Sears had also created and developed the line, I was curious and eager to take a look, but also very skeptical. Actually, I'm always skeptical, no matter who makes the products or where they're sold, but in this case it was hard not to make jokes. Sorry, Sears.

continued on page 12

Many of the hues, shades, textures, and products are inappropriate or just too heavy for most skin types or for a soft, natural look. For example, one of the foundations, Pan Stick, contains mostly petrolatum, carnuba wax, lanolin, and castor oil. To call this product thick and greasy is an understatement. There are three types of concealer, but the primary one, which comes in quite a nice range of colors, has an incredibly heavy, thick, dry texture that lives up to its designation as a concealer but lacks the ability to look inconspicuous. The wide range of eyeshadow and blush colors designed for use anywhere on the face are eye-catching and extremely adaptable, but

continued on page 14

In This Issue

Also by Paula Begoun:

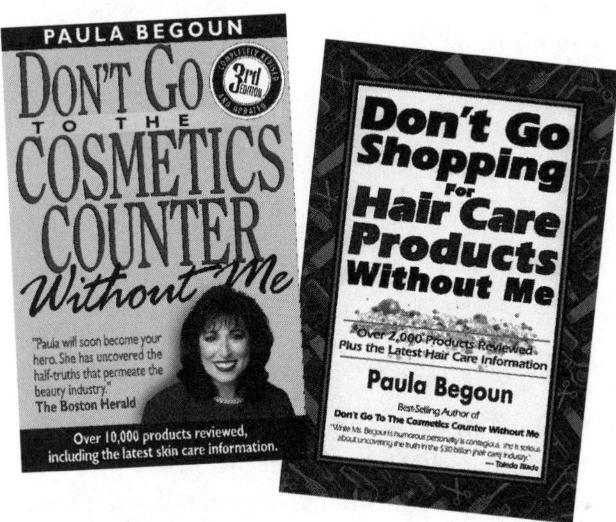

Don't Go to the Cosmetics Counter Without Me, 3rd Edition

$16.95 US

Don't Go Shopping for Hair Care Products Without Me

$14.95 US

To order any of these titles, please send a check for the total price of each book, plus $3 per book for shipping and handling/$4.50 US per book to Canada/$12 US per book to Australia, to:

Beginning Press
5418 South Brandon
Seattle, Washington 98118

To order call (800) 831-4088
Visa, MasterCard, American Express, and Discover accepted

Visit Paula at her Web site: http://www.cosmeticscop.com

Editors: Miriam Bulmer, Sherri Schultz, Kris Fulsaas, and Laura Kraemer
Art Direction, Cover Design, and Typography: Studio Pacific, Inc.
Printing: Publishers Press, Salt Lake City, Utah
Research Assistants: Kristin Folsom, Laura Kraemer, and Rachel Permann

Publisher: Beginning Press
5418 South Brandon
Seattle, Washington 98118

First Printing for this edition: November 1997

ISBN 1-877988-22-7
1 2 3 4 5 6 7 8 9 10

This book is distributed to the United States book trade by:

Publishers Group West
4065 Hollis Street
Emeryville, California 94608
(800) 788-3123

and to the Canadian book trade by:

Raincoast Books Limited
8680 Cambie Street
Vancouver, B.C., Canada V6P 6M9
(604) 323-7100

Table of Contents

TABLE OF **CONTENTS**

TABLE OF **CONTENTS**

Chapter Three—Sun Sense

Chapter Four—Understanding Skin Type

Chapter Five—Skin-Care Planning

TABLE OF **CONTENTS**

Chapter Nine—Body Care

TABLE OF **CONTENTS**

Chapter Ten—Problems? Solutions!

Chapter Eleven—Animal Rights

Appendix—Ingredient Dictionary

Note from the Publisher

The intent of this book is to present the author's ideas and perceptions about the marketing, selling, and use of cosmetics. The author's sole purpose is to present consumer information and advice regarding the purchase of makeup and skin-care products. The information and recommendations presented strictly reflect the author's opinions, perceptions, and knowledge about the subject and products mentioned. Some women may find success with a particular product that is not recommended or even mentioned herein, or they may be partial to a $250 skin-care routine. It is everyone's inalienable right to judge products by their own criteria, research, and standards and to disagree with the author.

More important, because everyone's skin can, and probably will, react to an external stimulus at some time, any product could cause a negative reaction on your skin at one time or another. If you develop a skin sensitivity to a cosmetic, stop using it immediately and consult your physician. If you need medical advice about your skin, it is best to consult a dermatologist.

Preface

Let Me Introduce Myself

I am the author and publisher of several best-selling books on the cosmetics industry: *Blue Eyeshadow Should Be Illegal* (which was revised four times and reprinted dozens more), *Don't Go to the Cosmetics Counter Without Me* (now in its third edition), and *Don't Go Shopping for Hair Care Products Without Me.* I am a syndicated columnist with Knight Ridder News Tribune Service and I have a regular column in the *New York Daily News.* Over the years my writing has been strictly based on my earnest desire to get beyond the hype and chicanery of the cosmetics industry and to disseminate straightforward information a consumer can really use to look and feel more beautiful.

I am not a cosmetic chemist, a doctor, or a scientist of any kind. My expertise is, like that of any other consumer reporter who covers such topics as food, cars, or toys, based on extensive research in the area I am writing about. What makes my situation unique is that I also have years of personal experience from working as a professional makeup artist and esthetician, and from selling makeup and skin-care products at department stores, salons, and my own stores.

I have used my reporting background to continually and extensively research the cosmetics industry over the past 14 years. I base all my comments on comprehensive interviews with dermatologists, oncologists, cosmetic chemists, and cosmetic ingredient manufacturers and on information I've gleaned from cosmetic industry magazines and medical journals. I am constantly reviewing scientific abstracts and studies. I do not capriciously or abruptly make any conclusions. Everything I report is supported by studies and information from experts in the field. Naturally, there are many who disagree with my assertions, and I do the best I can to present other points of view whenever I can. However, I assure you a great number of people in the industry agree with my conclusions, even if they can't do so publicly.

In many ways I am surprised that reviewing, researching, investigating, and questioning the cosmetics industry is what I do for a living. It never was my intent when I started out as a makeup artist and facialist. But a single-minded course of action and purpose has followed me since 1978, when I started doing makeup, as I've tried to uncover the truth inside the bottles and behind the sales pitches of the cosmetics industry.

At first my quest was personal. I had suffered with acne for many years. I visited over a dozen dermatologists, I tried hundreds of skin-care products from both inexpensive and expensive cosmetics lines, and still I had acne. How could that be? How could all the stuff I diligently applied to my skin, which salesperson after salesperson and doctor after doctor assured me would work, not work? Sometimes one worked a little, but not as well as I hoped and not for very long. And there were always side effects. Most products made my skin so red and irritated I thought it was going to fall off. Slowly but surely I worked my way through the confusion, and after much research and lots more frustration I began to recognize some fundamental problems with the cosmetics industry and the field of dermatology.

The cosmetics industry's information was little more than marketing mumbo jumbo. In the field of dermatology, research was lacking (at least in those days) and most doctors didn't have time to give patients the information they needed or to explain the limitations of treatment.

In truth, I started out wanting to be an actress, and being a makeup artist was only a way to pay the rent. In a very short time it became clear to me that I wasn't going to enjoy much success at acting, or at least I didn't have what it takes to persevere, but I did have what it takes to be a good makeup artist and skin-care consultant. My clientele quickly grew, as did my income. I definitely preferred a paycheck to struggling with acting auditions and rejections. Of course, that didn't mean everything was rosy. Along the way, when my free-lance makeup business was slow, I tried to supplement my income with work at department-store makeup counters. But each new job for a different cosmetics line resulted in my being fired.

My first dismissal was after an argument with the line representative, who wanted me to say a toner could close pores and a moisturizer could heal when I knew that wasn't true. (If a toner could close pores, everyone who used toners would have flawless, poreless skin, and if moisturizers could heal skin, no one would have a pimple or a wrinkle.)

Several months later I was involved in a brouhaha with several of the cosmetics saleswomen working at the other counters. If a customer wanted a particular type of product and I didn't think the product from the line I was selling was right or if my line didn't offer one, I would walk her over to another counter that I knew had the right product and sell it to her. That caused a nuclear meltdown. I was told to stay behind my counter and not touch another product from any line other than the one I was assigned! (When I recommended the woman walk over to the other counter herself, I would then get in trouble with the sales representatives from my line.) How ludicrous. A great product, five feet away, was out of my reach because it wasn't from my counter.

PREFACE

My final department-store cosmetics counter experience ended when I just couldn't take listening to the distortions and exaggerated claims anymore and decided to go out on my own. I opened my own makeup stores, Generic Makeup, in 1981. I didn't sell blue eyeshadow, wrinkle creams, or toners that claimed to close pores. Along the way, I hooked up with a business partner who was at first thrilled with my ideas and concept, mainly because of all the publicity they attracted.

In their own way the stores were rather controversial, which got me a lot of media attention. Eventually I was asked to make regular appearances on a local TV station in Seattle, KIRO-TV. I also started receiving some national and international TV and print exposure.

Eventually none of this pleased my partner. The department-store counters were bombarded by women buying blue eyeshadow, wrinkle creams, and toners, so shouldn't we sell them too? My philosophy was not to take advantage of the consumer the way everyone else was, and to my partner that was untenable. After all, if you saw women throwing away their money on those sorts of products, at prices ranging from $25 to $250 an ounce for items that cost $1 to $2 to produce, you wouldn't want a partner like me either. I sold my shares back to her in 1984 and stayed at KIRO-TV for the next two years. Sadly, the stores went out of business shortly after I sold them—but I learned a lot about investigative reporting and writing.

I left the TV station in 1986 after finishing my first book, *Blue Eyeshadow Should Be Illegal.* I decided to self-publish after I received several rejection letters from major publishing companies telling me that they liked my manuscript, but because I wasn't a celebrity or model, no one would be interested in my point of view. I disagreed. I believed lots of (OK, not all) women were tired of hearing useless information from models and celebrities who were born beautiful and knew the right managers to hire, but little more.

I was right, and I sold several hundred thousand copies of my first book! At that point I thought I would go on to something else, like writing the great American novel. I felt I had done my job and written down everything my research and experience in the world of skin care and makeup had taught me. I believed I had given the consumer what she needed to tackle the cosmetics industry with more balanced, complete information.

I was wrong. After I wrote *Blue Eyeshadow,* I received thousands of letters from women asking me, now that they knew how crazy the cosmetics industry was, what they should buy or what I thought of this product or that. It was one thing to have an overview of the cosmetics industry, another to have specific information about a product you are thinking of buying or being enticed to buy because it was formulated by some doctor or pharmacist, or had impressive studies demonstrating its outstanding effectiveness. (It's amazing how many bogus studies I've run into, performed on behalf of thousands of products.) That's when I wrote *Don't Go to the Cosmetics Counter Without Me.* (Besides, my sister, mother, and women friends wouldn't stop asking me to go shopping for makeup, skin-care products, or hair-care products with them, and I just couldn't keep up.)

The demand to know what works and what doesn't has grown, mostly because the industry has grown. The number of new product lines emerging every day is sheer madness. What with infomercial lines, multilevel direct marketing lines, home shopping network lines, new department-store and drugstore lines, and the endless parade of new product launches from existing cosmetic lines, my job was only beginning.

That brings me to this latest book. The cosmetics industry has gone through many changes since I wrote *Blue Eyeshadow.* In many ways it has gotten more complicated as research into skin and skin-care products has increased. My goal with *The Beauty Bible* is to compile and clarify all the new data and research to help each woman create the best skin-care routine for her specific needs, as well as the best makeup look in the fewest steps with the easiest and most effective techniques. I also want to separate fact from fiction, because the fiction spread by the cosmetics industry is nothing less than startling (it makes Mother Goose look like the Encyclopedia Britannica).

The amazing number of letters I receive from women asking me to continue doing what I'm doing and the wonderful thank-you letters I receive daily are gratifying and encouraging. Sometimes I absolutely need the encouragement. Cosmetics counters are not friendly places for me. As I have become better known, I often receive a cold shoulder and a quick comment like "You can get that information from calling the company" or "Let me speak to my manager first." Not exactly what you would call a cordial reception. But perhaps the most difficult part is keeping a straight face when I hear the crazy things cosmetics salespeople tell consumers. Combatting this endless parade of useless and bizarre information can be maddening. But it's my job, and it has been far more rewarding than I ever expected.

Giving Thanks

Although I complain profusely about the way cosmetics companies can invent or twist the truth about their products, and about the way some cosmetics companies won't grant me interviews, I want to give my heartfelt thanks to the companies that actually do provide me with information and interviews. I know this might seem like a strange departure, given that I don't always agree with what I'm sent or told, but these courtesies are welcomed and appreciated more than I can say. It is my intent to provide the best information possible, and whenever I can see things from the cosmetics industry's point of view it makes my reporting that much more accurate. Granted, it often adds fuel to my ire about false claims and misleading information, but it also helps me tell consumers when and where to find some wonderful products.

I tend to harp on the negative and crazy claims, prices, and poor quality, but the major reason I do what I do is because the cosmetics world does offer so many amazing products. The parade of superlative makeup and skin-care products is nothing less than exciting. I am hardly anti-makeup or anti–skin care. Far from it. I am in awe of how well most cosmetics work. Where would we be without the brilliant cosmetic chemists who make the exquisite products we use? Thanks to their astonishing skill we have moisturizers that take care of dry skin, mascaras that build thick, lush lashes without flaking or smearing, foundations that smooth out skin tone, sunscreens that protect skin from sunburn as well as from wrinkles and skin cancer, lipsticks that add elegant color and definition to the mouth, blushes that softly accent cheekbones, and, well, the list is endless.

I want to sincerely thank all the cosmetics companies who have provided so much of their time and information to me for this book, as well as for my newsletter and my other books. We often don't see eye to eye, but despite our differences more companies than ever have been generous and forthcoming with information and products.

I want to thank all cosmetic chemists everywhere who strive to produce better and better products that continue to make the beauty industry so incredibly beautiful. I also want to ask cosmetic chemists to do the best they can, whenever they can, to combat the insane marketing departments they have to work with. I know most of you don't believe even a fraction of what the advertisements, salespeople, infomercial hucksters, or editorials in fashion magazines say about the products you create. Your work is rooted in science, not hyperbole. I know you would be taking a risk. After all, creating products that no one buys is not going to get anyone a promotion, and the marketing department knows all too well what women want to hear, no matter how ridiculous. But try anyway, just to add a bit of fresh air into an otherwise very cloudy business.

CHAPTER ONE

In the Beginning . . .

Separating Good from Bad

Just after Adam and Eve ate from the Tree of Knowledge, as the story goes, they became aware of the difference between good and bad. I've often wondered if Eve didn't right then and there look at her naked body and notice all the cellulite on her thighs, the wrinkles under her eyes, and the dry patches on her cheeks, and think to herself that she was in desperate need of a manicure. Of course, Adam simply grabbed a fig leaf, gave himself a once-over, and declared he was "looking good!"—but that's another story altogether.

History and literature are filled with stories of a woman's need, at any age, to feel and look beautiful. Women expect—and are expected—for better or worse, to attain the nirvana of flawless skin and the elite status of classic or exotic beauty. What is so damnably frustrating about this ever-present feminine need is that perfection is fleeting and beauty is always being redefined. Contemplating the variety of ideals embodied by Kate Moss, Marilyn Monroe, Cindy Crawford, Elizabeth Taylor, and RuPaul is enough to give anyone a beauty of a headache.

Adding to the confusion is the cosmetics industry, which steps in claiming to champion a woman's desire to be beautiful, or at the very least attractive, and offering an arsenal of products that promise eternal youth, luminous skin, and enhanced sensuality. Women are eager consumers in this arena, ready and willing to buy the latest concoction that boasts of being able to close pores, erase wrinkles, heal blemishes, smooth skin, and eliminate irritation and redness. The cosmetics industry annually does $35 billion worth of business in the United States alone, and the primary consumers are women. Being attractive, whether it is genetically inherited or personally created, is a powerful statement for many women.

Readers who know my other books, *Don't Go to the Cosmetics Counter Without Me, Don't Go Shopping for Hair Care Products Without Me,* and *Blue Eyeshadow Should Be Illegal,* are already well aware of my love/hate relationship with the world of cosmetics and skin care. We all know there are an astounding number of truly effective beauty products available. I am in awe of the remarkable and varied items cosmetic chemists have created. If you want long, thick lashes, you can find wonderful mascaras that produce the desired effect. If you have dry skin, any number of moisturizers can provide soothing results. Did somebody say sunscreen protection? Voilá! Richly colored lips, more shape to the cheekbones, smoother skin tone—drugstores and department stores alike carry more than enough lipsticks, blushes, and foundations to add whatever is missing.

Yet the other side of the cosmetics coin can be devastating. Many products can irritate and hurt the skin, poor sunscreen formulations and photosensitizing ingredients can put the skin at risk for cancer and allergic reactions, heavy foundations can look like a mask on the face, the wrong lipsticks will bleed or peel off, and moisturizers can oversaturate the skin, causing breakouts or, worse, impeding the skin's healing ability. And what about the absurdly distorted prices that those inside the world of cosmetics laugh about behind the backs of unsuspecting, gullible women?

Protecting as well as supporting this insanity is an information system guaranteed to keep women deluded and deceived. Most women get their skin-care information from cosmetics salespeople (who are rarely, if ever, skin-care or makeup experts) and fashion magazines (which are supported by advertising for cosmetics). Neither of these sources has a reason in the world to tell you, for example, that a sunscreen, despite the fact that it is labeled SPF 15, may still put you at risk for skin cancer because it does not contain the only three ingredients approved by the federal Food and Drug Administration (FDA) that can block over 80% of ultraviolet A (UVA) radiation. (UVA rays cause cancer and wrinkling, while UVB rays cause sunburn.) Can you imagine *Allure* or *Vogue* publishing articles explaining that Borghese, Lancome, Pond's, or Oil of Olay sells products that expose your skin to serious sun damage? Not in this lifetime, even though that may indeed be the case.

Aside from the latest information about sun damage, there is an immense range of additional vital information the cosmetics industry and fashion magazines are reluctant to provide. For example, the two worst things a woman can do to her skin (besides not using sunscreen) are cause irritation and overmoisturize. I discuss both of these issues in more detail in Chapter Three, "Sun Sense," but here let me summarize a few points to explain why the cosmetics industry refuses to divulge certain information and misdirects consumers. For example, in regard to moisturizing the skin, the essential skin-care product practically every woman, regardless of age, believes she cannot and must not do without is moisturizer, and plenty of it. However, overmoisturizing the skin, or using a moisturizer when you don't need one, can actually turn off the skin's own immune/healing response. Saturating the skin with moisturizers, especially when several products are layered on, inhibits the skin's immune system from doing its job of healing. It's like putting a Band-Aid over a wound—the wound won't heal until you take the Band-Aid off and expose it to air. Exposure to air allows the skin's own healing process to take place. After skin is exposed to the sun without adequate protection, which causes a certain amount of damage daily, it won't heal or "repair" itself if it is oversaturated with a moisturizer!

("Skin repair" is a term the cosmetics industry loves to use in regard to the moisturizers and serums it sells; ironically, those very products may be getting in the way of the skin's healing.) What cosmetics line in the world wants you to know that a moisturizer may be the last thing your skin needs unless you have truly dry skin?

Irritation is another issue the cosmetics industry doesn't want you to know about. According to most of the dermatologists I interviewed for this book, principally Dr. Zoe Draelos, clinical associate professor of dermatology at Bowman Gray School of Medicine, any amount of repeated skin irritation can be damaging. Even more startling was her statement that even if a product with irritants doesn't make your skin feel irritated, it might still be causing problems. In other words, even if they don't cause your skin to burn or sting, the irritating ingredients can still break down and hurt the skin.

Irritation can stimulate oil production by activating nerve endings attached to the oil glands and it can kill skin cells, which can cause increased dryness as well as clogged pores. Irritation can also harm the skin's integrity by breaking down its protective barrier (the intercellular structure of the epidermis, the outer layer of skin), which, over time, damages the skin. Additionally, breaking down the skin's protective barrier can allow the introduction of bacteria, therefore risking breakouts.

What is and isn't irritating? This is a subject I've been warning women about for years. Potentially irritating ingredients include everything from essential oils (which are almost all potentially irritating and truly unessential) and SD alcohol (a cosmetic form of ethanol alcohol) to witch hazel, lemon, grapefruit, eucalyptus, menthol, peppermint, and on and on. However, despite the known risks these products have for skin, you aren't going to hear this kind of information at the cosmetics counters, in infomercials, from in-home salespeople, or in fashion magazines, because it would mean avoiding lots of the products these sources sell.

Remember, what you don't know can hurt your budget and your skin. Even if you have an unlimited budget, wasting money and hurting your skin is hardly beautiful. The idea that expensive means better is completely unproven and inaccurate.

A Completely Different Point of View

It isn't easy being a writer in a field that caters primarily to industry-friendly reporters, who say only nice things about the products being sold by the cosmetics industry and the models representing those lines. While I have trouble getting information or interviews from cosmetics companies, other beauty reporters receive an endless parade of products and press releases, so much so that they have tables of the stuff sitting around for their fellow employees to take.

What this means is that consumers need to be very skeptical about what they read in fashion magazines or newspaper articles involving skin care, makeup, body care, facials, spas, and any other aspect of the cosmetics industry. If an article doesn't cast a critical eye on a product or topic involving beauty or fashion, or if it buries the cautionary words in the middle of the report, be suspicious. When you think about it, how often do you see an article in a fashion magazine that doesn't have something nice to say about any skin-care or makeup product, or about any cosmetics line that happens to be one of its advertisers? About as often as you see an overweight model.

The majority of fashion reporters have their journalistic hands tied by the demands of the companies that advertise in the publications they write for. And there is little impetus to change things. If a magazine depends on advertisers, it is simply prohibitive to tick them off. When cosmetics companies spend thousands of dollars or millions of dollars a year advertising in a magazine, a writer cannot expect to criticize their products and stay employed. This commingling of editorial and advertising control results in gushing "news" stories that are little more than company publicity pieces and biased product recommendations. All the news that's fit to print—as long as it's what the cosmetics industry wants the consumer to know.

Our Studies Show . . .

Another ploy used in the world of cosmetics public relations takes advantage of reporters who are trying to be unbiased. Fashion magazines carry lots of reports and articles about the results of some new study by such-and-such a respected doctor, pharmacist, or chemist. Yet the reporter never poses questions about who paid for the study, how the study was conducted, whether the study had a broad enough scope to be significant, whether there is any independent corroborating research, and, most important, who benefits from the study. All that information is vitally important and relates directly to the study's validity and credibility.

Very few consumers, or reporters for that matter, are aware of the number of skin-care "research" laboratories whose only clients are cosmetics companies that want to use enticing statistics or validation of incredible claims as a marketing strategy. These research labs exist solely to provide pseudoscientific material for the cosmetics industry. That way, if the marketing copy says a moisturizer provides an 82% increase in moisturization or a 90% increase in the skin's water content, the company may very well be able to point to a study that says this is true. Whether the study is the least bit valid is another question altogether. Quoting these inconclusive, vague studies in a news story or ad can make them sound significant and meaningful, but in truth they are more often than not just more hype and exaggeration generated to sell products.

Here's a perfect example of how these feigned studies are done. Let's take a typical claim about a moisturizer providing a large increase in the skin's moisture content. Without some basic information about how the study was conducted, that percentage is meaningless because you can take almost anyone's skin, rub some alcohol on it or just wash it with plain soap, then put any moisturizer in the world on, and the skin would reflect anywhere from an 82% to a 200% increase in moisture content. (In fact, you can sit in the bathtub for 30 minutes and come out with your skin well saturated with water and have a 500% increase in its moisture content.) Furthermore, perhaps the test included only five or ten women comparing only two products, one with an unknown formula, which means that maybe brand A worked better than brand X, but what about compared with the 5,000 other moisturizers on the market? Maybe lots of those work just as well as brand A.

All that is very typical in these types of studies. In essence, the study sounds impressive but is virtually meaningless. It doesn't tell you anything about the product's effectiveness, or even whether that product is good for the skin (it turns out a high moisture content isn't), but it gives the cosmetics company statistics it can show off in its press releases.

I've seen this process at work firsthand, and it is frightening. Whoever is paying the bill hires the research lab. The lab is handed the products and told what to look for and what kind of results are needed—for example, proof of moisturization, exfoliation, smoothness, or some other parameter. Then the lab goes about proving that position. Rarely are these studies ever done double-blind, or using a large group of women, or showing long-term results, and rarely (actually never) are the results negative. More to the point, these studies are never published. Unpublished research is nothing more than sheer fantasy and illusion, completely unscientific and considered invalid by independent researchers. Yet consumers are led to believe this unverified information is fact when they read about it in editorials in fashion magazines and even, on occasion, in newspapers.

This same ploy is used quite effectively in brochures and ads. Many cosmetics counters hand out impressively designed, scientific-looking brochures showing how well a product works on the skin. You might see, for example, a microscopic close-up of a patch of skin paired with an explanation of why it looks bad. Beside it is another close-up of the same patch of skin after the product is applied. See how wonderfully the product worked? The deception here is that you are not given enough "before" information. For example, if the woman had acne, what was she doing before to take care of her skin? Was she using products that clogged pores or aggravated breakouts? Had she never used any effective skin-care products for acne? In that case, any basic skin-care routine for acne could make a difference. And was this the best result of the lot? Were there others who still had breakouts despite treatment? Just because information looks scientific doesn't mean it is.

Next time you see stories about test results showing younger-looking skin, new cell growth, or any other claim that sounds too good to be true, regardless of who is making the claim, stop and think. Ask yourself how many times you have heard this "perfect skin in a bottle" message before. Is this "story" about one study, or are there any corroborating studies? Does it sound too good to be true? You may also want to ask yourself how many more times you are going to swallow another exaggerated claim about a skin-care product, or spend money believing that you've finally found the "best" product available. (Do you really believe that gorgeous, childlike model in the picture looks like that because of the products being advertised?) Think about how many times you've been sucked in by a cosmetics ad, claim, or fashion magazine story, only to be disappointed again and again, until the next advertising campaign for a new product catches your attention. There *are* wonderful things that you can do to take care of your skin—lots! But there are also a ton of things that are an embarrassing waste of money.

How does the cosmetics industry get away with telling you things that aren't entirely true or quoting studies without any real substantiation? Funny you should ask.

They Don't Have to Prove Their Claims

Perhaps the most insidious aspect of the cosmetics industry is that the FDA doesn't require cosmetics companies to prove their claims. That means they get to say just about anything they want about their products without any substantiation or proof whatsoever. Pharmaceutical and over-the-counter drug regulations are infinitely stricter than those dealing with cosmetics. If a drug company makes a claim about what an antihistamine can do to prevent sneezing, it must contain particular ingredients in specified amounts to win approval from the FDA. The same is true for aspirins, antacids, decongestants, anti-inflammatories, and on and on in the world of pharmaceuticals. It is not true for cosmetics. A cosmetic company can say a product provides all sorts of alleged benefits, from firming to closing pores to repairing skin, yet the product can contain any combination of ingredients as long as they are approved for use in cosmetics, and the benefits don't have to be proven.

The only FDA restriction on cosmetics companies' claims is the legal prohibition of phrases that directly state or promise a permanent change in the skin.

Of course, there are a million ways to make something sound permanent to consumers without sounding permanent to the FDA.

What about the federal regulations concerning truth in advertising? That issue generally falls under the jurisdiction of the Federal Trade Commission (FTC) and the Federal Communications Commission (FCC), but it doesn't take much to get around these guys either. For example, I can describe at great length how miraculously my product works as long as I throw in phrases such as "appears to," "seems to," "feels as if," "looks like," "you may experience," and several variations on these themes. All of these phrases invalidate any promise of a product's performance. A company is not considered to be lying to the consumer when these kinds of terms are used because the purported results are subjective, not actual. It may "seem" like your cellulite has disappeared, or you may "appear" to look younger, or you can "experience" a clear complexion, but nothing has happened except that you may be convinced something has taken place. That's how cosmetics advertising gets around truth-in-advertising restrictions every time.

Also, spending $80 on a wrinkle cream or cellulite lotion gives a woman plenty of psychological incentive to see a difference in her skin. There are plenty of studies indicating that a woman will indeed feel her skin is doing better if she used an expensive product as opposed to an inexpensive product, even when the two products are identical.

Cosmetics companies give their claims a veneer of scientific compliance with words like "dermatologist tested," "noncomedogenic," "hypoallergenic," "designed for sensitive skin," "laboratory tested," and "our research shows." But those claims are still all smoke and mirrors, with nothing behind them but artifice and half-truths. None of those terms have an ounce of meaning. There are no regulations to provide a standard definition of those terms. There are no regulations to make cosmetics companies live up to their claims.

"Dermatologist tested" does not tell you which dermatologist or what he or she tested. "Noncomedogenic" sounds like the product won't cause blackheads, but is there any data on how that was determined? Assuming a test was done, was it done on the skin of someone who never had a blemish in his or her whole life? Surely the results would be radically different from a test performed on someone who suffered from acne.

"Hypoallergenic" and "designed for sensitive skin" are nonsense words that imply a product is unlikely to cause allergic reactions, but again there are no standards, so every company can make its own determination of what those words mean. I've seen lots of products that claim to be safer for sensitive skin, yet they contain plants, fragrance, camphor, alcohol, and myriad other ingredients that are known to cause skin reactions.

"Laboratory tested" and "our research shows" might be all well and good, but if the research was conducted by the company's own lab, it's not exactly independent or unbiased information. Furthermore, the test results may just have been the cosmetic chemists saying they like the product a lot. Although a lot of cosmetic testing goes on in the world, there is a stunning lack of it as well. Take the world of alpha hydroxy acids (AHAs). Avon launched its Anew line in the United States in 1992; by 1994 more than 260 AHA products were on the market, and now in 1997 there are well over 400. Has every line done extensive research on the effects of AHAs on the skin? Hardly. Are there any long-term studies to look at? None. Alpha hydroxy acids just haven't been around long enough to determine what happens when you use an AHA product consistently, month after month and year after year. For much of the cosmetics industry, that's just the way it is: the consumer is the guinea pig. I'll explain more about the specifics of AHAs in Chapter Two, "What Works and What Doesn't," but here I want to point out the emptiness of the term "laboratory tested."

AHAs are very popular, and the amount of research on this widely used group of cosmetic ingredients is limited. Other endlessly hyped cosmetic ingredients have absolutely no research. I've searched for abstracts (studies) that evaluate the effectiveness of such heralded cosmetic ingredients as bovine extract, spleen extract, placenta extract, melaleuca (tea tree oil), algae, wild yam extract, plant extracts of all kinds, exotic minerals, emu oil, milk protein, minerals, vitamins, and many, many more in treating aging skin or acne. Other than research commissioned by the companies that sell these ingredients or make products that contain these ingredients, there is nothing. The lack of independent research on them is pathetic. Despite the emptiness behind the promises of these wonder ingredients, and the fact that only minuscule amounts show up in absurdly expensive products, consumers desperately hope that this lotion or that cream may finally be the fountain of youth. Of course they aren't, and in fact they take consumers' attention away from ingredients and products that really might have a positive effect on skin, such as sunscreens, ceramides, glycerin, silicone oil, glycosaminoglycans, salicylic acid, benzoyl peroxide, magnesium, and alpha hydroxy acids, or from over-the-counter and prescription products that have lots of substantiation concerning their effectiveness, such as Retin-A, Renova, Differin (adapelene), topical antibiotics, Accutane, and cortisone creams.

The only part of the cosmetics industry that is closely regulated is the ingredient list. In the United States since 1978, in Australia since 1993, and in the European Union since 1997, mandatory ingredient lists have been required on every cosmetic product sold, whether it be makeup, skin care, or hair care. (Come on, Canada, what's taking you so long?) Ingredients must be listed in order from the most to the least, which is why water is almost always the first ingredient. Water accounts for at least 80% of almost any skin-care product's content.[1]

The ingredient list is the only place where a consumer can readily find the truth about what she is buying. Unfortunately, as accurate and truthful as it is, it is also the most difficult part of the label to decipher. There are thousands of cosmetic ingredients available to a chemist creating any of a wide variety of products. It's no easy task for the consumer to differentiate between highly technical ingredient names. Yet even if you had a good basic understanding of cosmetic ingredients, which some consumers do, amounts and formulation specifications are not discernible just from reading the ingredient list.

I absolutely don't want to dissuade anyone from reading ingredient lists. Quite the contrary. Becoming familiar with what cosmetics contain, especially wrinkle and acne products, can help counter some of the seductive glamour of showcased ingredients (such as plant extracts, exotic oils, animal extracts, minerals, vitamins, or other scientific-sounding ingredients) that turn up at the bottom of the ingredient list (which means they account for little more than 0.5% of the product). But the ingredient list provides just an overview. Some very good ingredients work best in very minute amounts, while others are useless if they aren't among the first on the list.

It's my job to help you figure out what doesn't work and what does, and the most effective quantities of the latter. Over the past 15 years I've continually reviewed and discussed formulary considerations with cosmetic chemists and pored over the available research on a wide range of cosmetic ingredients. Reading this book will help you learn what to pay attention to and what to ignore, so you can take better care of your skin and stop wasting money.

How the Industry Works

According to numbers provided by Datamonitor Cosmetics & Toiletries Database, over 1,700 new skin-care products were launched in 1996. The Lauder Company alone introduced several dozen new products in its three major lines: Prescriptives, Estee Lauder, and Origins. L'Oreal and its high-end sisters, Lancome and Biotherm, introduced another 40 or so. Of this small sample of new cosmetics brought to market in a one-year period, more than 30 were some kind of new moisturizer. Why launch 30 new products that are essentially the

---

[1] One way a cosmetics company can make it seem like their product contains something more than just plain water is to use the term "aqueous extracts of," followed by a long list of plants. It's basically plant tea, and that concoction is well cooked and preserved before it even gets into the product, which is again cooked and preserved. Even if these plants provided any benefit to the skin, their potency is eliminated before you ever get a chance to use the product.

same as many other products within the same line, or virtually identical to others on the market? It takes only a quick glance at the ingredient lists to notice that these "new" products aren't really all that new.

Most women believe these new products are created by profoundly brilliant cosmetic chemists, the best of whom work high up in the Swiss or French Alps, perfecting secret formulas and ingredients no one else knows about. (Women in the United States believe European skin care is automatically better than any American counterpart. Ironically, women in Europe hold American products in high esteem.) Almost as good as a foreign chemist is a doctor or pharmacist associated with a prominent university who, with rare medical insight into skin-care research, has concocted an astonishing new formula. Despite these thousands of different creation scenarios, what all these miraculous mixtures have in common are their promises to erase wrinkles; firm, tone, lift, or hold moisture in the skin; stop or reverse aging; stop acne; or end skin oil production.

Are these promises fulfilled? Occasionally, at least in one form or another—but not hundreds and hundreds of times over, and not with any discernible improvement with the launch of every new product or product line. (By the way, when a new line is introduced based on a new finding, why are there five to 20 products in the line? If one product will do the job, what is all that other stuff for? The answer has to do with the notion that if a little is good, a lot must be better, and now we have the marketing phenomenon known as line extensions, which I'll explain in the next section.)

To better understand how this endless procession of "new" products usually gets created, let's visit the inner sanctum of a cosmetics company—the meeting room. Here's how the cosmetics industry often works.

A New Moisturizer Is Born

A cosmetics company at one of its Monday-morning sales meetings decides it needs to bolster its bottom line by generating more sales and more interest in its product line. After discussing how best to achieve this goal, everyone agrees that introducing a new moisturizer is a good idea. Lots of women have dry skin and lots more believe that a moisturizer will ward off wrinkles, so consumers are out there just waiting for something new and different. But there are already thousands of moisturizers on the market; who needs one more? This is where the marketing department gets involved. Women may not need another moisturizer, they say, but if we make one that contains special vitamins, or plants, or a new scientific-sounding ingredient; or if we say it could enhance skin tone, or firm, or tighten, or lift, or erase wrinkles; or that it's best for sensitive, oily, or super-dry skin; and if we make it sound new and different, that would get attention and increase sales. And it would be even better if one product could have and do it all! Then the exact marketing direction is hashed out.

One cosmetic executive might say, "We just did a moisturizer for oily skin that also firms, so we can't do that again. A few months ago we launched a dry-skin moisturizer with vitamins, so that's out of the question. We haven't done a moisturizer with a new combination of plants and a scientific-sounding ingredient in a long time—let's do that. Estee Lauder just launched a moisturizer like that and it's selling like hotcakes; why not piggyback off their marketing campaign?"

Once that's established, the cosmetic chemist is told to create a new moisturizer that contains an exotic plant and impressive scientific-sounding ingredients. Now the process is in motion. The art department sets to work designing the bottles and boxes, and the advertising department writes the copy, and the lab is busy doing its thing. A few months later, the new product shows up at the cosmetics counter (or drugstore) in a beautiful new box emblazoned with stunning claims about what it can do for your skin. Is this new moisturizer really better for your skin? Is it better than the 20 other moisturizers the company sells or the thousands of other moisturizers being sold? Maybe, but probably not. Who has time to come up with something really new? It doesn't really matter, anyway; the important thing is that the new product is generating new sales. And at next month's meeting, this whole process starts all over again and a new product is created.

Sometimes this scenario works in reverse. A cosmetic chemist may develop a new moisturizer that he or she is really excited about. It really might be different from other moisturizers or acne products on the market. Maybe it contains a new ingredient that can help keep water in the skin, or it may have a new delivery system ("delivery system" refers to the way the ingredients are mixed together and are then absorbed by the skin). It may have a new plant extract from an exotic part of the world. The proud chemist presents it to the people in charge of retailing decisions, explaining what it can do for the skin. The group of marketing executives then decides if the product can be added to the line and what kind of "story" can be built around it. What is the competition selling, and can this compete? What kind of exotic ingredient does it contain? Is it something a woman can understand or care about? Does it have natural ingredients, vitamins, something new, something old with a new twist, or is it just the same old thing but with new claims? Most important, can this one product be splintered into new, coordinated products if the original sells well?

Good skin care is a very minor factor in the decision to launch a new product. Most new cosmetics are inspired by marketing considerations and what companies think they can convince a woman to buy.

Is there anything new under the sun? Are there Swiss scientists up in the

Alps producing secret new cosmetic formulations? Are physicians and pharmacists inventing brilliant skin-care products? Well, yes and no. I'm sure there are cosmetic chemists someplace in the Alps and medical doctors and scientists involved in skin-care research, but none of them are inventing miracles. (Even the remarkable skin-care products Retin-A and Renova, available only by prescription since their invention over 30 years ago, are hardly a miracle, just very effective skin-care products with some potential drawbacks.) Also, there's no such thing as a real secret in the field of skin care. Scientists change jobs like everyone else and take what they know with them. There are no patented secrets, because patent law requires full, total disclosure, down to the smallest molecule. Moreover, reliable scientific standards require corroborating independent research and, as I pointed out earlier in this chapter, truly independent research in the cosmetics industry is extremely rare.

The world of cosmetics constantly produces new, rehashed versions of old ingredients. AHAs, BHA, water-binding ingredients, emollients, antioxidants, benzoyl peroxide, and a host of anti-irritants show up in some great formulations, but also in lots of awful ones. Yet each product is wrapped in an elaborate package and accompanied by elaborate claims showcasing stunning models who assure you this stuff can make you beautiful. After taking in all this cosmetic mumbo jumbo, even the most sensible woman will randomly buy whatever sounds the best, without any clear understanding of what is inside that enticing bottle, tube, or jar. In all likelihood, her skin won't be any more beautiful and she may encounter problems and her checking account may soon be as empty as the claims behind the products.

If One Is Good, More Is Better

One of the best marketing strategies to keep you interested in a company's products is a technique referred to as line extensions, or spin-offs. The scheme is relatively simple and almost foolproof. We fall for it every time. A cosmetics company launches one or two new products. Sometimes the products are intriguing and unlike anything else on the market; for example, Revlon ColorStay Lip Color, Cellex-C from Anti-Aging International, Almay Revitalizer, Elizabeth Arden's Ceramide Time Capsules, Alpha Hydrox Lotion, Hydron (available via infomercials), and Avon Anew. Often they are just the same old stuff hiding behind a new name, with hardly anything unique or special to offer, such as Nivea Visage, La Prairie Age Management, L'Oreal Plenitude, Estee Lauder Verite, Borghese Cura Vitale, and Bobbi Brown Skin Care. The original product comes with an interesting story or angle on how it could be beneficial for some skin types (although the ads usually make it sound great for practically every woman alive). If it sells well, the cosmetics company capitalizes on the popularity of that product by creating more products based on the original.

The film and television industries thrive on spin-offs, and so do cosmetics companies. It doesn't mean the new products (think of them as sequels) are even vaguely as good or as interesting as the original, but that doesn't matter. Cosmetics companies know consumers are very likely to try other products with the same recognizable name.

Alpha Hydrox (one of the first companies to develop a reliable AHA product) started out with just two products (face lotion and cream); now, a few years later, the line includes more than 20 items, including products for the feet and products aimed at men. Practically every company adds to its bottom line with spin-offs. Elizabeth Arden's original Ceramide Time Capsules were wildly popular products. Soon, Ceramide Purifying Cleansing Cream, Ceramide Purifying Toner, Ceramide Time Complex Moisturizer, Ceramide Night Intensive Repair Creme, Alpha-Ceramide, and Ceramide Eyes Time Complex Capsules were added to this growing group of products. From a marketing standpoint these spin-offs are great line enhancers; from a consumer's viewpoint they are neither necessary nor worthwhile. Ceramide is a cosmetic ingredient that acts as a water-binding agent, much like mucopolysaccharides, collagen, or hyaluronic acid. All of those are components of skin and share a concentrated ability to keep water trapped in the skin—nothing more, nothing less. Including ceramide in a moisturizer makes sense, putting it in a cleanser doesn't, and Arden wasn't that wasteful. Although the cleanser and toner carry the Ceramide name, they don't contain any ceramides. The Ceramide Purifying Cleanser won't purify anything. It is a fairly standard mineral oil–based wipe-off cleanser with ordinary thickening agents to give it a creamy appearance, and it can leave a greasy film on the skin. The Ceramide Purifying Toner is a very pricey alcohol-based toner. Alcohol doesn't purify the skin, but it can cause irritation and dryness, negating the effectiveness of the moisturizer.

Cellex-C is another spin-off story that makes my head spin. (For more detailed comments on the Cellex-C sensation, see my newsletter and the latest edition of *Don't Go to the Cosmetics Counter Without Me.*) Just to sum up, the commotion about vitamin C as an anti-aging ingredient not only is exaggerated, but borders on preposterous. There is only one real study about the effect of applying vitamin C (specifically L-ascorbic acid) on the skin. Dr. Sheldon Pinnell from Duke University looked at the effect of sun exposure in relation to applying L-ascorbic acid (a form of vitamin C) on pig skin. It seems the pigs did not get very sunburned when exposed to the sun when they had this stuff on their back. L-ascorbic acid turns out to be a very good antioxidant and can help reduce sun damage, but it's exceptionally unstable. That's why Cellex-C Serum comes in a little brown bottle. When exposed to air, sun, or heat, it decomposes. At $70 an ounce, you want a product that lasts longer than a few weeks, but they don't tell you about this fact at the store.[2]

That's the skinny on Cellex-C: one product based on one study. But lo and behold, despite the fact that only Cellex-C Serum has the version of vitamin C used in Dr. Pinnell's study, the line has more than 20 additional products for all aspects of skin care. Even Dr. Pinnell has noted that the serum is the only product he researched. I imagine the company licensed to sell the product, Anti-Aging International, decided it didn't matter if the vitamin C is unstable or useless in other formulations and containers, or even completely unnecessary. What they fail to explain is why this line contains all these other products if the original Cellex-C in the little brown bottle is supposed to be so amazing, with mesmerizing before-and-afters. Why would you need AHAs, toners, and other wrinkle creams, if only one very expensive product is supposed to be doing all the work? There are some good products in this line, but the prices are stupefying, the claims are exaggerated beyond belief, and the notion that a combination of several products will make a difference on the skin when there is minimal evidence that even the original product works goes beyond misleading to farcical.

I don't want to point to Elizabeth Arden or Cellex-C as being the worst offenders; they aren't. I could point out many more, but they all read the same: one product begets a family of products based on marketing, not on good skin-care research. Line extensions are primarily a way to encourage more sales by piggybacking off a previous product's success, without necessarily creating new and better products.

Naturally Absurd

Put succinctly, there is no such thing as "all-natural," "pure" cosmetics. They don't exist and if they did, they would not be good for the skin.

Whatever preconceived or media-induced fiction you might believe about natural ingredients being better for the skin has no basis in fact or scientific legitimacy. Not only is the definition of "natural" hazy, but the term isn't even regulated, so each cosmetics company can use it to mean something different. If a company wants to call its products natural, it can, and it doesn't matter what they contain.

---

[2] An interesting side note is that, anecdotally, women are experiencing smoother skin from using Cellex-C. In light of the fact that a woman would never notice the effect of reduced sun damage on her skin (it takes years for sun damage to show up), how could this be? Plus, the study concerning Cellex-C only showed that a pig's skin didn't become sunburned. That's all well and good, but UVB radiation, which is responsible for sunburns, doesn't cause wrinkles or skin cancer. Does vitamin C have any effect on UVA radiation? No one knows.

So what is "natural"? Good question. It can mean anything and nothing. For most cosmetics companies it means including plant extracts in their formulations. The ingredient list may include "aqueous extracts," with a long list of plant names following. This is little more than tea water. What is the concentration of the plants in the tea? That is anyone's guess, but it is, at best, minuscule. What good is this tea water? That's another excellent question, for I've yet to see these remarkable, exotic concoctions packaged by themselves for skin care. Why is that? Because they are mostly ineffective. If they are so exceptional for the skin, and the other "unnatural" ingredients in the product are so insubstantial (you never see those ingredients talked about in advertising or brochures), why not just bottle the exotic plants and leave out all the other stuff? Why? Because without the "unnatural" ingredients, you would have a useless, moldy, smelly, unusable product.

The cosmetics industry doesn't like to publicize ingredients such as neopentyl glycol dicaprylate, cetyl alcohol, PEG 60 hydrogenated castor oil, stearic acid, polysorbate 40, butylene glycol, methylparaben, and potassium hydroxide, even though these account for much more of what's inside most cosmetics than a pinch of plant extracts, regardless of the claim on the label.

Even if an "all-natural" product did exist, you wouldn't want to use it on your skin anyway. Think about a bunch of plants, fruits, or vegetables sitting in your bathroom. What would happen in a very brief period of time if they didn't contain preservatives? They would become moldy and disgusting in just a few days. Skin-care products contain very "unnatural"-sounding preservatives, and that's great. According to many cosmetic chemists, a reliable preservative system helps avoid the risk of microbial contamination, which could cause problems for the eyes, lips, and skin. For most people, the possibility of an allergic reaction to a preservative is the lesser of the two evils.[3] But even that is only a small part of why "all-natural" is a bad joke on the consumer. So-called natural ingredients can themselves cause allergies, irritation, and skin sensitivities. Just think of how many people have hay fever, and you will start to realize just how unfriendly natural ingredients can be.

The notion that "natural" equals good skin care or better makeup will waste

---

[3] Women with incredibly sensitive skin will no doubt be interested to learn that some cosmetics companies are experimenting with preservative-free formulations. In Japan the Fancl cosmetics company offers a line of preservative-free skin-care products that come in tiny, hermetically sealed containers. After being opened, their products last about two to four weeks (probably more like two) before they risk becoming contaminated. The Fancl corporation is very straightforward and honest about the limited shelf- and bathroom-life of their products. According to a Fancl executive, one of the largest Japanese cosmetics companies was very concerned about the growing popularity of Fancl's preservative-free products and came out with their own preservative-free products. It didn't work well for this competing company, because they couldn't explain why their other products weren't also preservative-free.

your money and probably hurt your skin. I'm not sure if the majority of women who buy cosmetics are ever going to be able to believe this. The pressure to believe the lie about natural products being better for the skin is hard to resist, and women want to believe it. Cosmetics companies spend lots of money to reinforce their message about the benefit of "natural" ingredients through their ads, sales force, and brochures. Despite the corroboration from countless physicians, cosmetic chemists, and other scientists in a variety of academic research, it still isn't easy to counter the hype surrounding products claiming to be "all-natural" or "pure." It gets even more confounding as the "natural" sources become more exotic and eccentric, such as sea plants or foliage from the rain forest or herbs from India. Yet it is worth the effort, because women deserve to know the real story behind the cosmetics they are buying. Can every plant growing hold a miracle for human skin? The cosmetics industry would like you to believe it does.

What makes this natural craze so annoying and undesirable is that it perpetuates myths that can hurt a woman's skin. All of the following natural ingredients can cause skin irritation, allergic reactions, skin sensitivity, and/or sun sensitivity: allspice, almond extract, angelica, arnica, balm mint oil, balsam, basil, bergamot, cinnamon, citrus, clove, clover blossom, cocoa butter, coriander oil, corn oil, cornstarch, cottonseed oil, fennel, fir needle, geranium oil, grapefruit, horsetail, jojoba oil, lavender oil, lemon, lemongrass, lime, marjoram, melissa, oak bark, papaya, peppermint, rose, sage, tea tree oil, thyme, witch hazel, and wintergreen. The label might say "pure and natural," but you could be buying a purely irritating product that might cause an allergic reaction.

Natural ingredients are one of the most bogus, misleading components of the cosmetics industry because they focus attention on the wrong information. For example, while many women with sensitive skin know fragrance and perfumes are notorious for causing allergic reactions and skin sensitivity, they incorrectly feel that essential oils are safe because they are derived from plants. Yet essential oils are usually nothing more than volatile oils used most often as fragrance ingredients.

Furthermore, the notion that natural ingredients are better than synthetic ingredients is even more distressing, because it just isn't true. **While vegetable or plant oils may sound better for the skin, dimethicone and cyclomethicone (silicone oils) are actually far more beneficial and offer the most impressive benefits for the skin. But it's hard to glamorize and advertise a "synthetic," unnatural-sounding ingredient.** Dimethicone and cyclomethicone are basic, standard oils that feel like silk and show up in over 80% of all the skin-care, makeup, and hair-care products you buy. Yet you rarely hear about them because the cosmetics companies think consumers won't find them as sexy or as alluring as plants, or oxygen therapy, or cellular repair, or a thousand other marketing angles that have nothing to do with what really works for your skin.

I'm not saying there aren't some natural-sounding ingredients that are good for the skin, because there are, but the idea that they are still natural once they have been extracted from their source and mixed into a cosmetic is ludicrous. One of the more potent examples of how the natural craze gets in the way of good skin care and good information concerns alpha hydroxy acids. AHAs have gotten a lot of press over the past several years, and many women know that AHAs work as effective exfoliants for sun-damaged skin. Of the several AHAs used in cosmetics, lactic acid and glycolic acid are the most popular and the most researched. AHAs have been promoted as being natural because lactic acid is derived from milk and glycolic acid is derived from sugarcane, but "derived from" doesn't mean the original ingredient has anything to do with the extracted ingredient. Milk and sugarcane are not the same as lactic acid and glycolic acid. Rubbing milk or sugarcane on your face won't have the same effect as applying a product with lactic or glycolic acid, just as rubbing moldy bread on your body isn't the same as taking penicillin, even though penicillin is derived from moldy bread. (Beware of products that list sugarcane extract, or milk by-products, or some other food substance; they do not function like glycolic or lactic acid either.)

Companies like Aveda—companies based on an all-natural concept—do list the technical-sounding ingredients along with the natural sources. Although this appears to be helpful information, it still leads consumers in the wrong direction. For example, ammonium lauryl sulfate, a standard detergent cleansing agent, is listed on the Aveda ingredient label as being derived from coconut oil. Doesn't that make it sound pure and pleasant? Ammonium lauryl sulfate is the salt of a sulfuric acid compound, neutralized with an ingredient like triethanolamine. None of that is bad for the skin, and I wouldn't tell anyone to avoid ammonium lauryl sulfate, but it is the more accurate description of that ingredient. Associating it with coconut oil, a far-removed organic source, just makes for better (though misleading) marketing lingo.

One of the lesser-known aspects of skin care is that cosmetic ingredients can cause problems for the skin even if you can't feel the resulting irritation. Some of you may be thinking that you've used lots of products that contain natural (or synthetic) ingredients I've mentioned as potentially irritating, but your skin is doing fine. Unfortunately, according to several dermatologists, the skin doesn't have to look irritated to be irritated and damaged (a breakdown in the skin's protective barrier as well as a decline in the skin's immune/healing response). Irritation is a problem that the cosmetics industry is only now beginning to address.

Next time you're faced with marketing claims about natural being better for the skin, remember the following:

1. **Food-type ingredients in a product increase the need for additional preservatives to decrease mold and bacteria contamination.**
2. **Plant oils decompose faster than mineral oils and require higher concentrations of preservatives and fragrance.**
3. **Plant oils often contain fatty (saturated) acids that can clog pores and cause acne.**
4. **Food can feed the bacteria present in skin, increasing risk of breakouts.**
5. **Plant extracts are no longer plants, and the process used to do the extraction is not "natural."**
6. **Yeast or bacteria cultures in cosmetics can exacerbate rosacea and psoriasis.**

Can You Get What You Want?

Everyone wants younger, healthy-looking skin, with the goal of looking more beautiful (or at least the best you can). No one wants wrinkles or drooping skin, and no one wants to have blemishes. No one. I can make such a sweeping statement because obviously no cosmetics company in the world is selling products that will make skin look more wrinkled, saggy, or broken out. At least not knowingly. Does that mean you may unwittingly be buying products that harm your skin? Absolutely. If that makes you take a deep gulp, that's good—it should.

So can you get what you want for your skin? It all depends on exactly what you want. If you want the impossible, you will just be throwing money to the cosmetics industry and doing nothing for yourself. But if you want good skin care based on what is known to be feasible, yes, you positively can get close to what you want, or at least as close as is physiologically possible. The chapters in this book are aimed at helping you get the skin and the look you want, paying close attention to what is factually known about skin. No one has discovered the fountain of youth yet, Dorian Gray certainly does not exist, hormones that exacerbate the tendency to break out still rage on, and the sun still rises every morning and beams damaging ultraviolet radiation on our skin.

Wanting the impossible, believing skin-care products can effect radical before-and-afters, and presuming expensive means better all serve the cosmetics industry, but not you. Skin-care products that can do amazing things for the skin, and makeup products that can make a beautiful and powerful fashion statement, do exist. But understanding all your options and formulating a clear plan of action for yourself, in the face of all the mind-controlling advertising out there, requires approaching the subject of beauty with a little Zen realism.

A Little Less Desperation Would Help

Most women reach a certain stage in life and begin to worry about the impact age has on their skin, lifestyle, opportunities, and potential for being beautiful. When someone feels the ache of being a certain age, she quickly assesses her life, scrutinizes her skin-care arsenal, and decides she better start doing something to prevent any further breakdown or meltdown. What is that certain age? It turns out to be an ever-changing number marked by different milestones in a woman's life or emotions, but it always involves preventing or warding off a perceived point of no return. Some women reach it when they turn 18, worrying about how they will weather the transition from childhood to adulthood or how they will establish their individualism and identity, thinking if they don't do it now, they may never get the chance.[4]

Others hit their "certain age" marker at 25, concerned about how to be taken seriously or how to look sexier and more alluring, because opportunities related to career and finding a significant other may be slipping by. A large number of women hit the "certain age" wall between 32 and 40, when youth seems to be a vague memory and wrinkles start appearing. Some women wait until 50, but virtually every woman at some point commences worrying about what is happening to her appearance and then turns to makeup and skin-care products to assuage that concern or fear.

This "certain age" phenomenon is most vivid for women (particularly baby boomers) who are focused on their dread of aging or their intense hatred of breakouts or, horror of horrors, both at the same time. It doesn't take much to convince a woman who wants to erase wrinkles or fight blemishes that there are products capable of such a feat, because lots of products do lots of wonderful things for the skin. They can't alter aging or cure acne, but that doesn't stop women from anticipating that the next product will do the trick. And eventually it might—there *are* products that work, but finding them is like throwing darts at a list of stocks, hoping you hit the right one. It is the intensity and purchasing power of women fighting wrinkles and acne that makes the "certain age" phenomenon such a boon to the cosmetics industry.

Then there is that rare specimen of woman who never reaches a certain age and never worries that she might. This uncommon group is divided into two personality types. The first personality type is a woman who feels the same at 50 or 60 as she did at 30, only better. This woman simply loves life, celebrating

[4] What stands out the most about this particular age group is that in their attempt to make a statement about how unique and different they are, they enthusiastically turn to the daring trend of the moment to display their singularity—and end up looking much like everyone else their age. Young women in this age group currently tend to pierce various parts of their body, shave their head à la Sinead O'Connor, and/or wear Dracula-like makeup.

every moment to its fullest; she exercises, follows a healthy diet, and pays attention to her appearance on the basis of her own personal lifestyle and her own idea of beauty, rather than that of some magazine or television show.

The other personality type who never reaches a certain age is at the other end of the spectrum. This type of woman has no zest for life and feels incapable of dealing with any part of her appearance. She is trapped by an inability or reluctance to do anything to celebrate her goals or her potential for creating a beautiful visage.

I always champion a balance in life from the former perspective. I don't want to be a woman who doesn't acknowledge her age, but I also don't want to be constrained or frightened by it. I don't want to be so concerned about fitting in or getting attention that I cover my body with tattoos and holes. I don't want to be so worried about looking sexually attractive that I don't pay attention to any other part of my identity. I don't want to be so fearful of the media's interpretation of beauty that I run out and buy every new product that promises to erase or cover wrinkles and blemishes or slavishly follow the latest fashion trend.

I see no special benefit in being any age other than the age you are, as long as you are physically fit. Every age should be celebrated, but that takes self-esteem and self-confidence, exercise, and a healthy diet, and you won't find any of that in a cosmetics bottle or jar. If you can understand and believe the concept that beauty is a health statement and an issue of self-worth and individual identity, you will save a great deal of time and money.

I am most sensitive to the intense rush women feel about trying every new makeup, skin-care, and fashion trend espoused by fashion magazines that are strictly designed to establish shopping frenzies. This gets in the way of women in all age groups. (How many times are they going to try to bring back blue eyeshadow?) Many women approach cosmetics with an almost reverent attitude of blind faith. Their motto is "Sell me anything that will make me look better. Sell me anything that will stop wrinkling. Keep me beautiful so men will find me attractive." Giving the cosmetics industry so much credit and power is a huge mistake. This is how women turn the flashy hype of the cosmetics industry into hopeful self-delusion.

It isn't that makeup and skin care don't serve a very important purpose in a woman's life. They absolutely do, and wonderfully; it just depends who we want to be in control of it. There needs to be a balance between what is advertised to us and what we decide to buy. That takes a keen eye and a genuine sense of who we are, who we want to be, and how we want to get there. With that in mind we can better tackle the cosmetics counters and determine what works for us and what doesn't.

Thou Shalt . . .

Feeling and looking beautiful is a wonderful, satisfying, joyous process as well as a state of mind women can revel in with much pleasure and reward. Yet all the delightful and beautiful possibilities can get zapped by frustration caused by poor information and broken promises. Is there anything quite as irksome as spending $70 on a lavishly hyped wrinkle cream or $200 on a whole new skin-care routine, only to end up with more problems than you started with and none of the changes you were hoping for?

The truth is, beauty isn't easy (I wish it were effortless, but we all know better) because human skin and contemporary definitions of beauty are complicated topics. Skin-care problems from both external and internal sources can be exceedingly technical and difficult to understand. Skin is the body's largest organ, and the only one that exists primarily on the outside. That's a lot of area to take care of. Also, skin isn't static: it can change from day to day, month to month, season to season, and year to year. And then there's the skin's intricate, complex structure and its dependence on hundreds of elaborate, integral chemical processes. All this makes it an understatement to say that skin care is complicated. Yet skin is one of the first things people notice about us. Our skin tells the world where we stand in terms of beauty and age. Skin displays the ravages of time, via sun damage, gravity, and genetically determined signs of aging, well before any of us want to see them. In our culture, flawless and wrinkle-free skin is an obligatory component of beauty. And let's not forget that whole region from the neck down.

There are ways to tackle all of this, but the first step is to acquire a clear understanding of how the so-called "beauty" industry works. Let's begin at the beginning with some basic guidelines that can help you get through most of this information. I call them "The Ten (Plus Four) Commandments of Beauty." Get to know them before you go shopping at another cosmetics counter, see another infomercial, have a friend introduce you to a new multilevel cosmetics line, or read another fashion magazine. Once you've taken them to heart, you will have a better perspective on what you are really buying at the cosmetics counters, what these products can and can't do, whether what you are using is worth the money, and, most important, whether any of this can hurt your skin.

The Ten (Plus Four) Commandments of Beauty

Actually, there are a lot more "thou shalts" and "thou shalt nots," and I go through each and every one of these throughout this book, presenting the information you need to make an educated decision about your skin care, body care, and makeup.

1. THOU SHALT NOT believe expensive cosmetics are better than inexpensive cosmetics. Women who spend more money on cosmetics do not have better skin than those with a tighter budget. Many expensive lines own inexpensive lines, ingredients listings don't differ between inexpensive and expensive lines, and cosmetic chemists are not chained to one company.
2. THOU SHALT NOT believe there is any such thing as a natural cosmetic (or that natural means better).
3. THOU SHALT NOT believe in miracle ingredients that can cure skin-care woes, but thou shalt believe there are great products in all price ranges.
4. THOU SHALT NOT covet thy neighbor's perfect skin (or believe her perfect skin came from a particular product or a particular cosmetics line; skin is more complicated than that).
5. THOU SHALT NOT believe everything a cosmetics salesperson tells you. (Cosmetics salespeople are not there to tell you their products suck.) Read the ingredient list, try the product on, and be willing to return what doesn't work or fails to live up to the claim on the label, while also being very, very skeptical.
6. THOU SHALT NOT use the tiny applicators that come packaged with eyeshadows and blushes.
7. THOU SHALT NOT believe in the existence of anti-wrinkle, firming, toning, lifting, or filling-in creams, lotions, or masks that can permanently erase wrinkles. (I wish it were so, but nothing on the horizon besides surgery can do that. I'm praying that this changes, and I'll let you know the second it does so we can all have truly wrinkle-free visages without the help of a surgeon.)
8. THOU SHALT NOT be seduced by every new promotion, new product, or new product line that the cosmetics industry creates.
9. THOU SHALT NOT get a tan. Sun is your enemy, not your friend; it is the primary reason that skin wrinkles and develops skin cancer.
10. THOU SHALT NOT buy a cellulite cream, nor shalt thou assume you can dissolve fat from the outside in, because you absolutely cannot. Any product that could would be regulated as a drug and be extremely dangerous and risky to use. Where would the fat go? Into the bloodstream? The lymph system? The liver? The heart? Certainly not where it goes when it is naturally metabolized. Anyway, if these products did work, who would be fat?

11. THOU SHALT NOT see pictures of pubescent, anorexic models (who spend two hours getting their hair and makeup done and another two hours posing while the photographer and a corps of assistants determine the most flattering lighting, after which the resulting picture goes through a battery of digitally enhanced touch-ups and adjustments) and believe you will get the same (or even similar) results from using the products being advertised (unless you happen to be pubescent and a model and can stay in the right lighting all the time).
12. THOU SHALT NOT buy products from an infomercial or from a home shopping network, especially when the praise goes on and on for over 15 minutes with no opposing information. You are receiving a bizarrely one-sided point of view. It isn't natural for anyone to ever applaud a skin-care product. Ever.
13. THOU SHALT NOT believe words and phrases such as hypoallergenic, noncomedogenic, for sensitive skin, dermatologist tested, exclusive formula, increases moisture content (by some astronomical percentage), or any other gross, unsupported generalization about a product.
14. THOU SHALT NOT buy cosmetic hormone creams assuming that they can replace dietary sources of plant hormones or medically prescribed hormone therapy.

The ultimate commandment is: Thou shalt be an informed consumer, because what you don't know can cost you dearly in terms of your skin, appearance, and money.

Judging a Book by Its Cover

How I evaluate skin-care formulations deserves more explanation. The best analogies I can think of are the ingredient list on prepared or processed food products, and information on the nutrition content of whole foods. When it comes to my diet, I start by judging food on the basis of its ingredient list or nutrition content. Information about fat, sodium, preservatives, coloring agents, calories, and many other details are spelled out in the ingredient list or in diet books. Without that information, regardless of taste (everyone has their own bias), you would never know what you are putting in your body. You could be causing yourself harm by eating more fat than you should, or eating more preservatives than you should, or skimping on vitamins, fiber, or protein, and on and on, leading to a variety of health problems.

Food labels are incredibly important, and so are the labels on skin-care products. If a Duncan Hines cake mix contains 100 calories per serving rather than

500 calories per serving, that's fundamental information for deciding whether it's good for you. If a makeup product says it is for sensitive skin but contains ingredients known to cause irritation or breakouts, that is crucial information. If a skin-care product sells for $100 but contains the same ingredients as a product that costs $10, that is important information. If a product says it is good for breakouts but contains alcohol and peppermint oil, it is good to know it could hurt your face and actually cause more breakouts. The ingredient list helps you sort through the jungle of choices. Besides, it is a far better starting point than basing decisions strictly on advertising mumbo jumbo.

I actually test a large percentage of the products I review, especially makeup products. I have purchased over $100,000 worth of cosmetics and I spend a great deal of time at the cosmetics counters. I use, and test, a lot of makeup and skin-care products, relying on my years of experience and research. But whether the product worked for me doesn't tell consumers what they need to know about a product's effectiveness; it tells them only what works for me or what I like. Unless our skin types and personal preferences are identical, what I like or what I am allergic to is useless information for you. A consumer needs much more information than that. That's why I establish guidelines for each type of product and technique I recommend.

I have been taken to task by cosmetic chemists for the way I break down cosmetic formulations in my book *Don't Go to the Cosmetics Counter Without Me.* Several have suggested that my typical description—"This product contains mostly water, water-binding agent, silicone oil, thickening agents, plant extracts, plant oils, vitamins, and preservatives"—is just too simplistic. And they are right, it is simplistic. The procedure a cosmetic formulator goes through to create a product is much more complicated than that. However, no consumer would have the tolerance to put up with the extremely technical vernacular of the scientific world in explaining a cosmetic formula. I've asked many times if there is a better alternative, and no one had any suggestions, other than allowing the cosmetics companies to disseminate their misleading information.

For now, this is the best way I can think of to help someone understand what she is buying. It is certainly more informative than the marketing language used to sell 99% of the cosmetic products out there, including things like "[this product] represents the ultimate advancement in cosmetically reversing the aging process" or "the molecular structure of [this product] uniquely inhibits aging, delaying and diminishing lines, wrinkles, and age spots," even if it contains nothing new or unique to live up to even an iota of this claim. **As long as the cosmetics industry continues to blow itself out of proportion, I will continue to use the information I have at my disposal to bring it back down to earth.**

I explain at length later in Chapter Five, "Skin-Care Planning," exactly what I expect from each kind of product for each skin type. Once you have all the information, you can make your own decisions about what is best for you.

Advertising Victims

While insecurity and lack of consumer information prompt most women's cosmetics buying, it is fueled by pervasive, endless advertising. Cosmetics advertising generates sales in the billions and billions of dollars. If you don't understand how advertising works, you will always be a victim of its wiles and contrivances. Yet most consumers make decisions about what they are going to buy based strictly on advertising. Is it any wonder that the advertising industry in just the United States is a multibillion-dollar business? Procter & Gamble alone spends $1.3 billion annually to advertise its products to the American public. L'Oreal spends about the same. These companies pay these vast sums for advertising because they want (and get) more sales. Revlon doesn't sign Cindy Crawford to a multimillion-dollar endorsement contract just because they like her face, and Lauder isn't giving Elizabeth Hurley a fortune just because they think she's pretty. It's because these companies know certain faces can sell billions of dollars' worth of products.

We may think we recognize the influence advertising can have on us, and even feel we are above this kind of blatant manipulation. But whether we like to admit it or not, we are greatly influenced by the power of advertising.

As you flip through fashion magazines or watch television, notice that a typical ad for makeup or skin-care products showcases a beautiful young model. The underlying message is that if you buy the right makeup or skin-care products, you will be beautiful, have a good body, win male attention, eliminate wrinkles, reap praise from those you know, enjoy increased fun, and radiate sex appeal just like the model. That's why Revlon ads display Cindy Crawford's face more prominently than the products Revlon makes, and why Elizabeth Hurley overshadows Lauder's products in Estee Lauder ads. Successful advertising often stresses the benefits of *using* products made by a particular company, not necessarily a specific *product.* That isn't always the case, but it is a primary scenario in the world of cosmetics.

Although gorgeous models are an especially obvious advertising tool, the technique of persuading consumers to buy is limited only by the creativity of Madison Avenue (the advertising bastion). One basic tenet of the business is repetition, repetition, repetition. When a new product is launched by a company, it is very typical for it to be promoted via radio, television, newspapers, magazines, counter displays, and promotional literature. With these constant reminders, it soon becomes apparent, either subconsciously or consciously, that you are missing out on something if you don't have whatever it is you've been hearing about. (Repetition as a reinforcer is most evident in the world of infomercials, but more about that later in this chapter.)

After choosing a pretty face to go with its products and fixing on a strategy of steady repetition, a company needs to ensure its longevity by creating the impression of superiority to other companies. Establishing a solid reputation in the mind of the consumer is a significant goal, although superiority is only a perception. Cosmetics companies spend billions of dollars to promote their logos as symbols of reliability and value. Once a woman has confidence in a company's ability to produce a good product—for example, Revlon's ColorStay lipstick—she can be easily persuaded that the other ten products with the ColorStay name are just as good. Whether that's true is another story, but the perception is all that counts.

Another consumer issue, price, has its own tricky, elusive attraction. It may motivate more decisions to buy than any other appeal. The magic words "sale" and "discount" are directed at consumers with great frequency and in all price categories. Clothes with designer labels such as Donna Karan, Chanel, and Ralph Lauren can be found on sale (eventually) in the most chic department stores. But when it comes to cosmetics, discounts are to be found only in drugstores, through in-home sales, and on infomercials. There are no discounts at the department-store cosmetics counters (discounts have a "cheap" connotation that expensively priced cosmetics companies want to avoid like the plague). Instead, high-end cosmetics companies maintain the image of exclusivity by offering "gift with purchase" or "purchase with purchase" deals. The "something-for-nothing" appeal of this bizarre marketing deal has women waiting in line as if they really were getting something for nothing.[5]

In essence, the more expensive cosmetics companies very quietly, though quite plainly, control prices. After all, if Nordstrom had a sale on Estee Lauder products, what would Macy's do? Macy's would have to cut its prices, and so would Lord & Taylor, and then Marshall Fields, and then Bloomingdales. Can you imagine the competitive cosmetics retailing that would get established at the department stores? The "gift with purchase" would pale as a consumer in-

[5] The products in these gift or bonus purchase sets are not by any stretch of the imagination the value they claim to be. The products all cost pennies to manufacture. The most expensive part is probably the makeup bag they come packaged in. (And how many of these can you collect? It would be cheaper to just go buy a nice bag.) Most of the preselected colors are unusable—either too bright, too shiny, too dark, too light, or just not your colors. It looks like you're getting a lot of different things to take home and experiment with, and on occasion you are, but a lot of the products in these sets are things you probably shouldn't be wearing or using anyway. Much of it ends up being wasted, which is no bargain for anyone. Also, most of the products in these "purchase with purchase" or "gift with purchase" promotions are trial size, not full size, so the real value is that the company is getting you to try their products at your expense.

centive. Everyone would just wait for sales, and the glamour and status of shopping the counters would evaporate. It would be great for the consumer who shops sales regularly at the department stores, but the cosmetics companies, which keep a tight rein on the department stores, think of it as a nightmare that could become reality all over the country. Keep in mind that price fixing (although the cosmetics companies would never call it that, because it brings up antitrust questions) is quite illegal. Yet it is business as usual at the cosmetics counters.

Another powerful advertising tool in the cosmetics industry is the celebrity endorsement. Celebrities are visible everywhere in infomercials and fashion editorials (information about which celebrity is using which new product or skin treatment racks up lots of sales) because we as consumers equate acting ability or celebrity status with knowledge and integrity. An endorsement by someone with a well-known face carries weight. But is what a movie star uses on her skin in any way relevant to your skin-care needs? Does a world-famous model's beauty, fame, and money mean she knows something you don't? Enticing as it is to believe that listening to celebrities can get you better skin and a better look, that's not the way it is.

First of all, actresses and models don't all use the same products (or the same plastic surgeon). They use lots and lots of different products in all price ranges from a vast array of lines, and, like all women, they can be fickle. What they use today may not be what they use tomorrow. Celebrities look for "perfect" products as much as the next person and are as subject to being misled and wasting money as anyone else. Besides, what someone else is using doesn't necessarily have anything to do with your skin-care or makeup needs. If there is any lesson to learn here, it is that a celebrity whose name is attached to a specific line has signed some type of lucrative contract, and is not endorsing the products because she loves them.

Aside from all these standard advertising ploys—celebrity endorsement, impossibly perfect young women (groomed and photographed by the best in the fashion world), and repetitive advertising—there is an underlying message that is hard to slough off. Cosmetics advertising is frequently fear advertising. Fear of wrinkles, acne, or just being out of date is a strong motivator for women who would otherwise not be taken in by all the other bells and whistles used to stimulate sales. Pay attention to ads that make you feel worried or anxious about your skin and appearance. They have a compelling influence over women of all ages and drive buying through fear, not empowerment. It's not that you shouldn't be concerned or motivated to deal with your skin and appearance, but when advertising generates angst and instigates action on your part, you are being manipulated, not educated.

Be aware of the vast difference between the information provided in advertising and objective information. Advertising is one-sided. There are no negatives in ads, except in regard to the competition's products. The truth about almost all products, whether in the cosmetics industry or some other industry, is that they all have their pros and cons. A consumer's job is not to be swayed by advertising. It is the task of the company paying for the ad, or the salesperson selling you the product, to portray the product in absolutely glowing, positive terms. **It is, however, your job to search out as much impartial information from independent sources as possible. You might still buy the product, but at least you will have some facts to base your decision on and not just pretty pictures and catchy words.**

As far as cosmetics are concerned, the only candid information to be found is the ingredient list. Of course, that's the only part of the package that never gets featured in the magazine or on television, yet it is the only place that absolutely tells the truth.

How Cosmetic Advertising Misleads

The number of things we are told about skin care and beauty concerns is nothing less than astounding. To start thinking in terms of reality, facts, and balanced information, we must learn to recognize and ignore the baseless, unfounded claims that are constantly bandied about in the guise of serious information. You may have run into the following terms and sales pitches for myriad skin-care and makeup products. These come-ons entice purchasers, even though they are vague or illogical.

"Anti-aging." Ah, if only it were true. As one cosmetic surgeon explained to me, "If any of these anti-aging products worked, or even did a little of what they claimed, wouldn't I be out of a job?"[6] Thousands of skin-care products make promises about removing wrinkles or preventing the skin from aging. They contain a hodgepodge of ingredients and formulations. There is no consistency in any of them. Yet they all claim to stop aging, and still no one stops getting wrinkles or sheds a wrinkle. Where does the truth lie? The sun causes skin to wrinkle (as does gravity pulling the muscles of the face down); that accounts for 95% of the aging we see on the skin, something all dermatologists

---

[6] The rest of the doctor's quote: "If anything, younger and younger women are coming in to medically erase wrinkles because that's the only thing that really makes a long-term difference. Women can hardly help themselves when it comes to anti-aging products because they'll try anything in the hopes of staying young or looking more beautiful. But they rarely do what it really takes, which is staying out of the sun. Yet even if they do start staying out of the sun, they can't undo what they've been doing to their skin since they were babies, namely going out in the sun without protection. That's why I became a cosmetic surgeon: what I do as a cosmetic surgeon will never become obsolete—never."

and cosmetic chemists agree on. Marketing departments don't publicize this information; promising the impossible makes money.

"Insulates skin from premature aging factors so it's free to repair itself." It sounds very impressive, but all this particular product contains to back up that statement is a sunscreen. Unfortunately, it's not a very good sunscreen because it doesn't contain UVA-blocking sunscreen agents. UVA rays are the ones that cause skin cancer and wrinkles. If a product doesn't contain avobenzone, titanium dioxide, or zinc oxide, it can't protect against the sun's UVA radiation. Sunscreens that do contain UVA protection can prevent continuing damage. Sun damage is like any injury but, while the skin has some capacity to repair itself, it can't if you continually reinjure it.

"Closest to your skin's own strengthening lipids." Lipids are fats, and skin contains lipids: the sebum your skin secretes as oil is a lipid, and there are lipids in the layers of skin between the cells. If you put a lipid that resembles skin lipids into a skin-care product, that's nice, but lots and lots of ingredients can do that, everything from glycerin to ceramides to silicone oil, mineral oil, and waxes. If you put on almost any moisturizer in the world, it does help the lipids in your skin do a better job, and the expensive product can't do a better job than the inexpensive product. Moisturizers make the skin feel better and help keep moisture in the skin, period.

"Dermatologists gave us permission to make this line available to the public." Dermatologists do not vote on skin-care products, nor do they have to give permission to sell a product. This is supposed to sound like dermatologists love the products from one specific line, but I've yet to get any consensus from the dozens of dermatologists I've interviewed in regard to any cosmetic.

"Soothing botanicals." Botanicals are simply plants, such as herbs and flowers, or plant extracts in the form of oils or juices. Is any of that soothing? There *are* some soothing botanicals such as green tea, kola extract, bisabolol (from trees), licorice root (glycyrrhetinic acid), and burdock root. But the preponderance of natural ingredients, from lemons to strawberries, lavender oil, and jojoba, can be problematic for lots of skin types either as irritants or because they can clog pores. I can't tell you the number of products I've found making claims about being good for sensitive skin, even though they contain a host of irritating ingredients.

"Independent tests confirm up to 45% reduction in visible lines and wrinkles, as well as significant firming and smoothing." I called to ask if I could see these independent tests. I was told I couldn't, that they were secret. If that's the case, why quote them at all? If a test were truly independent, it would be open to public review just as all scientific research is.

"Soon expression lines appear smoother." What you think "appear smoother" means is one thing; what it means literally is something else. Dry skin can look "superficially" wrinkled; if you put on moisturizer, the dry skin can absolutely look smoother, but the effect is gone the next day. If you have dry skin and you don't reapply the moisturizer, the wrinkles come back. A moisturizer won't get rid of wrinkles, but then, the ad doesn't say the product will eliminate wrinkles, it just appears to. That claim can be attributed to any and all moisturizers.

"Superficial lines." Watch out for the word "superficial"; it is a powerful tool when used in cosmetics advertising. "Superficial lines" really refers to the temporary, transient lines caused by dryness, not those caused by sun damage (sun-damage wrinkles are hardly superficial). Most products could make elaborate claims about smoothing superficial wrinkles and they would not be lying to you. Superficial wrinkles go away when you put on any moisturizer, and that is wonderful. But—I repeat, *but*—superficial wrinkles are not the ones you are worried about. Permanent wrinkles, such as laugh lines, furrows between the eyes and on the forehead, and expression lines, are not eliminated by the use of a moisturizer unless it contains irritants that temporarily swell the skin. The word "superficial" is misleading because it doesn't really refer to the lines and wrinkles women are most concerned about.

"Start today and see a young tomorrow." First, this line doesn't say that "young" has anything to do with you; rather, it has to do with tomorrow being young. So exactly what is a young tomorrow? The implication is that tomorrow you will see a younger you. That's not what it says, but that's the impression you are supposed to get. Even if the phrase did say "see a younger you," how much younger are you supposed to see yourself tomorrow? Five minutes? An hour? A day? "See a young tomorrow" suggests something will happen to your wrinkles, but that is not actually what is being said; it's only what you hope is being said.

"Helps neutralize free radicals." It sounds convincing, yet there is no way to know if free radicals are being neutralized on the skin because that can't be measured. You can observe free-radical damage in a petri dish, but you can't see it taking place on the skin. Besides, how much of an ingredient is needed to combat free radicals, and how long does it last on the skin? No one knows.

"Just for your ultra-delicate eye area." The advertiser may want you to use the eye cream only around your eyes, which means you have to buy a face lotion separately, but the ingredients of these products are rarely different enough to warrant the extra expense. There is no reason an eye cream can't be used on the face and a face lotion can't be used around the eyes. The only time a special eye cream would be necessary is when the skin around the eyes is different from the skin on the rest of the face, which may require a more or less emollient moisturizer.

"Calms fine lines." I never knew wrinkles needed calming. Were they over-excited in the first place? What this suggests is that if your skin is stressed out, it must look more wrinkly. There is no proof at all that stress causes the skin to age. Sun ages skin, age ages skin, smoking ages skin, and other biochemical factors in the cell age skin, regardless of how stressful your life is. If anything, most women think of the sun as soothing and calming, and yet it is incredibly damaging to the skin!

"Makes dark circles seem to disappear." There's that word "seem" again—watch out for it. There are no creams that can eliminate puffiness or dark circles. However, dry skin can seem puffier and make naturally dark skin tissue look darker. Any moisturizer applied over an eye area that is dehydrated will make it "seem" to be less dark and puffy. Another cause of dark circles is surface circulation showing through the thin skin around the eyes; that can't be altered by skin-care products either.

"Dimpling seems to virtually disappear." Aside from the word "seems," the word "virtually" is also a disclaimer. According to the dictionary, *virtually* means "in effect, but not factually." So this statement doesn't really say that anything is going to happen when you put this product on. Dimpling refers to cellulite, which cannot and should not be altered from the outside in. If these products did work, a woman would never have to diet, and she could use the product to break down fat in every part of her body, and then no one would be overweight or have cellulite. If fat could be eliminated via some external process, it would be seriously dangerous for the body and pose critical health concerns.

"Nighttime repair." The suggestion here is that somehow a cream can help increase cell reproduction and undo skin damage. It's not possible, though it would be nice if it could be. Cosmetics can't change the way cells reproduce. You can do some impressive things with a moisturizer and create smoother, healthier-looking skin, but it is all temporary. Stop using it and things will go back to the way they were. If you could change the way cells reproduce, no one would have wrinkles or sun damage, and no one would get skin cancer.

"Nourishing hydrobeads release vitamins and minerals." You can't feed the skin from the outside in. Vitamins and minerals applied on the surface of the skin don't work in the same way as the vitamins and minerals you swallow. In order for vitamins and minerals to have an effect on the skin, they must be digested and combined with a vast array of other nutrients before they are converted to a form the body or skin can use. "Hydrobeads" sounds like a special delivery system that can somehow transport these vitamins and minerals into the skin. It can't. Literally, hydrobeads means "beads of water." Big deal. There are a lot of these "microbeads" running around in cosmetics nowadays. When I visited a cosmetic chemistry laboratory at the University of Cleveland under the supervision of Dr. Randy Wicket, his students were making moisturizers with colorful microbeads swirling through a gel matrix. Very pretty to look at, but all of them knew the stuff served no benefit for the skin.

"All at once the past is forgiven, the present improved, the future perfect." This doesn't refer to anything specific, but it is wonderfully seductive. Sometimes ads don't say anything about what the product really does; they just imply that the product will do something, anything, that may be good for the skin. The present can be improved but you can't undo the past, and, unless the product contains a good sunscreen with UVA protection, you can't affect the future.

"Microtargeted skin gel-rebuilding the skin's appearance." "Microtargeted" is a good word. It sounds like this gel will zap just the area where you need it to work. If you have a wrinkle right next to your eye, no other area will be affected by the gel, right? That is what "microtargeted" seems to mean. But the ad doesn't say that, even though you are supposed to jump to that wrong conclusion. The term could mean anything. Plus, there is no evidence you can rebuild skin with cosmetics.

"Test results reveal the cream beneficially affected the appearance of the skin surface." Whose test results? In almost every case the cosmetics company is quoting its own results, which are not substantiated by any other source.

"Natural bonding materials slow down loss of critical moisture." You know what these bonding materials are? Hairstyling agents, plasticlike ingredients that put a microscopic layer over the skin that helps keep water from evaporating. Hairspray ingredients show up in lots of skin-care products these days. This is a decent way to keep moisture in the skin, but making it sound impressive is at best stretching the point.

"Dramatically diminishes wrinkles by penetrating the top layer of skin to create a balloon effect, pushing the skin out from beneath the surface." I had a tough time deciphering this one. But after reading the ingredient list, it was obvious that all the product could do was to irritate the skin, which would make it swell. Swollen skin can temporarily look less wrinkled. Of course, this ad doesn't mention that many dermatologists warn against using products that irritate the skin, because irritation can damage skin, which eventually makes wrinkles worse. Ironic, isn't it, that many of the very products advertised as diminishing wrinkles can possibly make them more pronounced because of chronic irritation?

"Works with the microcirculation of your skin." "Works with" is always a good phrase, but exactly what kind of work is being referred to? "Microcirculation" also sounds very impressive. Yet technically, all creams can affect the microcirculation of your skin. If the idea is to stimulate circulation, then rubbing any cream onto the skin will do that. It isn't the cream doing the stimulation, it's your fingers rubbing the cream into your skin. But suggesting in an ad that—product or no product—all you need to do to stimulate circulation is massage your skin wouldn't sell anything.

"Penetrates deeply into the layers of the skin." "Penetrates" is a very impressive though imprecise word. Almost any cosmetic ingredient, if its molecules are small enough, will penetrate the skin, though the molecular structure of most cosmetic ingredients is too large to penetrate the skin. When cosmetic ingredients are capable of penetrating the skin, the word "layers" is frequently added to confound you. Layers of skin are so microscopically small, they are negligible. A cream can penetrate millions of layers and still not have traveled anywhere. And even if the cream could penetrate the skin deeply, it would be partially absorbed and flushed out.

"The skin's ability for self-rejuvenation is helped." The skin can self-rejuvenate (up to a point) if we don't get in the way of that process with sun damage, smoking, or irritating the skin. You can't rejuvenate the skin if you continually damage it. Yet this product does not have a sunscreen or any warnings about irritation or smoking.

"Deep cleansing." This term has always baffled me. How deep is deep? Sounds like a dentist cleaning your teeth. I can vividly hear the sound of a drill trying to get into your pores. If a product could clean deeply—I mean *really* deeply—you would be bleeding and no one would ever have blackheads because you would eliminate them through "deep cleansing." In this case, "deep cleansing" probably means "thorough cleansing," which is fine. But cosmetics companies encourage the belief that deep-cleansing products can get into a pore and eject a blackhead. There are ways to dissolve the stuff inside a blackhead, but "deep cleansing" won't.

"Gentle to the skin" or **"Good for sensitive skin."** Products described as "gentle to the skin" often contain ingredients that absolutely can cause irritation—a lot of it. As with the term "hypoallergenic," there are no guidelines or specifications about what constitutes a gentle product. If you don't read the ingredient list, you won't know you're buying something that's neither gentle nor good for sensitive skin until you put it on your face (and even then you may not know because irritation is not always evident on the surface of the skin).

"Designed to restore the skin's natural moisture balance." Moisturizers add moisture to the skin and help keep it there, but they can't alter how the skin behaves. This clever marketing copy implies you won't need to continue using this moisturizer because it teaches your skin how to be moist on its own. That is hardly the case for any skin-care product. You can't retrain skin. Cosmetics can't change your body's hormones, your genetic coding, years of sun damage, or other health concerns, which are the things that greatly affect the skin.

"Cellular protein nourishes the skin to visibly tighten and tone." Even if cellular protein could nourish the skin, which it can't, protein is too large a molecule to get past the surface of the skin. You can't feed the skin from the outside in. Nourishment is a very complicated process that does not rely on a single chemical, vitamin, mineral, or food. It requires an intricate digestive process that delivers site-appropriate chemical substances (thousands of them, not just one) to where they are supposed to go. Protein sounds good, but by itself, especially when applied to the skin's surface, it does nothing for the human body and skin.

Excerpt from Cosmetics Counter Update

Dear Paula,

You always calm me down from a frenzy of desire brought on by advertisements. Here's a new one: an anti-wrinkling pill. Have you heard of this? (I have enclosed a copy of the full advertising packet.)

Of course, I know enough from your works not to be enticed by the latest or most expensive AHA cream or moisturizer with antioxidants. Especially not when Alpha Hydrox can give me an effective product for about $10.

But what about this pill? It claims it "replenishes collagen; rebuilds elastic fibers." "The same formula used in the Scandinavian studies." I remain skeptical, but I would greatly appreciate your comments.

Susan, via e-mail

Dear Susan,

I know I shouldn't be shocked by this kind of blatantly guileful advertising, but this one makes me just want to scream. Unfortunately, many women will waste their hard-earned money as this insanity builds a deceived following. First of all, there are no studies that support the contentions in the ad—not in Scandinavia, not anywhere. Furthermore, if this is an anti-wrinkle pill, how did they get the before-and-after pictures the ad portrays: a woman with a face that's half wrinkly and half smooth? If it's taken orally and the effects are systemic, how did it happen to work on only one side of her face?

There are many reasons why this is nonsense besides the two points I mentioned above. Collagen is only one of the many skin components that deteriorate and make skin look older. If this product affects only collagen, you would not get the benefits shown in the ad. If you did get this benefit, why would it work on the face only? If it's taken orally, wouldn't it affect collagen all over the skin, so that anyplace you have depleted collagen or sagging, wrinkled skin would get lifted? Wouldn't your breasts stand up, your sagging backside become firm, and on and on?

Perhaps more to the point, if this pill did work, it would be classified as a drug, but the ad clearly states it is a cosmetic. That means no proof of claims is required. Also, no safety date is required unless someone complains. That's after the fact, not before as with prescription and over-the-counter drugs.

This product doesn't deserve anyone's attention, but I understand the seductiveness. Please, do not give these people, or any other company for that matter, any more incentive to lead the public around by their fear of aging.

The Crazy Things Cosmetics Salespeople Say

Separate from the advertising mumbo jumbo, there is an entire realm of appallingly inaccurate or just plain wrong information being disseminated on a daily basis by cosmetics salespeople all over the world. These false sales pitches are tomorrow's new myths, spun before a captive audience. Here are my latest favorites, but I have to admit these only skim the surface.

"In order for the products to achieve dramatic results you must use all of them; the skin must be properly conditioned to accept all the products in the line in order for any of the products to work." This is one of my favorites because its purpose is to convince you to buy all the products from one line. It is a classic sales technique. In essence, what you are being told is that the line's wrinkle cream won't work unless all the other products are used first, so don't bother buying the wrinkle cream unless you are going to buy everything. In my years of reviewing skin-care routines, I have never seen a cosmetics line with products so unique that you couldn't substitute a dozen other products for them, and many that would work better. Further, every cosmetics line has products you should avoid because they contain irritating ingredients, or inadequate amounts of sunscreen, or moisturizers that oversaturate the skin. The term to note here is "dramatic results." What the cosmetics company considers dramatic results may be dramatically different from what you would really like to see the products do—even if you use all of them.

"Our ingredients are high quality; that's why they are so expensive." It would be nice if that were true, but I can't get any cosmetics company to give me proof of it. I've asked for the names of their suppliers to find out what grades of products they are selling and if they do have inferior grades that go to some companies but not others. From what I've been able to find out on my own after talking to several cosmetic-ingredient manufacturers, the grades of cosmetic ingredients don't vary that much, and everyone buys cosmetic-grade ingredients, which are all high quality. For example, DuPont is one of the largest suppliers of glycolic acid to the cosmetics industry, and it supplies the same thing to everyone.

"You need to wear makeup because it acts as a barrier between your skin

and pollution." It's just not true. Perhaps the more opaque, solid particles in foundations, powders, and lipsticks can reduce the skin's exposure to the sun's rays, but that's not pollution. Inorganic pollutants such as smog, car exhaust, and other industrial fumes can be absorbed right through makeup and moisturizers.

"See how smooth it makes your skin feel—that's the vitamins and plant extracts working." Take some vitamins or plants like chamomile, lemon, or peppermint; rub them on your skin; and then tell me how that makes your skin feel. You wouldn't feel any difference (unless you have an allergic reaction), because it would have no effect at all. Besides, the amount of vitamins and plant extracts in cosmetics is so minute as to be undetectable by your skin. The ingredients that make the skin feel smooth are usually the standard oils, waxes, emollients, and slip agents (glycerinlike ingredients that slip over the skin and help give it a smooth feeling) that show up in product after product.

"Layering different moisturizers one over the other gives you the benefit of each one's specialized purpose." The only benefit derived from layering moisturizers is to the cosmetics company that was able to convince you to buy more than you need. Skin does better with less. Too much moisturization is bad for skin because it can turn off the skin's natural immune/healing system. Plus, the more products you use, the more skin-care ingredients you are applying[7], raising your risk of experiencing an allergic reaction.

"We use only natural ingredients; synthetic ingredients are bad for your skin because they are fake and made from gasoline." I have yet to see any cosmetic that is "all" natural. Some synthetic ingredients are awesome for your skin, and they are in every skin-care and makeup product on the market, regardless of their claim about being all natural. Synthetic ingredients are derived from many sources, but they all start as natural because everything comes from our environment; nothing is created via alchemy. Petrolatum and mineral oil are the only popular skin-care ingredients that are a by-product of the gasoline industry, but not only are they remarkably good skin-care ingredients, they are also recognized by cosmetic chemists the world over for being superior emollients and completely harmless. Why these two ingredients get a bad rap from so-called natural skin-care lines is a mystery. You're better off having petrolatum or mineral oil in your moisturizer than a plant any day.

"You need to use facial masks and give yourself regular spa treatments that

---

[7] The average cosmetic contains 25 to 40 ingredients. If you use a cleanser, toner, three different moisturizers, foundation, concealer, blush, powder, and two eyeshadows, your skin is exposed to somewhere between 100 and 440 cosmetic ingredient variations. That's intense. Is it any wonder women have allergic reactions to cosmetics?

include steaming to pull toxins out of the skin and remove debris from the pores." There is nothing lurking around in one's skin and pores that can be pulled or sucked out of the skin. In all likelihood toxins are present in the skin cells, but they cannot be removed by skin-care products. (If scientists ever do figure out how to get toxins out of skin cells, you probably could reverse some important aspect of skin aging, not to mention how the entire body ages, but they haven't identified even a fraction of the toxins that might be causing cell damage and genetic mutation.) What does need to be removed from pores is cellular debris (dead skin cells) that fill the pore, along with wax and tiny hairs that have built up in there. That takes more than an occasional mask to remove; it takes daily effort and salicylic acid and sometimes prescription drugs such as Retin-A and Differin. If these masks could do what they claim, no one would have clogged pores or wrinkles, and that just isn't happening. By the way, you also can't sweat out toxins or debris from your pores; the only thing sweat contains is sweat.

"A famous scientist [doctor, chemist, pharmacist, dermatologist, or whatever—I've heard it all] created this formula and it is only now available to the public." Lots of doctors and chemists are involved in all kinds of products in the world of cosmetics, but all cosmetics contain standard cosmetic ingredients. They can't contain anything else or they would be regulated quite differently.

My favorite example of this type of claim is Estee Lauder Creme de la Mer. What a story accompanies this very costly little cream *($150 for one ounce)*! It was created by Max Huber, a NASA aerospace physicist, supposedly to take care of burns he received in an accident. He sold and marketed this product himself. After his death, his daughter continued selling the cream until recently, when Estee Lauder purchased the rights to manufacture and distribute it.

As enticing as this dramatic story sounds, the reality is that this very basic, and I mean *really* basic, cream doesn't contain anything particularly extraordinary or unique, unless you want to believe that seaweed extract (sort of like seaweed tea) can somehow be worth this much money or that it can in some way heal burns and scars. Even if it could heal burns, heat and sunburns don't have much to do with wrinkling; UVA radiation is what causes most wrinkling, and those aren't the burning rays. According to Susan Brawley, professor of plant biology at the University of Maine, "Seaweed extract isn't a rare, exotic, or expensive ingredient. Seaweed extract is readily available and used in everything from cosmetics to food products and medical applications." Creme de la Mer contains mostly seaweed extract, mineral oil, petrolatum (similar to Vaseline), glycerin, waxlike thickening agents, plant oils, plant seeds, minerals, vitamins, more thickeners, and preservatives. How expensive can it be to stick some seaweed and vitamins in a cosmetic? According to the cosmetic chemists I've interviewed, it costs pennies, not hundreds of dollars.

This scientific silliness began back in the early 1980s, when Dr. Christian Barnard, who pioneered heart transplant surgery, was recruited by a cosmetics company to endorse an anti-aging cream. The cream contained a new ingredient called glycosphingolipid (GSL). An ad campaign was launched and Barnard was quoted in the ads as saying, "When environmental damage is repaired, many of the normal functions of the skin cells return, allowing the skin to look younger." As it turned out, glycosphingolipid was merely a good lipid (fat or oil) and a water-binding agent, but nothing more, similar to many other cosmetic ingredients, such as hyaluronic acid and mucopolysaccharides. It does not affect the skin cells or make them act younger (meaning they don't reproduce like younger skin cells do). Barnard's career was never the same after that, and the FDA made the company behind this claim, as well as others that had copied this endeavor, stop.

"The reason you have oily skin is because you don't have enough moisture in your skin. Your skin produces excess oil to protect it from moisture loss. If you had enough moisture in your skin it would stop producing oil. That's why it is so important for someone with oily skin to wear a moisturizer." What nonsense! Oil production has nothing to do with the state of dryness in your skin. If that were true, wouldn't someone with dry skin have her oil production turned on? Women with dry skin do not increase their oil production when they don't wear a moisturizer. Oily skin appears to be primarily produced by genetic inheritance and hormonal production, but no one knows exactly why some people have oily skin and others have dry skin.

"Just because the surface of your skin is oily doesn't mean the underlying layer of skin isn't dry and in need of moisture." I could help a large number of women eliminate their complaints of oily, combination, or acne-prone skin if I could just get them to stop using moisturizer. Moisturizer is the most abused skin-care product, because unless you have dry skin you absolutely don't need it. There is nothing protective about moisturizers: they don't stop stress, they can't prevent pollution from getting to the skin, they can't feed the skin, they can't thwart sun damage (unless they contain sunscreen), and they can't permanently alter the skin's structure. If your skin has a dry layer it can be a result of using drying soaps, cleansers, and toners that contain alcohol or other drying ingredients (like lemon or grapefruit), or of using too much moisturizer, which prevents skin from sloughing off naturally.

"This moisturizer is perfect for someone with oily or combination skin because it is oil-free." I can't tell you the number of products touting this claim when they indeed contain oils, or waxes that feel oily, or other ingredients that can clog pores. They may not be oils you recognize, like plant oils or mineral oils, but they are nonetheless in there, with names you don't understand. Saying a product is oil-free gives you no information about what it may or may not do to the skin. What is most confusing is that ingredients known for causing breakouts may not leave a greasy feel on the skin. Surprisingly, one of the greasiest ingredients, mineral oil, has been shown in study after study not to cause breakouts, although it can still feel greasy. Go figure. The fewer skin-care products a woman with oily or blemish-prone skin uses, the better off her skin will be.

As a general rule, because they can leave a greasy feeling on the skin, it is best to avoid any and all oils in skin-care products, including silicone oils, if they are high on the ingredient list. Women with oily skin should avoid any ingredients ending in triglyceride, palmitate, or myristate, and ingredients such as jojoba (jojoba oil and wax can cause breakouts), lanolin, beeswax, candelilla wax, carnuba wax, cocoa butter, shea butter, and tallow (found mostly in soaps). These can all clog pores or leave skin feeling greasy. Keep in mind that there are a host of ingredients that can aggravate oily skin and acne while actually feeling cool and drying on the skin, including alcohol, menthol, lemon, and mint.

"The soya protein in this product helps strengthen lashes." There are no cosmetic ingredients that can strengthen lash hair, but especially not protein. Protein from any source doesn't cling well to hair, and the molecules are too large to get inside and shore things up.

"The sage, lemon, and grapefruit in this product help normalize skin oils." Lemon and grapefruit can irritate skin and stimulate oil production, but that's about it. Plus, oil in the skin is regulated primarily by hormone production, and there are no plants you can rub on your face to alter that.

"By using this product at night you can prepare the skin to offset the visible effects of daytime aggression." There is nothing you can do for your skin at night to change or reduce the effects of sun damage (that's the only daytime aggression you should worry about skinwise).

Brand-Name Addiction

Since I began evaluating cosmetics, the question I am asked most frequently is "Which product line do you like the best? What do you think of Lancome, Estee Lauder, Mary Kay, or hundreds of other lines?" That was the major reason I wrote *Don't Go to the Cosmetics Counter Without Me.* By actually reviewing each line, I could point out specifically what we already know is true: every line, regardless of price, has good and bad products. Brand-name loyalty does not make any sense. Lancome makes great mascaras and some great foundations, but several of its toners contain alcohol, its sunscreens don't all have UVA protection, some of its eyeshadows are too shiny, and its skin-care products are overpriced. Clinique has some very good foundations, sunscreens, and a wide variety of other products, but its eyeshadows are all shiny, its toners are mostly alcohol and one contains acetone (that's nail polish remover), and its TurnAround moisturizers (which contain the exfoliant BHA, salicylic acid) are not the right pH, so they can't turn around anything. Revlon has some great foundations, decent matte eyeshadows, good mascaras, excellent blushes, and terrific lip pencils, but its ColorStay foundation goes on way too thick, its ColorStay eyeshadows are tricky to use, and its skin-care products are almost nonexistent and mediocre (they don't have an SPF 15).

We already know this to be true. Yet the success of the major product lines in establishing brand-name loyalty is astonishing. It is particularly apparent in how a woman responds to questions about what brand of makeup she is currently using. The answer usually reflects the amount of money she has spent on the product. A customer usually whispers or acts embarrassed when she admits to using a drugstore brand, but if she's using an expensive brand you can hear her across the room. The reality is that the cost of a cosmetic has nothing to do with whether it will work for you. I have used both inexpensive and expensive makeup that looked wonderful and was good for the skin, as well as inexpensive and expensive makeup that looked awful and was bad for the skin.

Another point about brand-name loyalty is that when we buy a product from a particular cosmetics line, the company has not necessarily manufactured that product. Many of the eye pencils offered by different companies come from the same manufacturer in Germany. Many eyeshadows and blushes sold by different lines come from the exact same labs. Skin-care products are often manufactured by contract labs all over the world, including China and India.

Years ago, just after I opened my first makeup store, I visited one of the manufacturing plants that was wholesaling its makeup to me. As they proudly showed me around their facilities, showing me rows and rows of material and machinery, we passed an area where they were assembling eyeshadow tins. At the end of this conveyor were boxes labeled with most of the major cosmetics brand names. They obviously wanted me to know that I would be selling the same stuff these big shots were selling. They were right—I was impressed. I was also pleased to know firsthand how things really happened.

What I have just described is the reality of the cosmetics industry. I'm hardly the first person to discover this. The television show *60 Minutes* did a segment on this very issue, and Ralph Nader has argued the point on numerous talk shows and in his own book on the cosmetics business, as have other consumer reporters. The package doesn't tell you anything about the product's value, and the price doesn't tell you anything about the quality—how it will go on the skin or how long the effect you're looking for will last.

I have also heard the claim that you need to buy all your skin-care products from one line because the products are designed to work together. That may be the company's intent, but it doesn't hold up. Lots of skin-care products contain ingredients I would not want anyone to use on her face, or they can clog pores or cause skin sensitivities.

Why is it, then, that a particular brand of cosmetics is so expensive compared with a less expensive brand made by the same manufacturing company? In the final analysis, price is determined by what the market will bear. If you're willing to pay $25 for a foundation because you believe you'll look twenty-five dollars' worth better, they'll sell it to you for just that. Hopefully, by now your ideas about brand-name loyalties have changed. Don't just take my word for it! Go to any library and check out a copy of *Drug and Cosmetic Industry* magazine or *Cosmetics & Toiletries* magazine and read about the manufacturing of cosmetics and cosmetic ingredients, or read the *Journal of Cosmetic Dermatology.* These periodicals reveal how the cosmetics industry really works.

Infomercials—The Evil Empire

I may be the only person in the world who has a recurrent dream that all women change channels every time an infomercial comes on the air. Of course, that is sheer fantasy on my part. The charisma of the salesperson/celebrity/doctor, the stunning before-and-afters, and the heartfelt testimonials always drive viewers to buy. Objective information is never part of the sales pitch anywhere in the cosmetics industry, and this is painfully so in the field of infomercials.

For as long as I have been researching and monitoring the cosmetics industry, I have been most amazed by the overly enthusiastic rantings and the ardent, rapturous claims espoused in infomercial after infomercial and on shopping channel after shopping channel. They are all, with their slick settings, attractive celebrity hosts, authoritative-looking doctors, and breathtaking before-and-after shots, shockingly redundant. This is little more than snake oil, but it all sounds so good women can hardly help themselves. Infomercials and shopping channel pitches are no worse than other kinds of advertising, but they go on for such long periods of time, the hype just grows and grows like Pinocchio's nose.

I wish I could divulge everything I've heard via the people I've met and interviewed in the infomercial business about what goes on behind the scenes, but none of it is substantiated. (I got the information from what I consider to be a reliable source, but I couldn't get corroboration. Without a second reliable source repeating the exact same story, I feel it would be unethical to share what I've learned. I use this standard rule about substantiation in all my books and newsletters.) For example, I would love to let you know about two very popular skin-care infomercials in which the celebrity spokeswomen both carried on at length about the quality of the products, yet neither had even seen them before they walked on the set the day of the shoot. Or about another very popular skin-care infomercial that cost about $5 million to produce but lost a huge amount of money when more than 40% of the products were returned by disappointed consumers. I've also personally seen the process of how in-home shopping channels choose the skin-care products they will put on the air. The person responsible for getting these products on the air admitted to me that they couldn't do anything about how useless or poor in quality the cosmetics they sold were or the exaggerated claims made by the people selling the products. I was told that if the spokesperson is entertaining enough and appears to have a good pitch or angle, that is enough to get the product some air time.

I've often wondered how many more infomercials women will swallow about miracle skin-care products, skin-care regimes, and makeup products before they start to yawn (or laugh) and keep their money in their pocket. On the other hand, it is sadly true that women have an insatiable appetite for being misled by every slickly positioned sales pitch they hear. From Victoria Principal, Ethocyn, Hydron, Forever Spring, Adrien Arpel, and Marilyn Miglin to Mon Amie, H+, Murad, Dr. Mary Lupo, ProActiv, Serious Skin Care, Dr. Feder, and on and on, there isn't one that lives up to its claims. I'm not saying there aren't some truly good products in these lines, but the majority of the claims and adulation for all these are manufactured and fabricated for the audience's entertainment. Which is exactly what infomercials are, entertainment, and they should not be taken as fact or information. (I've reviewed all of the above lines in either my book *Don't Go to the Cosmetics Counter Without Me,* third edition, or previous issues of my newsletter, *Cosmetics Counter Update.*)

Why We Believe

I'm often asked why we believe all of this foolishness, given the copious amounts of information to the contrary. I wonder sometimes too, but our willingness to believe has little to do with being foolish. It is much more complicated than that, from both an emotional and a sociological perspective. I believe there are extremely compelling reasons why we get taken in time after time by empty, meaningless ads and claims.

Reason No. 1. For the most part, skin-care products and, more specifically, wrinkle creams feel good and take very good care of skin. We all need to clean our face, and many of us have to fight dry skin, oily skin, or combination skin. One way or another, without skin-care products we would be left with more problems than we started with. Soap all by itself, for the majority of women, leaves the face dry and irritated. Even though many toners contain irritants, they at least take off that last layer of makeup, which can clog pores. Moisturizers (wrinkle creams are, after all, just moisturizers) can be an essential part of taking care of dry skin. So the reason we buy the stuff in the first place is because a great number of these products take great care of our skin. They don't perform the miracles they suggest; they aren't worth the big bucks they frequently cost; but, in general, they do help. The fact that lots of skin-care products perform well can lead someone to believe that another brand or price range may perform better yet.

Reason No. 2. Even though most skin-care products do work, they also just as often fail miserably. Women frequently buy the wrong products for their skin type. Sometimes the formulations are so irritating and poorly conceived that they cause complications, making matters worse, or they simply do not eliminate the skin problems they were bought for. That's why women are in constant search of the right products. They believe the right ones for their skin type are out there somewhere, if they could only find them. Skin problems are a recurrent headache. It is the rare individual who doesn't have to be concerned with acne, wrinkles, dry skin, oily skin, irritation, or a combination of them. Anything but perfect skin seems to be what we all have, but perfect skin is what we are all after.

Most women think the major questions to ask about skin care are "Which products will be best for my skin?" and "Which products work and which ones don't, and where do I find them?" The questions themselves show where the problem lies. The search should not be so much for the right product, but for the right (and wrong) ingredients. If you just look for products but don't know what's inside, you could be buying the same formulation over and over again without really changing what you are doing for your skin. Once you understand that even with the most expensive products you can overmoisturize the skin while trying to eliminate dryness, irritate the skin in the name of drying up acne, or make oily skin worse by using so-called oil-free moisturizers, you will be way ahead of the game.

Reason No. 3. Beauty myths die a long, hard death. Once we believe something about our skin, it is very hard to change our mind. I discuss many myths throughout this book, but they are almost endless. Letting go of myths isn't easy. It takes information, and some of that information is boring, technical, and hard to grasp. But once you've mastered some of the basics, none of the bogus facts you hear or see will catch you off guard again.

Reason No. 4. Everything the ads, brochures, and cosmetics salespeople tell us sounds very convincing. Given the amount of money cosmetics companies spend on packaging, promotions, and advertising, it should. Just remember that all that glitters is not gold. The glitter and shine at the cosmetics counters sure looks like gold, but it rarely, if ever, is. Do not be convinced again and again that because something "sounds" good, it is, or that expensive means better, because it isn't.

Reason No. 5. It is very difficult to believe that cosmetics companies want to take advantage of us when what they are selling seems so beautiful and attractive and comes in such stunning containers. This desire to trust in a company's higher purpose is part of what we all want to presume. It is tiresome to be cautious about everything. And the spokesmodels for these companies look so convincing and sweet; surely they wouldn't lie to us.

The truth is, cosmetics companies have one purpose, and that is to sell their products. That is their bottom line. Whether they do anything else is less important than that one objective. Many companies do make good products, and there is nothing wrong with selling products. But to assume that a company is in business for the good of the consumer and that, as a result, they really do sell miraculous formulas or everything in their line is automatically good, is unwise.

Reason No. 6. We want to believe that what they tell us is true. It is reassuring to assume that the $10 or $50 or $150 you just spent is somehow going to take care of your skin-care or makeup problems. Surely all those scientists and dermatologists must have invented something by now.

We also want to believe that there are wrinkle creams that get rid of wrinkles and astringents that close pores and lipsticks that last all day, but it is important to be skeptical. If wrinkle creams can work, why do any of us have wrinkles? If astringents or toners can close pores, why do any of us have open pores? If lipsticks really can last all day, why must we constantly reapply them? It is OK to accept reality, because being realistic will not make you any less beautiful or prevent you from taking good care of your skin.

Reason No. 7. The cosmetics companies aren't really lying to us. They aren't exactly telling the truth, but even the most extreme ads hedge their promises and claims with vague language that doesn't really say anything specific. When you see an ad for a wrinkle cream that reduces fine lines, restores suppleness, and rejuvenates the skin, you must remember that any moisturizer can make that claim and not be lying. The rest is all exaggeration and nonsense, but the basic quality of the product is often intact.

Reason No. 8. Salespeople are well trained to sell you their products. They can be very skilled in subtle but effective sales techniques. Their best sales tactic is to reinforce a woman's insecurity. This emotional battleground is the salesperson's best weapon and the one the consumer is least equipped to avoid or resist. See if these routines sound familiar:

(1) The salesperson reminds the consumer that she is not as beautiful as she

could be because she isn't yet using the salesperson's products. The salesperson offers a lipstick and says, "This color would look much better on you."

(2) The salesperson helps the consumer notice all the problems her skin is having (after all, she's the expert—she's supposed to notice these problems). She may ask, "Aren't you concerned about how dry your skin is, particularly around your eyes?" or "You aren't using a moisturizer [shocked reaction]? Everyone needs a moisturizer to protect their skin from the environment, stress, hormones, or makeup."

(3) The salesperson suggests that if a woman continues to make the same skin-care mistakes over and over, she will pay for it down the road: "You can't start too soon using this product, because it can only get worse if you wait, and then it may be too late to do anything about it."

It is essential to know that cosmetics salespeople are not necessarily trained in skin care or makeup; they are trained to sell products. Assuming these people have a scientific or even a basic knowledge about skin is a serious mistake. A 1992 study by the city of New York's Department of Consumer Affairs assessed the statements and claims made by cosmetics salespeople and stated that "more than one in three [cosmetics salespeople] stretched the truth beyond recognition, making claims the company attorneys would never allow." Another one-third gave ambiguous or cryptic responses to skin-care questions, and the rest just recommended products.

The only way to defend yourself against these sales techniques is with a strong sense of self-esteem. Security in who you are is important in life—and at the cosmetics counters. If you are willing to accept the idea of being rescued by the products being sold to you, you are at the mercy of a good sales pitch. You must recognize right now that there are no answers inside these glittering, slick boxes and jars—that what you need is information from independent sources (not fashion magazines or salespeople) that can help you to understand your skin and recognize what cosmetics can and can't do.

I admit that I repeatedly come down fairly hard on cosmetics salespeople. It isn't that I haven't met some wonderful cosmetics salespeople, because I have. Many times these remarkable women and men have given me insights into the cosmetics industry that otherwise would have been impossible for me to obtain. I would also like to acknowledge from experience that, for the most part, particularly at department stores, selling cosmetics is not an easy or lucrative way to earn a living. Unfortunately, I have also had some difficult encounters with cosmetics salespeople. I have listened to and overheard hundreds of crazy conversations about skin care and makeup application that are nothing more than sales pressure and incorrect information. Because it is generally hard to differentiate between sales technique and valid information, it is safe to assume that you are far more likely to encounter salesmanship than factual information when buying skin-care or makeup products.

Reason No. 9. It's hard to question advice from a cosmetics representative. It isn't customary for women to refute what they hear, either directly or indirectly. Asserting your doubts and scrutinizing what you are told when dealing with cosmetics salespeople (or any salesperson) is difficult, but once you do, you will start noticing the information being doled out is baseless and mostly unbelievable. As you start questioning what you hear, the salesperson inevitably gets caught in the pretense and fumbles about, trying to find a plausible explanation. I wish this was as easy as it sounds, but it can be tricky. I can't promise you'll receive a pleasant reaction when you imply you don't believe what you are being told. My suggestion is to take it one step at a time. The next time you are at a cosmetics counter, try a few probing questions or ask to see the ingredient list when they start explaining the wondrous potion inside. Once you do, you will be less likely to leave feeling oversold. The more information you have, the less susceptible you will be to the hype and fantasy the cosmetics industry confronts us with everywhere we turn. Once you've finished reading this book, you will know more than most of the women and men selling makeup and skin-care products.

Reason No. 10. Fashion magazines make everything the cosmetics industry sells look and sound amazing. Their editorial comments 90% of the time glorify cosmetics, with only occasional, buried hints of objectivity. Cosmetics companies have a stranglehold on the way fashion magazines present information on skin care and makeup. What makes this so pathetic is that reading fashion magazines is a primary way women get advice, news, and reports on their beauty needs. Gloria Steinem, in an article in *Ms.* magazine, once explained why she would no longer accept advertisements for cosmetics. She said her advertisers demanded that their ads be placed near compatible and positive editorial stories; that they must not be near material that challenged the nature of the product; and that stories in the entire magazine must not contain anything the advertiser found objectionable or displeasing. That concisely explains why you never see a negative article about the cosmetics or fashion industry in the pages of fashion magazines.

Whom Should You Believe?

Wouldn't it be easy if the answer was to just believe me and then be done with it? Not that I don't want you to believe what I'm saying, but it is still your job as the cosmetics consumer to figure out exactly what you are going to do about the information you receive, whether it is from me or the cosmetics companies. When it comes to beauty decisions, that is no easy task. There is not much reality or rationality associated with makeup and skin care. Yet without a firm basis in reality and rational thinking, there is no way to approach your skin-care or makeup needs in a reasonable, sober light. What I mean by reasonable and sober is keeping your feet on the ground and your head out of the fluffy clouds of babble that accompany cosmetics. It doesn't mean that you can't attain an image of beauty or glamour you're comfortable with; it just means you will do it more easily and with more confidence once you know how to separate fact from fiction.

The first battle is trusting what you already know to be true. From mascara to astringents, no cosmetic can do anything earth-shattering for you, no matter whose name is on the label. And one company does not have all the right products for you, or the best secret formulas. Each and every cosmetics line has good and bad products, and even the great products (of which there are many) can have drawbacks.

What I mean by facing "reality" about cosmetics is best illustrated by an example that has nothing to do with cosmetics. I think that shopping for cosmetics is much like shopping for a beautiful pair of shoes. The salesperson brings out this absolutely gorgeous, to-die-for pair of high heels of red Italian leather, studded with multicolored rhinestones that fan out from the pointed toe and continue back to the elegant three-and-a-half-inch heel. Your feet slip into them like Cinderella's into the glass slipper. As you turn in the mirror, admiring the way they look, your entire profile is reflected like something out of a magazine ad. It's amazing what a pair of shoes can do for your appearance.

Unfortunately, the storybook never followed Cinderella home immediately after the ball. We were told that she ran home at midnight because of her fairy godmother's warning. The truth is, dancing in those glass slippers made her feet swell and ache so much she couldn't wait to get home. The dreamy look in her eyes when she was dancing with Prince Charming wasn't because of the prince, it was from thoughts of soaking her aching corns in hot soapy water. And the slipper she left behind wasn't a mistake: she would have gladly left both of them, but she couldn't get the other one off!

Get the picture?

Every time I shop for makeup, do my own makeup, or do someone else's makeup, I try to remember this image. The difference between the way we look without makeup and the way we look with a good makeup application is indeed dramatic. I would be the last person to deny the power of beautifully applied makeup or how lovely skin-care products can feel on the face and body. But makeup requires a daily repeated effort to apply it, keep it looking fresh all day long, and finally wash it off at night. Wearing makeup involves some give-

and-take, along with the expense. You must discover your best cosmetic options based on the most and least of what you can expect from your makeup.

CHAPTER TWO

What Works and What Doesn't

Cellular Renewal

Worry over the skin's slow but inevitable deterioration is a hot topic at the cosmetics counters and in fashion magazines. To fulfill women's hopes of reversing "environmental damage" (which is really only a fancy way to describe sun damage—toxins in the environment may play a part, but no one yet knows how or why) by "generating healthy cell growth" (in other words, the way that younger skin cells reproduce), the cosmetics industry sells a vast array of products promising to do just that. Everything from alpha hydroxy acids to plant extracts, marine extracts, animal extracts, vitamins, and now salicylic acid is sold claiming to provide new, smoother skin by exfoliating the old skin cells while creating new cell growth.

This idea of stimulating cell growth has some basis in a rational scientific context, but as usual the cosmetics industry distorts a grain of truth into a mountain of misinformation. You're supposed to conclude that AHAs, BHA, or any other ingredients that can really exfoliate dead skin cells will also stimulate the production of new skin cells and new collagen, making skin finally "look younger." (I discuss antioxidants and Retin-A later in this section, because their effectiveness in this arena deserves special attention.)

Exfoliating the skin does provide a great deal of benefit. As mentioned earlier, skin cell production slows down with age or sun damage. That can leave older, dried-up cells on the skin's surface longer than is normal. Skin cells can become misshapen, sticking together unevenly, causing problems with moisture content, and producing a dry, dull, and extremely flaky layer of surface skin. All of this builds a very good case for exfoliation, but it doesn't support the notion of cellular renewal. Removing dead skin cells helps pave the way for plumper, healthier skin cells to surface, which can make a huge difference in the appearance of the skin. When this takes place, skin thickness improves (the flat, misshapen cells are replaced by round, moisture-filled, smoother cells), moisture content goes up (the old, flat, dried-up cells are gone), and the skin functions better (oil flows more easily out of the pores, and blackheads and blemishes decrease now that the dead skin cells that got in the way are gone). All of this is true. But, as you might expect, many of the other claims circling around cellular renewal are more fiction than fact.

Cell renewal is a normal, inherent process all skin goes through. New skin cells are generated in the deepest structures of the skin, then migrate up to the skin's surface, changing their shape and size as they go. At the end of their life cycle, at the surface, the flattened and dried-up cells are shed. Healthy, newly produced skin cells make this trek to the surface over a period of about 28 to 45 days. What happens to skin cells during this time can greatly affect the skin's appearance.

What can go wrong with skin cells as they are born, die, and shed? Depending on your age and skin type, a lot. In most women under the age of 40 with normal skin, new skin cells are generated and move upward, through the layers of the epidermis, with a complete turnover taking place every 28 to 45 days. **But for some women, particularly older women and women affected by sun damage, smoking, genetic abnormality, or the presence of unknown toxins in the skin cells, that process is not always smooth, and problems happen along the way that can affect the appearance of the skin.** When skin cells turn over sluggishly, the turnover process can take much longer, leaving dead skin cells on the surface longer. These dead skin cells that are hanging around longer than they should have a dull, flat, thickened appearance and a grainy, coarse texture.

While genetic abnormality (such as autoimmune-related skin disorders) is not a controllable factor, you can avoid sun damage, abstain from smoking, and avoid toxins (although we don't know what toxins are affecting skin cells, so we don't really yet know which ones to avoid). Even if a woman could do everything right, there still exists a genetically preprogrammed turn-off point where all skin cells in the body stop reproducing as they did when they were young. Remember, all cells are regenerated again and again. For a good deal of our lives we continue producing new cells, but as genetic aging (our natural life span) takes place, the process simply slows down, almost to the point of shutdown. No one knows how to turn around this cellular slowdown—no one—so don't believe the cosmetics industry when they claim to have the answer.

Cell regeneration and migration from the lower layers of skin to the surface has nothing to do with the way skin wrinkles. Cellular renewal does not affect the collagen and elastin fibers that support the skin, nor does it affect the intercellular structure between the skin cells (where substances like glycerin, hyaluronic acid, ceramides, and glycosaminoglycans reside), all of which do greatly affect the skin's appearance. Collagen and elastin deteriorate when exposed to sun over a period of time, and this is a primary cause of wrinkles, but the production of collagen and elastin is not related to the regeneration and movement of skin cells. The substances that exist between the skin cells (as opposed to the skin cells themselves) seem to be affected mostly by aging and possibly by sun damage.

Dermatologists as well as cosmetics experts agree (and they rarely agree) that most skin types need help with the process of shedding skin cells. The disagreement exists over whether new skin cells can be generated by using cosmetics or pharmaceuticals. Can you generate new skin cells? And if you can, can you generate enough to make a difference? Without question, you can make a difference in the appearance of skin by helping skin cells on their journey through the layers of skin via cosmetics that use AHAs or BHA. But the only legitimate, peer-reviewed, published studies that document increased production of anything (namely, collagen) concern the topical tretinoin products Retin-A, Renova, and Micro-Retin-A, and it took two years before any measurable difference was detected. No one is sure why the collagen was created. In the meantime, ignore the claims about cellular renewal, because it just isn't possible, at least not the way we want it to be possible. **Besides, when it comes to exfoliation, there is a fine line between helping the skin cell "turnover" process and causing irritation that can damage the skin.**

Repairing Skin

The term "skin repair," much like "cellular renewal," is one we will hear well into the next millennium. It is best to come to terms with this trend now, or it will cost you lots of wasted time and money in the future. Repairing skin means many things to many different cosmetics companies, but the overall picture the consumer is supposed to have is that you can repair skin damage via some healing process that mends skin.

If skin wrinkles because of damage that causes the skin to break down (and that is indeed what takes place due to sun exposure, genetic aging, and trauma to the skin), then by repairing that damage you should be able to stop wrinkling and potentially even reverse the process. **To some extent that logic is absolutely valid (and lots of researchers in many medical disciplines, from oncology to dermatology, are pursuing this angle), but translating it into reality is far from possible right now.** If it were possible to obtain those results from a cosmetic or a prescription drug, we would all invest our hard-earned savings in the company making it, because it would truly be a miracle product.

When skin is damaged there are indeed ways to help repair it, but not the ways the cosmetics industry recommends. Vitamins, plants, and other bogus ingredients can't feed the skin from the outside, and they can't bandage skin and sew it up. The first step in skin repair is absolutely to stop causing more damage: stay out of the sun, stop smoking, avoid secondhand smoke, don't overirritate the skin, and avoid saturating the skin with too much moisturizer. All those things can make skin damage worse and get in the way of the skin's natural healing response. The best thing you can do for the skin is to stop hurting it rather than administering more skin-care products.

The Two Major Skin-Care Concerns

Wrinkles and blemishes are, by far, the dominant skin-care concerns for a large majority of women. Looking for answers to these two skin-care woes often results in lots of cosmetic sales. Yet the cosmetics world may be the last place you should be focusing your attention. I believe the best place to start when dealing with any skin-care topic is with information.

The twin headaches of wrinkles and breakouts are accompanied by two pervasive myths that not only hurt skin but also perpetuate a never-ending cycle of product-buying mistakes. The first myth is that dry skin and wrinkles are associated; the second is that you can dry up blemishes (a corollary to the second one is that a blemish can be spot-treated). Neither of those myths is true in the least! Dry skin and wrinkles are *not* associated and blemishes *cannot* be dried up or spot-controlled!

The Myth About Blemishes

What about drying up blemishes? Water is the only thing you can dry up, and a blemish has nothing to do with being wet. Skin cells do contain water, and when you dry up the skin, you cause the skin to flake, which won't stop breakouts but can cause irritation and add another predicament to your skin-care grief. Blemishes *can* be aggravated by oil production, which needs to be reduced and/or absorbed. Absorbing oil on the skin or in the pore (or breaking down the oil) is a process radically different from drying the skin. Moreover, you can't "zap" zits. A blemish takes about two to seven days to go away (depending on the depth and size), no matter what you do.

A blemish is produced in several stages that take place far beneath the skin, inside the pore over a period of time. Deep in the pore, weeks before you ever see a blemish, sebum (oil), dead skin cells, and bacteria interact to start forming a blemish. You can reduce the redness and inflammation caused by a blemish, but what you need to do to get rid of blemishes must take place continually and methodically, over an uninterrupted period of time. You need to consistently do what you can to reduce oil production (such as using a gentle skin-care routine and a facial mask of milk of magnesia), remove dead skin cells (such as using an AHA or BHA lotion or gel), and disinfect the site (with 2.5% benzoyl peroxide or a topical antibiotic). I discuss this routine more completely in Chapter Six, "Special Battle Plans for Blemishes."

The Myth About Wrinkles

I understand how difficult it must be to overcome the bombardment of moisturizers claiming to take care of wrinkles and dry skin, yet it is completely false that dry skin and wrinkles are related. **How do we know dry skin and wrinkles are not associated? Because after slathering on tons of moisturizers and wrinkle creams and lotions over the years, women still get lots of wrinkles.** Even women who use expensive products still get wrinkles and make appointments with a plastic surgeon. Moreover, kids with dry skin don't have wrinkles, and women with oily, sun-damaged skin do have wrinkles. Scientifically, we know dry skin and wrinkles are not associated because when you look at the skin under a microscope there is no physical evidence that the two are linked. Dry skin may look more wrinkly, but that doesn't mean those wrinkles are permanent.

The dilemma is that, in fact, dry skin does look more wrinkled and—here's the crux of the confusion—wrinkled skin looks better with a good moisturizer on it. That's how we get sucked into this myth about wrinkles and dry skin. A woman with oily skin has her own built-in moisturizer (that's basically what moisturizers are: oils or oil-like ingredients and water), which helps her skin look smoother without the aid of a moisturizer.

The truth is, moisturizing the skin does not have any long-term effect on wrinkles. It doesn't mean moisturizers can't make wrinkles less apparent, because they absolutely do, but the notion that these soothing creams, lotions, gels, and serums do anything to change the skin is wishful thinking fostered by constant reinforcement from the cosmetics industry. But the cosmetics industry tells us lots of things that aren't true, and this myth seems more believable as we get more worried about wrinkles.

It Really Is Irritating

I started my career as a cosmetics consumer advocate by warning women about the damage being done to their skin by irritating skin-care ingredients. Over the years my fears about irritation have been confirmed and reinforced by many dermatologists and cosmetic chemists. Indeed, irritation is a bigger problem for the skin than even I had suspected. As many already know, irritation can stimulate an already overflowing oil production by activating nerve endings attached to the oil gland; it can dry up skin cells that need to retain water; it can cause increased dryness, which adds to cell debris, which can clog pores; it can cause breakouts like a diaper rash over the skin; it can cause redness; and it can bring out surfaced capillaries on the face. In short, irritation is hell on the skin.

It also appears that irritation can destroy the skin's integrity by breaking down its protective barrier, which, over time, damages the skin's structure and impairs the skin's natural immune/healing ability. Additionally, breaking down the protective barrier can allow the introduction of bacteria, therefore risking breakouts. Even more startling is the histological evidence that even if your skin doesn't feel irritated when you apply a cosmetic or skin-care product containing irritants, it is still being irritated and the skin breakdown is nonetheless taking place. That means if a product contains potentially irritating or sensitizing ingredients, the irritating ingredients can still harm the skin, even if it doesn't sting or burn. Not paying attention to the irritation potential of ingredients can be damaging to the health of your skin.

Stopping Oily Skin

How active your oil glands are is regulated by hormones and genetic predisposition. Likewise, genetically speaking, oil glands are more abundant in certain areas of the body like the nose, chin, forehead, upper back, and chest. It isn't surprising, then, if your oil glands are predetermined to produce more oil and your hormones are busy activating them, that those areas would register the most problems. While the oil glands are controlled by hormones and inherited traits, they can also be further stimulated by irritation, which increases the activity in the pore. Unfortunately, there is little you can do to alter genetically determined traits and hormonal activity. Accutane and birth control pills are the only way to truly change those functions and I discuss those alternatives in Chapter Six, "Special Battle Plans for Blemishes." For now the reality is that you can't dry up oil, you can only dry up water. Trying to dry up oil will only cause more problems by promoting irritation, redness, and inflammation and drying up the skin, which causes a dehydrated layer of skin.

The good news is you can absorb oil and calm down oil production. Being gentle to the skin is a basic way to start calming down oil production. All of the skin-care products and regimes I recommend help to promote little to no irritation of the skin. Perhaps more important is to not add more oil or oil-like ingredients to the skin. That doesn't mean just avoiding ingredients with names like "oil" but avoiding ingredients like triglycerides, myristates, palmitates, and fatty acids (which most plant oils contain), which are similar to the oil produced by the oil gland.

When it comes to absorbing oil, most women think of turning to clay masks, but they are not as effective at absorbing oil in comparison to using a facial mask of milk of magnesia. I know this sounds strange, but it is simple enough to test for yourself. Plain milk of magnesia (no mint or cherry flavors), just like you buy at the drugstore for an upset stomach, is just liquid magnesium. Magnesium, like clay, is an earth mineral but, unlike clay, it has some disinfecting and anti-inflammatory properties and can absorb more oil for its molecular weight than clay can. Plus, lots of clay masks contain irritating ingredients that can cause problems for the skin. That makes milk of magnesia a superior way to absorb oil without drying out or irritating the skin.

Emotional and Environmental Stress

Plenty of emotional and environmental stresses bombard your skin all the time. Some you can easily control, and some are much more difficult to manage. An intense work schedule, a frenzied home life, endless bills, your car breaking down unexpectedly—all can potentially affect the skin. Heat in the summer (or in a sauna or a Jacuzzi), cold in winter, sun, wind, and pollution are all forceful drying agents. Many companies suggest that their products can fend off all those external skin bullies. Sometimes they can. Moisturizers beautifully counter the drying effect of outside cold during the winter and dry heat[1] during the summer or in arid climates. Sunscreens with an SPF of 15 that contain avobenzone (Parsol 1789), titanium dioxide, or zinc oxide can prevent wrinkling, skin cancer, and sunburn. But while sunscreens help to prevent wrinkles and moisturizers help to prevent dryness, there are no products that can reduce the effects of emotional stress on your face or form a force field over the face and keep environmental enemies off your skin. It would be great if skin-care products could keep air pollution off the face, but if polluted air can get through your skin, a most formidable barrier, it can easily get through any moisturizer or foundation. Stress is a problem, but topical products aren't going to calm your nerves or solve your work problems. Massaging on a product may be relaxing, but it's the massage, not the product, that makes the difference.

Heat Is a Problem

As good as heat feels, both wet heat and dry heat can cause problems for the skin. For years, I have been recommending washing the face with tepid water because hot water burns the skin and cold water shocks the skin, and both leave it irritated and dry. These two temperature extremes can overstimulate nerve endings in the skin and oil glands, injure skin cells, dehydrate the skin, and cause capillaries to surface. Extreme temperatures in any form cause problems for the skin, but heat is the more attractive alternative (most people avoid a cold shower or bath).

Dry heat is clearly dehydrating. Whether the dry heat comes from a dry sauna or an arid desert climate, it pulls water right out of the skin cell. That's bad for any skin type, but especially for someone with dry skin.

Wet heat is a bit more deceptive. We all know how great the skin feels ini-

---

[1] By the way, during the winter, a humidifier in your room or home can go a long way toward reducing dry skin problems.

tially when you exit a hot shower, Jacuzzi, or sauna. It feels plump and saturated with water because the skin absolutely loves drinking up all the water it can. After even a short soak in a tub of water, your skin can swell and become engorged with water. When you leave a bathtub and your fingers are all thick and wrinkly, it isn't because they are dry, but because they are distorted and swollen with water-saturated skin cells. Because the surface layer of skin likes water so much, hot water can enter the skin, stay there, and cause a burnlike reaction. As a general rule, if water feels hot to the touch, it's too hot for the skin, especially the face. Be very skeptical about facial treatments that involve the use of heat or washing your face with hot (or cold) water; they could be causing more trouble for your skin than you want.

Can You Heal or Prevent Scarring?

A lot of women want to know if applying aloe, vitamin E, or a variety of marine plants from algae to seaweed will help heal scars. I would like to suggest an entire battle plan to minimize scarring as much as possible. Although aloe, vitamin E, and algae can't hurt a scar and may indeed be helpful, what is more important is the overall way you treat the scar from its beginning, when the skin is injured, to the end, after it has formed.

Skin's unique but unfortunate response to injury is scarring. But skin, almost miraculously, also regenerates quickly, essentially renewing itself in two to four weeks. Depending on your genetic makeup and the depth of the injury, scarring can range from a slightly reddish discoloration to a thick, raised red or darkened scar (described as hypertrophic or keloidal) to serious disfigurement. Regardless, how you initially take care of a wound makes all the difference in the world.

Whether it is caused by acne, getting cut, or an operation, when skin damage first occurs you should allow the area to "breathe" as much as possible. Do not gunk it up with creams, lotions, or vitamin E capsules. Rubbing creams and lotions on a wound can damage fragile skin in the first stages of healing. Keep the damaged skin clean (but don't overclean it); using a liquid antibacterial soap from the neck down or a disinfectant like 3% hydrogen peroxide from the neck up is fine for keeping bacteria away. At this stage a little pure aloe vera or a very sheer lightweight moisturizing gel is just fine, but "little" is the operative word here. In the beginning, keep the injured site out of sunlight altogether, as opposed to loading up on sunscreen. Heavy creams will suffocate the skin and prevent it from healing. Once the wound is healed, keeping it out of sunlight as much as possible or protecting it with sunscreen is imperative. Considering sun damage is a wound of sorts, that is especially true for the face. Sun damages skin and doesn't promote healing, regardless of how good it feels. Smoking is a skin destroyer and will also prevent healthy healing,

After the wound has healed you can use slightly more emollient products with antioxidants (such as vitamin E, or pure vitamin E) to keep free-radical damage at a minimum. Sunscreens in a light moisturizing base are essential, not only to keep the skin moist but to allow the skin to continue healing. There is some evidence, although the relevant studies used small samplings, that AHAs, Retin-A, and Renova can significantly reduce the appearance of scarring by exfoliating the skin and stimulating cell turnover. Exfoliation can reduce the thick, discolored appearance of scar tissue. Retin-A and Renova over time *may* help generate collagen production to possibly shore up some of what was lost from the injury. (Some studies have indicated that Retin-A and Renova can improve the appearance of stretch marks, but "improve" is a loaded word here. Stretch marks treated with Retin-A or Renova did not disappear, but they were reduced to some extent—about 14% shorter and 8% narrower.)

Exfoliation, antioxidants, and sunscreens can all help to minimize scarring after the skin has healed. None of them will get rid of a scar, but the possibility of reducing the appearance of a scar is not to be ignored. Basically, there are no miracle skin-care ingredients or products when it comes to healing skin or reducing the appearance of scars. Instead, practice good skin care: don't overmanipulate the site, protect it from the sun, keep the area disinfected, keep heavy emollients off the skin, and, as much as possible, let the skin handle its own healing process.

Even though you have done all you can to help heal the skin, thicker raised scars can set in. Fashion magazines have been sporting ads for a product called **ReJuveness** *($39.50 to $295, depending on the size ordered),* which supposedly fights this type of scarring. ReJuveness and products like it are nothing more than pliable sheets of silicone, quite similar to the silicone oil used in so many skin- and hair-care products because of its texture and water-binding properties. It is not clear how these sheets of silicone oil work. They may increase the amount of water in the scar, and continuous rehydration of scars may soften the tissue, making it more elastic and pliable, and thus encouraging the flattening process. But work they do, and rather successfully (although I use the word "successfully" with caution).

Silicone sheets appear to be most effective for hypertrophic or keloidal scarring. As wonderful as this sounds, there are disadvantages. Users purchase one relatively inexpensive sheet of silicone that is worn over and over again. The sheet must be kept clean, which requires some amount of care and maintenance time. The sheet must be worn over the scar for prolonged periods of time, and you might not want to wear one on your face or other exposed parts of your body, at least not during the day. Also, the silicone sheet can stick to the skin (wearing a camisole or T-shirt over the sheet can help), and skin reactions such as rashes or irritation can occur.

To make things even more difficult and uncomfortable, you have to wear the sheet for long periods—for hours at a time, over a span of at least two to nine months—in order to see a difference. But patience pays off: the longer you wear it, the more likely it is that the scar will dissipate to some extent. Of course, these sheets work best over new scars, but they can make a difference with old ones too. Even acne scarring—thick, raised scars, not pits—can be reduced if the scars have been around for less than 16 years. As wonderful and hopeful as this all sounds, be aware that the word "reduce" is imprecise. Do not give these a try if you are hoping for extraordinary results, as the advertising implies. Dr. Loren Engrav, associate director and chief of plastic surgery for the University of Washington burn unit at Harborview Medical Center, explains that the "silicone strips are standard treatment for helping dissipate scars, and though the results may be good, they are absolutely not a miracle."

Some women buy the sheets to use over stretch marks, but there is no clinical evidence that this product will have any effect on them whatsoever, and the Silk Skin company will not guarantee its product for this use. These sheets use a flattening process, not a raising process, which would be required for stretch marks.

If you have serious scarring, I encourage you to check out ReJuveness, at (800) 588-7455 in the United States and (800) 361-0778 in Canada. It isn't for everyone, but if you are willing to be persistent, it is definitely worth a try.

What About Scars from Acne?

The best way to prevent scars is to not do anything that makes matters worse. Untreated or improperly treated acne is likely to cause the worst scarring because the problem is never mitigated and the skin has no chance to heal. Attacking blemishes, creating deep scabs and sores that take a long time to heal, gunking up the skin with too many facial products, avoiding the use of effective disinfectants to reduce the presence of blemishes, not exfoliating the skin to help remove dead skin cells, smoking, manipulating the skin, and not staying out of the sun can all help exacerbate scarring. At the outset, if you are good about not picking and oversqueezing blemishes, scarring can be greatly reduced. Yet even the most meticulous state-of-the-art acne skin-care routine can still result in scars. Most acne scars do fade with time, but that can seem interminable when the face is yours.

Once acne and breakouts have been reduced or eliminated, the brown, pink, or purple discolorations left by acne lesions can fade a great deal in about two to three months, depending on your skin color. You can speed up that fading by continuing the use of a product with AHAs, BHA, or Retin-A (which are all helpful in the treatment of acne and breakouts anyway). You might also consider a professional salicylic acid or glycolic acid peel to improve the appearance of surface scarring (these peels are unwarranted for scarring if the acne is still active). Just don't expect an AHA or BHA peel to improve the appearance of deep scarring.

Once acne has healed, small areas with shallow scars or pit-type scars can be injected with collagen to lift the depression. For larger areas of the face, laser resurfacing is absolutely the treatment of choice. The days of dermabrasion, when a wire brush or sanding apparatus was used to plane the skin, are long gone. Dermabrasion had a multitude of nasty side effects, including bleeding, high probability of pigment problems, and an undesirable change in skin texture. Laser resurfacing has fewer side effects (no bleeding, low probability of skin discoloration, improved skin texture), and the final results are much better.

Skin-lightening lotions with hydroquinone or other skin-lightening ingredients do not work well, if at all, on acne scarring. These lotions prevent melanin production; they do not have much effect on the color of scars.

Stop the Moisturizing Mania

Not everyone needs or should be using a moisturizer, especially women with oily, combination, or acne-prone skin! And women with dry skin need only one moisturizer (not including sunscreen). That sums it up. As we approach the next millennium (and it's getting closer all the time), I can't think of one skin-care product that is more misunderstood, misused, and abused than moisturizer. How did things get so out of hand? The only answer is that things tend to get out of hand in the world of cosmetics.

I like more moisturizers than I dislike (putting aside the nasty debate over cost versus performance), but because most women overuse moisturizers, they can cause some pretty surprising skin problems. A lot of women (maybe most) still cling to the erroneous belief that moisturizers somehow prevent wrinkles. Not just moisturizers with a high sun protection factor (SPF), which do stop further skin damage if they contain titanium dioxide, zinc oxide, or avobenzone, but all moisturizers. The mistaken notion that dry skin is more prone to wrinkles than oily skin remains firmly implanted in the mind of the consumer, and that's on top of all those claims about firming, toning, repairing, and lifting the skin with all sorts of creams, gels, and lotions.

The only reason to use a moisturizer is if you have dry skin or wrinkled skin you want to look smoother (moisturizers can smooth over, not change, wrinkles).

If you don't have dry skin, there is no reason to use a moisturizer. If you have oily skin or skin that breaks out, the worst thing you can do is use a moisturizer of any kind. It's that simple. What happens when you overuse a moisturizer? Pores get clogged and blackheads can develop; dead skin cells get trapped and have a harder time naturally sloughing off, which can leave the skin looking dull; and you run a higher risk of getting patches of dermatitis, increasing the number of breakouts, and creating your own combination-skin predicament. Additionally, oversaturating the skin can turn off the skin's own immune/healing response. Overdoing moisturizers can actually prevent the skin from repairing itself.

Interesting fact: You may have personally experienced the dry climate aboard an airplane, and it is dry: flight attendants frequently complain about battling dry skin. That is a problem, but it does not cause wrinkles. Rather, the force of gravity against a flight attendant's skin every time a plane takes off or lands stretches the skin and compounds wrinkling. Flight attendants also have easy access to more tropical holidays than most and end up with skin-aging tans. Dry skin may not feel great in those cramped cabins, but it isn't what is aging the skin. Along with this issue of dry skin on airplanes, you may have heard that spraying the face with a mist of water is good for the skin. It isn't. It may feel refreshing, but unless you use something over the face to seal the moisture in the skin, it will evaporate almost instantly. If you do spray a mist of water over the skin, quickly apply a light layer of moisturizer over it. Now, doesn't that feel better?

How Do You Know If You Need a Moisturizer?

Dry skin is technically a condition caused by a lack of moisture in the skin's top layers combined with a breakdown of the intercellular protective barrier (the substances that fill the area between skin cells) and an inadequate supply of lipids/oils from the oil gland. If the oil gland isn't doing its job—helping form a protective barrier composed of lipids and other chemical substances that guard and insulate the skin, preventing moisture from evaporating or being used up by the skin cell—you may need a moisturizer to help.

Generally, you can assume that, if you are using a gentle skin cleanser and no other irritating skin-care products, and your skin still feels dry 20 to 30 minutes after you wash your face, you should use moisturizer. (It is critical to make sure the dryness of your skin after cleansing isn't caused by the products you are using.) If your skin feels tight, dehydrated, taut, or uncomfortable from dryness by midday or at the end of the day, it is essential to use a moisturizer. If you have fine lines that improve with the application of a moisturizer, especially around the eyes, that is a great reason to use a moisturizer. Just keep in mind that it is best to use the most lightweight moisturizer possible that helps make a difference. If none of these problems are present, you don't have dry skin, so don't use a moisturizer. (Obviously, sunscreen is another story.)

I know giving up moisturizer may be hard to do, but think about it the next time you reach for one. Ask yourself if your skin really needs this or if it would be better off with an AHA product or a lightweight moisturizer for just around the eyes instead. You can even try a simple experiment to see if your skin does better by using moisturizer only on the dry spots or wrinkled areas rather than applying it all over. (Again, this presumes your skin-care routine is not drying out your skin.)

It's important to note that several skin conditions can look like dry skin but are not, and they may be exacerbated by the use of moisturizers. Eczema, seborrhea, rosacea, early signs of skin cancer, psoriasis, sun-damaged skin, and overuse of heavy moisturizers can all resemble dryness but are not helped by using a moisturizer. Eczema requires a cortisone cream; seborrhea, rosacea, and psoriasis require prescription topical medications to control the condition; skin cancer demands immediate medical attention; and sun-damaged skin is better off with an alpha hydroxy acid product to help exfoliate skin. Overusing moisturizers can not only mask these problems, it can cause breakouts, make the skin appear dull and thick (by holding down skin cells and preventing exfoliation), and inhibit the skin's natural immune/healing response.

How Moisturizers Work

While cosmetics companies carry on at length about all the miracles their moisturizers can perform, in reality moisturizers work primarily in one of three rather simple ways. Some moisturizers are designed to encourage skin cells and layers of skin to retain water by using ingredients that attract water from other sources in the environment. Other moisturizers are designed to prevent water loss by providing an occlusive film on the skin's surface to prevent water loss via evaporation. Finally, moisturizers can fill in the gaps between skin cells that cause the skin's surface to break down, allowing moisture loss and reduced healing response. Most moisturizers are designed to perform all three of these functions by including ingredients that function hygroscopically (attract water from other sources), ingredients that function as humectants and water-binding agents (ingredients that retain water), barrier ingredients (which prevent water loss), and emollients (which duplicate the skin's lipid structure). Thousands of ingredients handle those jobs very nicely. Cosmetic chemists use this almost unlimited variety of options to create a mind-boggling assortment of combinations and permutations to help skin stay moist, soft, soothed, smooth, elastic, and intact.

As wonderful as this all sounds, and it is wonderful, moisturizers are necessary only if your skin isn't functioning as it should. Most skin knows exactly how to keep the right amount of water inside, how to lubricate itself with oil from the oil gland, and how to keep the intercellular layers intact. Skin can forget how to do its job if it is bombarded with cigarette smoke, sun damage, irritating skin-care products, overscrubbing, or hormonal changes.

Should You Exfoliate?

It may seem incredibly contradictory to tell you that, despite the risks of irritation, an essential skin-care need of many different skin types is to do something irritating to the skin. If you have dry skin, oily skin, blackheads, acne, sun-damaged skin, flaky skin (not caused by a skin disease or a skin disorder), or a rough surface texture, those problems are best handled by products that may cause irritation, specifically those that exfoliate and slough off dead skin cells from the surface of the skin. (Disinfectants are also essential for treating acne, and they can be irritating; see Chapter Six for more information about the pros and cons of those.) How can this be? If irritation is so bad for the skin, why would you use a skin-care step that involves irritation? There is a rationale to all this that does make sense.

There is plenty of evidence that irritation is bad, but there is also plenty of evidence that some irritating products help skin. The balancing act is to find which irritating products can help skin (such as AHAs, BHA, Retin-A, or Renova), then use the mildest yet most effective form for your skin type, and do it as infrequently as needed to get positive results. Exfoliating the skin is extremely helpful for many skin types and skin problems; the goal is to use products with the least impact on the skin while still providing the best results.

It seems almost antiquated to discuss the issue of exfoliating and sloughing the skin, but it is still a primary, beneficial part of skin care. The only skin types that need to stay away from exfoliation are those with extremely sensitive skin or older skin, and those with skin diseases or disorders such as rosacea, eczema, dermatitis, or seborrhea.

Exfoliating Oily Skin

Let's start with oily skin or clogged pores. One way a blackhead or blemish occurs is if the oil gland (pore) produces too much sebum. Sebum is a soft wax that should liquefy when it reaches the surface of the pore, spreading a thin, imperceptible protective layer over the skin. When too much sebum is produced, the liquefying process can get backed up. Add to that problem a tendency for skin cells that should be naturally sloughing off to instead fall inside the pore and get stuck. The more skin cells that build up in the pore, the more oil will be held back from flowing easily out of the pore, and the result can be a blackhead or a blemish.

Skin cells that should be shedding on a regular, daily basis are being held back. One of the things that keeps the cells from sloughing off is that self-same oil (sebum). The oil works as an adhesive, preventing the shedding skin cells from going where they are supposed to go—off the face. One of the ways to keep pores from getting clogged is to help skin cells shed as freely as possible so they don't get trapped inside the pore. The more you keep skin cells exfoliating in a normal manner, the less cell debris can fill up the pore.

Exfoliating Dry Skin

The reason to exfoliate dry skin is different from the reason to exfoliate oily, blemish-prone skin, though the objective is the same: removing dead skin cells that are not shedding normally. Skin can be dry for many reasons, including lack of moisture, built-up dead skin cells that don't easily shed, and abnormal skin cells that adhere to each other in a way that prevents normal exfoliation and normal moisture retention. (Dry-looking skin can also be caused by moisturizers that are too emollient and hold dead skin cells in place, preventing healthy shedding. In those situations the surface of the skin feels "greasy" or moist, and the underlying layer feels dry.) Helping dry skin shed dried-up, dead skin cells can make room for less dry, plumper (moisture-filled) skin cells to come to the surface, which can lend a fresher look to the skin. It also allows moisturizers (the less and lighter, the better) to more easily penetrate the skin because there are fewer dried-up skin cells in the way to block absorption. Exfoliating helps the dead surface skin cells shed at a more normal rate to make room for the lower layers of newer skin cells. (For dry skin it is also helpful to efficiently remove dead skin cells to reduce the chance of pores becoming clogged and creating blackheads and whiteheads.)

What Type of Exfoliating Products to Use?

For many skin types, the issue is not whether to exfoliate, but what you should use and how often. The question then becomes, "How much irritation is necessary to do the job?" Now that's a tricky question.

There are a lot of exfoliating products out there waiting to peel the money from your pocketbook as well as the skin from your face. Scrubs, soaps with exfoliating ingredients, toners, facial masks, facial peels, abrasive sponges, washcloths, and facial brushes are all designed to exfoliate. Overkill (as in killing the skin) becomes an issue when your skin-care routine includes more than one exfoliating product or if the one you are using is too strong. In the world of consumerism, if a little is good, a lot must be better, and the cosmetics industry is right there with a host of products. Ignore them; it takes only one product to do the job, and your task is to choose the best product for your skin type.

Generally speaking, I do not recommend exfoliating facial masks because often, in addition to the exfoliating ingredient, they also contain a number of other irritating ingredients. Also, exfoliation works best when done consistently, while facial masks tend to be used irregularly and infrequently. (For a discussion of glycolic acid facial peels, see Chapter Seven, "Cosmetic Surgery." This is an area where even dermatologists and plastic surgeons are getting carried away, overdoing things and possibly putting the skin at risk.)

Facial brushes and washcloths are options, but I find they are both almost impossible to keep clean, they tend to exfoliate unevenly, they exfoliate only on the very surface of the skin, and they are not as effective or as gentle as other alternatives. Abrasive sponges, such as loofahs, are way too irritating from the neck up, and are also very difficult to keep clean.

Cosmetic scrubs can be a good way to remove the dead surface layer of skin, but there are difficulties with these types of exfoliants too. Many of them contain sand, bits of fruit pits, seeds, and other gritty abrasives that can be unnecessarily irritating. These abrasive fragments are not of a uniform shape and can literally cut the skin. In addition, cosmetic scrubs often contain thick waxes and creams so you can smooth them more easily over your skin, but these waxes can clog pores and leave a film over the face. Some scrub products also contain harsh ingredients such as peppermint, menthol, eucalyptus, alcohol, and roughly ground scrub particles that are simply unnecessary and overly irritating. The problem with all mechanical scrubs—even the one I recommend, namely plain baking soda or baking soda mixed with Cetaphil Cleanser[2]—is that you can easily end up scrubbing off more than is healthy for the skin. You need to exfoliate, but how to do that gently is the question.

Cosmetic scrubs and facial masks were the most popular and best ways to exfoliate the skin until the arrival of Retin-A for sun-damaged skin in 1987, Renova (which is Retin-A in a moisturizing base) in 1996, alpha hydroxy acids (AHAs) in 1992, and beta hydroxy acid (BHA, also known as salicylic acid) in 1995, although BHA has been around for decades as an acne treatment. If you

---

[2] If you do like using a mechanical scrub, baking soda is much better than the scrubs you buy in the drugstore or at the cosmetics counter. Baking soda by itself is an anti-inflammatory agent—it can reduce redness, irritation, and itching. For example, if you got a bee sting, you wouldn't rub it with honey and almond pits or scrub a washcloth over it, but you might use a poultice of baking soda to reduce the swelling. Finally, baking soda is not a grit suspended in a cosmetic base. Cosmetic scrubs often contain preservatives, coloring agents, and fragrances that can irritate the skin and waxes that can clog pores. For the money (89 cents for a medium-size box), you can't find a scrub product on the market that works any more efficiently to exfoliate the skin, and when used with Cetaphil Cleanser it is gentle enough for dry skin.

are interested in exfoliating, these are the major, if not only, players to consider. Before we get down to the nitty-gritty behind these very nongritty but effective exfoliants, let's clear up some of the mystery surrounding them.

AHAs and BHA

Surely by now everyone has heard about alpha hydroxy acids (AHAs), the most amazing cosmetic skin-care ingredient of all time, and beta hydroxy acid (BHA), which runs a close second. (There is only one beta hydroxy acid, salicylic acid, but there are a variety of AHAs.) They aren't amazing because they can perform miracles on the skin. What makes them so remarkable is the number of products they have spawned over the past four years, many, though definitely not all, of which have the ability to improve the appearance of the skin. More than any other cosmetic ingredient, AHAs have created an industry unto themselves. Since Avon launched Anew, one of the first mass-distributed AHA products on the market, in 1992, AHA products have appeared by the hundreds. What can this small group of acids do? How do they differ from BHA? You would think they are nothing short of a supernatural phenomenon. In reality, AHAs and BHA have both been around for years and years, but their growing use as effective exfoliants for many different skin types is indeed supernatural.

Most of the companies producing these products, as well as independent sources including dermatologists, plastic surgeons, and cosmetic chemists, claim that regular use of AHAs or BHA can make skin smoother, diminish wrinkles, and unclog pores. Quite a lot for a group of ingredients derived from such sources as wintergreen leaves, sugarcane, and milk, or synthesized from a mixture of formaldehyde and monoxide. The bottom line is, do these exfoliants work? The good news is that many of the AHA products on the market, from drugstore brands to infomercial products, department-store lines, and those sold at doctors' offices, do to some extent live up to those basic claims. But once the cosmetics companies fire up their marketing smokescreens, the whole topic gets exaggerated and quite confusing. It's not easy to undo the pretense, but it can be done.

There are five types of AHAs on the market: glycolic, lactic, malic, citric, and tartaric acids. The most commonly used AHAs are glycolic and lactic acids, because of their special ability to penetrate the skin. As mentioned above, there is only one beta hydroxy acid (BHA), salicylic acid.

What these acids can do is "unglue" (or burn off) the outer layer of dead skin cells and help increase cell turnover by removing the built-up top layers of skin, allowing healthier cells to come to the surface. Removing this dead layer can improve skin texture and color, unclog pores, and allow moisturizers to be better absorbed by the skin. Because AHAs affect the top layers of skin, they help to improve the appearance of sun-damaged skin, dry skin, and thickened skin caused by a variety of factors, including abnormal cell growth, smoking, heavy moisturizers, and sun damage. (Sun damage causes the top layer of skin to become thicker, creating a dull, rough texture and appearance on the surface of skin. AHAs nicely cut through this thickened exterior, revealing the more normal-appearing skin cells underneath.) Because AHAs and BHA work in a chemical rather than a physical process, they can produce better results than cosmetic scrubs, which work only on the exposed surface of the skin.

The fundamental difference between AHAs and BHA is that AHAs are water-soluble, while BHA is lipid-soluble (oil-soluble). This unique property of BHA allows it to get through the oil in the pores and exfoliate the built-up skin cells inside the oil gland. AHAs are much less able to do this because they can't get through the fat content of the oil (sebum). Therefore, BHA is indicated for use where blackheads and blemishes are the issue, and AHAs are more suitable for sun-damaged, thickened, dry skin.

I wish the discussion of AHAs and BHA could end here. I wish you could find a good AHA product by looking for glycolic or lactic acid on the ingredient list if you have sun-damaged, thickened, dry skin. Or, if you tend to have blackheads or blemishes and want to find a good BHA product, you would only need to look for a product that contains salicylic acid. But, alas, it isn't that simple. AHAs and BHA are effective as exfoliants only at certain concentrations (the quantity of the ingredient present in the product) and very specific pHs (the acidity or alkalinity of a product).

An AHA and BHA Scorecard

When it comes to AHAs and BHA, the crucial information is not only the name of the ingredient but its concentration in the product, as well as its pH level (in order to be effective, AHA and BHA products must have a low pH—in other words, be more acid than alkaline). Dr. Walter Smith, in a paper on AHA and BHA products and their effectiveness published in the *Cosmetics and Toiletries Ingredient Resource Series,* and supported by other studies on the issue, suggests that AHAs work best at concentrations of 5% and above and at pH levels of 3, their effectiveness diminishing as you go past 4.5. BHA works best at concentrations of between 1% and 2%, and an optimal pH level of 3. Both AHAs and BHA lose their effectiveness as a product's pH level goes up and the ingredient's concentration goes down. This is so central to the subject of exfoliation and cell turnover, it bears repeating: **AHAs work best in a 5% to 8% concentration, with a pH level of 3 to 4; BHA works best in a 1% to 2% concentration, with a pH of 3.**

If the cosmetics industry isn't forthcoming about pH and percentage for a BHA or AHA product (and most companies aren't), how can you tell if it provides decent or effective exfoliation? You can't. I've rated many of them in my book *Don't Go to the Cosmetics Counter Without Me,* but as a general rule it is best if the AHA ingredient is either second or third on the ingredient list. That makes it likely the product contains a 5% or higher concentration of AHAs. It is also important that a pH-balancing ingredient like sodium hydroxide or potassium hydroxide be somewhere on the list; these two are the most popular ingredients (you need so little) used to create a good pH. Glycolic acid and lactic acid are the two AHAs with the most research behind them and should be the ingredients to look for. There are others, but these are the most popular. Tartaric, citric, and malic acids are also AHAs and may perform in the same way, but there hasn't yet been enough research to make any conclusive statements, and it is felt they don't penetrate the skin as well as glycolic and lactic acid.

For salicylic acid, because such a small amount is required, it is fine if the ingredient is located toward the middle or end of the ingredient list, but the presence of sodium hydroxide or potassium hydroxide is helpful to identify an attempt at establishing a good pH. (Of course, you can always do what I do—test each product with a pH strip—but that is hardly practical for most women.)

Aside from exfoliating the skin when the concentration and pH level are right, AHAs also have water-binding properties. They can provide an added benefit by helping to keep water in the skin at the same time that exfoliation is taking place. BHA, though it provides more-penetrating exfoliation and therefore could be more irritating, may actually reduce irritating side effects because it is derived from acetylsalicylic acid, which is the technical name for aspirin, and aspirin has anti-inflammatory properties.

Another difference between AHAs and BHA is their duration. AHAs have a drop-off rate: their ability to exfoliate decreases over time (which is also true for Retin-A). BHAs, on the other hand, continue to exfoliate at a constant rate. (According to Dr. Walter Smith, writing in the May 1995 issue of *Cosmetics & Toiletries,* salicylic acid keeps the stratum corneum—top layer of skin—in a state of high turnover; AHAs' effect decreases once the stratum corneum has been exfoliated to a certain level.) Constant exfoliation may cause long-term problems on the surface of the skin by maintaining a permanent level of irritation.

Many experts, including Dr. Albert Kligman, the inventor of Retin-A, suggest that it is best to use any chemical exfoliant (AHA, BHA, Retin-A, Renova) on a consistent basis for about six months to a year and then reduce usage to alternate weeks or months, such as three months of daily usage and then three months of no usage, and so on. There are no studies confirming Kligman's theory of usage, so it's up to the consumer to experiment to see what feels best. But alternation is an option, and probably preferable to moving up to stronger percentages of AHA, which will increase exfoliation but also risk unnecessary skin irritation.

Keep in mind that none of these AHA or BHA products, regardless of concentration, pH, or type, can prevent aging or change a wrinkle. These products can smooth the skin, improve texture, unclog pores, and give the appearance of plumper, firmer skin (because more healthy skin cells are now on the surface), but when you stop using them, the skin goes back to the way it was before you started. Researchers theorize that AHAs, and possibly BHA, can increase collagen and elastin, much as Retin-A and Renova can. But this is only theory, and there is no research to prove it.

AHA/BHA Nonsense

As cosmetics companies jump on the AHA/BHA bandwagon with both feet, the consumer is left in the lurch with an array of genuinely ineffective, bad products. Some of these products can be purchased at drugstores and cosmetics counters; others are available through aestheticians, physicians, infomercials, and in-home sales. What makes this crowded field so troublesome is that so many cosmetics companies supply grossly misleading or completely inane information about their products.

Particularly annoying is the fact that many companies announce proudly that their products contain AHAs or BHA, but say nothing about (or even refuse to tell consumers) how much AHA or BHA is in the product, even though this basic information is the key to knowing what you are buying and has everything to do with a product's effectiveness and potential for irritation. They also aren't going to say anything about the product's pH level, but that is as important to know as the concentration.

Chanel's consumer relations department first told me their Day Lifting Refining Complex contains glycolic acid, but it isn't in the ingredient list; when asked, they said the name of the ingredient and the percentage used are confidential. Of course, the ingredients aren't confidential; they have to be disclosed on the ingredient list. My best guess after reading the list is that Chanel's product contains about 3% lactic acid and about 1% or less salicylic acid, but the pH makes it ineffectual as an exfoliant.

Revlon introduced its Revlon Results with Alpha ReCap at the height of the AHA craze. Surprise: despite its name, Alpha ReCap doesn't contain one smidgen of AHA. It did contain a very good water-binding agent, but if you wanted the exfoliating effects of AHAs, you were out of luck.

Estee Lauder's Fruition was one of the first department-store lines to launch an AHA product. It was an overnight success, but not because of its AHA content: Fruition contains less than 2% AHA. At that percentage AHAs are little more than good water-binding agents. That isn't bad; it just isn't what makes AHAs and BHA such fascinating ingredients. Consumers must have complained, because last year Lauder launched Fruition Extra, which contains a decent amount of AHA and has a good pH. It's absurdly expensive for what you get, and of course the company never bothered to explain why consumers now needed Fruition Extra if the original Fruition was supposed to be so amazing and wondrous for the skin.

Clinique's TurnAround products, which all contain about a 1% concentration of BHA, have a pH of around 5. That makes them completely ineffective as exfoliants. In reality, TurnAround can't turn around even one skin cell.

Then there are the AHA sound-alikes, including sugarcane extract, mixed fruit acids, fruit extracts, milk extract, and citrus extract, and the BHA sound-alikes, like wintergreen extract. You may think you've purchased a better, more natural AHA or BHA product when you see these less technical, more familiar names, but that absolutely isn't the case. Without knowing exactly what type of AHA or BHA ingredient you are buying, there is no way to know exactly what you are putting on your skin or how effective it really is. Although glycolic acid is derived from sugarcane and lactic acid from milk, that doesn't mean sugarcane extract or milk extract has anything to do with glycolic or lactic acid. Simply because a product contains sugarcane extract doesn't mean what has been extracted from the sugarcane is the acid. Even if it is the acid that has been extracted, you can't tell how concentrated it is, and what about the pH? It's all too vague and meaningless, making it impossible to determine what you are really buying. Be very suspicious of any product that claims an association with AHAs or BHA but contains a variety of sound-alike ingredients.

What About Higher Concentrations of AHAs?

I am very concerned about the introduction of products with higher percentages of AHAs, particularly those from a cosmetics line called M.D. Formulations, sold by doctors and salons. M.D. Formulations sells AHA products at 10%, 15%, and 20% concentrations in appropriate pHs of 3 to 4. Increasing cell turnover can be taken too far, however, and many cosmetic researchers and dermatologists worry that the increased irritation and exfoliation caused by higher concentrations of AHAs can actually hurt skin. Without more evidence showing genuine benefit from higher concentrations, and no such evidence exists at this time, I am not willing to recommend that anyone put her skin at risk in that way. Most likely the positive results women may perceive with higher concentrations of AHAs come from the swelling and edema they cause. That may diminish the appearance of wrinkles and make the skin feel smoother, but it is most likely not best for the long-term health of the skin.

If you use a well-formulated AHA product (5% to 8% concentration, with a pH of 3) but you don't "feel" it working on your skin, that doesn't mean it isn't working. Quite the contrary. It is indeed working—without causing your skin any discomfort or irritation.

How Do You Use AHAs or BHA?

Depending on your skin type, AHAs or BHA can be wonderful skin-care tools. In the past, because of the pH issues, many experts recommended applying the AHA or BHA (in a lotion or cream for dry skin, or a liquid or gel solution for oily skin) to your face or any other area 15 minutes after cleansing, and then waiting 15 minutes more before applying any other product such as foundation, sunscreen, or additional moisturizers. The 15-minute wait between product application was to avoid neutralizing the effect of the acid component of these ingredients. The concern was that other products you might use, such as soap or moisturizers, are slightly alkaline, and they could negate the effectiveness of the AHA or BHA. Waiting 15 minutes would allow your face to return to its own acid balance, which does not adversely affect the AHAs or BHA. Nowadays, that is not the worry it once was. Unless you are using bar soaps, which tend to have a high pH (over 7), the other skin-care products you are using most likely have a low pH and will not interfere with the effectiveness of the AHA or BHA.

Strictly based on your skin type and skin-care needs, you can apply an AHA or BHA product once or twice a day, and depending on your skin's sensitivity you can apply either of these around the eye area, keeping them off the eyelid and away from the eye itself. Apply the AHA or BHA product after the face is cleansed and after your toner has dried (if you are using one). Once the AHA or BHA has been absorbed, you can apply any other product, such as additional moisturizer, eye cream, sunscreen, and/or foundation. It is not essential to wear moisturizer over an AHA or BHA product. That totally depends on what type of skin you have, how it reacts to the AHA or BHA product, and what kind of base the AHA or BHA is in. Some AHAs and BHA come in moisturizing bases, and most skin types do not require another moisturizer.

I generally recommend using AHA or BHA in a gel or liquid form so you don't have to apply a moisturizing base all over where you don't need it. That way the AHA or BHA goes on first and the moisturizer goes over it only where the skin is dry or taut. Never purchase an AHA or BHA product that includes other irritating ingredients; AHAs and BHA can be irritating enough by themselves, and there is never a reason to add more irritation, especially when it provides no benefit for the skin. The only reason the irritation from AHAs and BHA is allowable is because their ability to exfoliate is useful for solving many skin-care problems.

I never recommend cleansers that contain BHA or AHAs, for several reasons. First, if they are in a water-soluble cleanser, you run the risk of possible contact with the eyes, which can cause irritation. Second, AHAs and BHA work on the skin or the pores when they have been absorbed. When they are in a cleanser, they get rinsed down the drain before they can work. (Some companies shockingly recommend leaving the cleanser on the face for several minutes so the AHAs or BHA can be absorbed into the skin, but that means the detergent cleansing agents would be left on the skin for longer than necessary, and that absolutely can cause unwanted irritation.) Finally, the skin needs only one good exfoliant, and that's it. Overexfoliating will further irritate the skin, and the long-term effects of that are unknown.

In terms of sunscreens, it would be great if an AHA or BHA product had a good SPF rating (at least SPF 15, with FDA-approved UVA protection). That way, if you wanted to use an AHA or BHA product during the day along with a sunscreen, you would have to use only one product instead of two. **As this book goes to press, none of the sunscreens currently on the market contain an effective concentration of AHAs or BHA with a proper pH level as well as an effective SPF formulation (SPF 15 with avobenzone, titanium dioxide, or zinc oxide). Until that happens, sunscreen needs to be a separate step from the application of AHAs or BHA (or Retin-A and Renova, for that matter).**

However, even if they do come up with an AHA or BHA product in an effective sunscreen, I would still suggest keeping the AHA or BHA application separate from the sunscreen. Sunscreen needs to be applied every day and all over. You may not want to apply AHAs, and definitely not BHA, all over the face. Furthermore, what do you use if you want to apply the AHA or BHA at night? You don't need sunscreen ingredients on the face at night. For AHAs there's also the issue of altering application after a six-month period to one month on and one month off.

As you search for an AHA or BHA product, cosmetics salespeople will tell you to use theirs along with their complete program, including two or three other moisturizers, toners, cleansers, eye creams, throat creams, and lord knows what else. Be prepared for the hard sell when it comes to AHA or BHA products. Many cosmetics companies treat them like the fountain of youth, and they are not. They do not stop wrinkling; they merely smooth the surface skin for as long as you continue to use them. Some companies deal in specialty AHA products that contain higher percentages (from 8% to 15%). However, higher percentages may guarantee higher irritation, and there is little research indicating what kind of risk or harm that might pose over time. Be aware that many, many AHA and BHA products are poorly formulated, with ineffective concentrations and high pHs. The purpose of AHAs and BHA is to exfoliate the skin. They can do that only at the appropriate concentration and pH. An AHA or BHA product that has a low concentration and a high pH may feel good on the skin, but it is good only as a moisturizer. That isn't bad, but it won't exfoliate the skin.

By the way, many AHA or BHA products designed for oily skin contain alcohol. I do not recommend these because of the risk of increased irritation and sensitization they pose. Likewise, someone with oily skin or breakouts will have problems with an AHA or BHA product that comes in a moisturizing base, because the ingredients may make the skin feel slick and can clog pores. Oily skin types need to look for AHA or BHA products in a gel or liquid form that are irritant-free (meaning no alcohol, plants, fruit extracts, or witch hazel) and do not come in a moisturizing base. More of these are becoming available, but the pickings are still relatively slim if you're looking for a good, reasonably priced AHA or BHA product that won't adversely affect oily skin types. (See Chapter Five, "Skin-Care Planning," for specific product choices.)

As a general rule, you should not use additional exfoliating products such as cosmetic scrubs, washcloths, and facial masks (clay or drying masks) if you are using an AHA or BHA product. Also, stay away from overdoing exfoliation. Lots of cosmetics companies put AHAs and BHA in everything they make. Remember, the skin can handle only so much irritation; one effective exfoliant is all that is necessary for anyone's skin.

Frequently Asked Questions About AHAs

What does the FDA say about AHA and BHA products? The majority of AHA products, even the professional-strength versions and facial peels performed by both salons and physicians (except for the prescription-only Lac Hydrin-12), are currently classified as cosmetics (meaning proof of claims, safety data, and substantiating data are not required), and that's exactly where the manufacturers would like to keep them. Safety reviews and legal standards are almost nonexistent for cosmetics manufacturers. Safety testing for drugs is vastly more stringent. According to Dr. John Bailey, the FDA's director of colors and cosmetics, his department has an active interest in AHA products. His main concerns are (1) What are the effects on people with sensitive skin? (2) What are the long-term side effects? (3) What levels of concentration are safe and effective? These are good questions, but it will take some time before the FDA has all the answers.

When it comes to BHA, there are fewer concerns about safety, because salicylic acid has been used as an exfoliating treatment for blemishes for a long time. When listed as an active ingredient on a product label, in concentrations of 1% and 2%, BHA is not a cosmetic but an over-the-counter drug, and tightly controlled by the FDA. There is plenty of documented evidence that BHA, when used for controlling blemishes, has no long-term consequences and can be effective. However, BHA is now being used for sun-damaged and dry skin, and there is no research indicating how it affects those skin types over the long haul. BHA is not considered an over-the-counter drug by the FDA when used in nonblemish, dry-skin, or anti-wrinkle products. As strange as that sounds, if BHA is used as an exfoliant for sun-damaged or dry skin, the FDA considers it a cosmetic and requires no proof of efficacy or long-term safety. Don't ask me why—that's just the way it is.

Are there any side effects? Should I take any precautions? Most people experience a tingling or slight stinging sensation when they use AHA or BHA products with appropriate concentrations and pH. Some people have had minor to severe flaking and redness. Minor reactions are to be expected, given the nature of AHAs and BHA. However, long-term irritation, redness, flaking, or patches of dermatitis are not healthy for the skin, and if any of these symptoms occur, you should stop using the product, reduce the frequency of application, or consider a more gentle (less concentrated) product. Listen to your skin: if it gets very dry and flaky, use an additional moisturizer for a period of time until the skin calms down and gets used to the new level of exfoliation. If it gets red and irritated, use the product less frequently, though still regularly (perhaps once a day, or two or three times a week). If it still gets very dry and irritated, consider stopping altogether. Severe irritation is not the goal or the desired result. As you probably already know, it is imperative that you wear a sunscreen every day, one with an SPF of at least 15 that includes avobenzone (trade name Parsol 1789), titanium dioxide, or zinc oxide to protect from UVA damage. Exfoliating the skin leaves it more vulnerable to sun damage and requires mandatory, maximum protection every day.

What about the data indicating that some products claiming an 8% concentration of AHAs really contain just an 8% concentration of a 70% solution of AHAs? The issue of concentration is one of the trickiest parts of the AHA equation, because there are no unified regulations. In their undiluted form, AHAs are crystallized and therefore hard for a cosmetics formulator to use. Most cosmetic chemists use a 70% solution of AHA, which means 70% pure AHA to 30% water (and other trace ingredients). Most companies that quote a percentage are referring to concentration from a 70% solution, not a 100% one. Thus, most, if not all, 8% AHA products actually contain a 5.6% concentration (8% of 70% is 5.6%). Is that misleading? Should we be looking for an 8% concentration from a 100% solution? Probably not (and, in any case, the cosmetics companies don't have to tell us what kind of raw material they are using, which means there is no way to know for sure). A 70% solution of AHA is fairly standard in the cosmetics industry, and an 8% concentration of that is completely adequate for exfoliation.

Which type of AHA or BHA product is best: lotion, gel, cream, or liquid? That depends on what your skin needs and the ingredients in the various products. Gels and liquids that contain alcohol can irritate the skin and cause more problems. (Alcohol can allow deeper penetration of the AHA or BHA, which could be good for a stronger initial impact, but it also increases the possibility of unwanted side effects.) These should be avoided at all costs by all skin types. Gels and liquids that contain no other irritants besides the AHA or BHA are best for someone with normal to oily skin. Creams and lotions slow down absorption of the AHA and BHA, but they also cushion the skin and protect it from possible irritation. AHA or BHA creams and lotions are best for someone with dry skin; however, applying a separate liquid AHA product and then a moisturizer allows some flexibility. For example, you could alternate the AHA or BHA gel or liquid product with your moisturizer—using the AHA or BHA every other night or applying the moisturizer only where you have dry skin, so you don't overmoisturize.

What about the long-term effects of these products and the notion of skin fatigue? There isn't much information about the long-term use of AHAs or BHA on sun-damaged or older skin. The available research indicates that within a few months AHAs stop working the way they did when they were first used. Is that good or bad? AHAs exfoliate the top layer of skin that has thickened because of sun damage or simply because some people produce more top layers of skin than others. Once that top layer has been exfoliated, AHAs no longer have the same effect, and that may be beneficial for the skin. This turn-off point does not exist for BHA. Because BHA continues to have the same effect, there is a potential for skin fatigue. Skin fatigue is what happens when the exfoliated skin grows back faster, becoming thicker again, almost like building a callus, even if you continue using the product. However, not everyone agrees with this concern about skin fatigue. Many dermatologists feel that BHA has been around forever with no negative results. What is certain is that if you stop using AHAs or BHA, the skin reverts to its original state, slowly, over a period of time. Using AHAs regularly for a while and then alternating regular applications appears to be the key to keeping skin smooth and exfoliated. The same seems to be true for BHA, although when it is being used for blemishes and acne, and not for sun-damaged skin, there is no reason to alternate applications.

AHAs vs. BHA

According to the March 3, 1997, issue of *The Rose Sheet,* a cosmetics and pharmaceutical industry newsletter, and an article that appeared in *The Journal of Geriatric Dermatology,* Dr. Albert Kligman provided information about a study he conducted comparing AHAs to BHA. Kligman based his approval of BHA over AHAs on two studies: one was a 21-day irritation study and one was a study that involved looking at before-and-after photographs of "hundreds of women" over a 12-week period. The women in one study were treated with either 1.5% or 2% salicylic acid (BHA) or a proprietary (established but unnamed) glycolic acid (AHA) cream. Observers rating the results found the women using the BHA product had a statistically significant improvement in the appearance of their skin. It goes without saying that these two studies were limited in scope; 21 days isn't much time, and comparing salicylic acid to one AHA product is not exactly a broad-based comparison. Still, given these test results, there are several reasons to consider a BHA product or peel instead of an AHA product or peel (and vice versa).

It takes less BHA than AHA to obtain exfoliating results. AHAs require at least a 5% concentration for exfoliation to occur, while BHA is effective at concentrations of 1% to 2%. Percentages of BHA are clearly listed on acne products because it is required by the FDA. But when BHA is used in antiwrinkle products, its concentration is not required on the label, and cosmetics companies (such as Clinique, Oil of Olay, and Neutrogena) that use salicylic acid in wrinkle products carefully leave off the percentage. Listing of AHA percentages is not required by the FDA in any product, and only a few companies list the concentration on their label. BHA is a single ingredient with no variances (at least not yet), which makes ingredient lists less ambiguous for the consumer, while many ingredients can be listed as AHAs (even ones that are completely noneffective).

BHA requires a slightly lower pH to be effective than do AHAs. AHAs are effective as exfoliants in a pH of 3 to 4.5, while BHA is most effective at a pH of 3. A pH of 3 can be irritating in itself, but irritation is a risk with all types of exfoliants. In a formula even a fraction above a pH of 3, BHA provides little to no exfoliation whatsoever. But even though concentration and pH levels for both AHAs and BHA are important, even more so for BHA than AHAs (something most studies agree on), it is absurdly difficult to ascertain exactly the pH of any specific BHA or AHA product. From that standpoint alone, it is almost impossible to make a wise consumer decision as to which is the best product.

Looking at the most visible BHA products, Oil of Olay Daily Renewal Cream has a pH of 3 (its cleanser also has a pH of 3, but I don't recommend BHA or AHAs in a cleanser because of possible contact with the eyes) and so do the two

Almay Time Off Revitalizer products. Clinique's TurnAround products have a pH of 5 to 6, so though they may be good moisturizers, they won't work as exfoliators.

BHA is lipid-soluble (fat-soluble) while AHAs are water-soluble. BHA can better penetrate a pilosebaceous unit (a hair follicle and oil gland) to remove the skin cells lining the structure and help unplug the pore. That is why salicylic acid shows up in so many acne products. If you could be sure that the pH of a particular acne product containing salicylic acid is low enough, it would be a definite consideration for someone who tends to break out, especially if it uses a liquid or gel base (a moisturizing base may clog pores). On the other hand, AHAs interact better with the watery intercellular layer of skin, helping those layers of dead skin to turn over, and may be better for sun-damaged skin. However, any amount of exfoliation can help skin, and the effect of too much exfoliation isn't clear.

BHA may cause less inflammation than AHAs. BHA is related to aspirin. Because salicylic acid is a derivative of aspirin (acetylsalicylic acid), it has been demonstrated that BHA retains some of aspirin's anti-inflammatory properties. Some physicians prefer salicylic acid facial peels to glycolic acid peels because salicylic acid has less irritating side effects than glycolic acid.

According to studies by Dr. Walter Smith, AHAs seem to have a turn-off point, while BHA keeps exfoliating. For someone with acne and clogged pores, BHA (in a low enough pH and in a 1% to 2% concentration) may be more effective than AHAs. This is due to BHA's ability to penetrate the sebum in the pore, exfoliate the cells in the pores, and provide constant cell turnover. The major question about both AHAs and BHA concerns the long-term effect of these ingredients at the right concentration and pH. Is there any long-term benefit for the skin in constantly exfoliating it? Is continued exfoliation helpful or hurtful in the long run? For now there is no conclusive answer, but even Procter & Gamble, in the press release for its Oil of Olay Age Defying line, states that "long-term irritation is not healthy for skin because it damages skin's natural ... moisture barrier and [ability to] protect itself from sun damage." I strongly agree and worry about the effect of too much irritation on the skin.

What about products that include both AHAs and BHA? Good question. There is no information about the effectiveness of these products in terms of what percentages are helpful for each group of ingredients. It may be a way to cover all your bases, taking into consideration AHAs' superior action on the surface of the skin and BHA's superior ability to exfoliate inside the pore. But theory does not in any way mean proof, and you don't want your skin to be the guinea pig for this one.

Bottom line: Most consumers like the way their skin feels after exfoliating. Until all the information is in and the cosmetics industry decides to be more forthcoming with specific information about products, try to use only those products that you know meet the criteria for effectiveness. I'll do my best to find out that crucial information, but for now, getting these critical numbers from the cosmetics industry is like pulling teeth.

Retin-A, Micro Retin-A, and Renova

After discussing AHAs and BHA at length, I do not want to play down the considerable importance of this group of prescription-only skin-care products, because they are major players when it comes to exfoliating the skin and actually changing the way skin behaves. If you have sun-damaged, dry, wrinkled, or acne-prone skin, you are most likely familiar with the name Retin-A. Most of you probably recall the hoopla that erupted regarding Johnson & Johnson's little-known acne drug Retin-A (tretinoin, or retinoic acid, a derivative of vitamin A, in a gel or a matte cream base) when, back in 1987, a study released to the media seemed to show that acne was not the only thing this prescription drug could tackle. Rather dramatic before-and-after pictures seemed to indicate scientists had finally found the fountain of youth. All forms of the media had a field day with this one. Every news channel, talk show, newspaper, and fashion magazine featured pictures from the study and interviews with Dr. John Voorhees, the doctor who performed the study, and Dr. Albert Kligman, the inventor of Retin-A.

If this kind of media blitz had been in the form of advertising, it would have been illegal, because prescription drugs can't be advertised without a vast range of restrictions and constraints. Drugs of any kind are tightly controlled by the FDA, with strict guidelines as to what the manufacturer can and cannot say about the product. (At that time, Retin-A was approved for use as an acne medication only. If an individual doctor wanted to let a patient use it for wrinkles, that was fine, but it was not sanctioned by the FDA, and the company could make no claims to the contrary.) Free publicity was another story altogether.

All that media coverage helped sales of Retin-A soar into the millions, which didn't hurt Johnson & Johnson's stock price either. What was the bottom line after the dust settled and all the prescriptions were filled? It turned out that the study that generated all the publicity was paid for by Johnson & Johnson, the study was too small to be significant, and many women who used Retin-A were not necessarily enthralled with the results, at least not when it came to a change in their wrinkles, and the risk of irritation was fairly high.

Now it is almost ten years later, and in that time Johnson & Johnson has labored long and hard to produce studies that would convince the FDA that Retin-A should be approved for use as a wrinkle cream. The result: the FDA has approved a version of Retin-A called Renova (which is simply Retin-A, tretinoin, in an emollient base for use as a wrinkle cream). That makes Renova the first medicine ever approved by the FDA for the treatment of sun-damaged skin, meaning wrinkles.

Should you run right out for your new Retin-A or Renova prescription? Well, the press release I received from the FDA in regard to wrinkles wasn't all that thrilling. Only a small percentage of users, about 16% in one study and fewer than that in another, were pleased with their results. More than two-thirds thought the results were mediocre, and another third experienced no change in their skin's appearance.

Despite all this marketing strategy to gain consumer attention for these topical prescription skin treatments, tretinoin just won't erase wrinkles, but it can do remarkable things for the health of the skin. Unlike AHAs and BHA, which unglue skin cells, helping them slough off to reveal healthier skin cells underneath, tretinoin works, for the most part, in a radically different manner. Tretinoin works by exfoliating the skin just the way AHAs do, but on a deeper level. Tretinoin has the ability to locate receptor sites on the skin cell that accept certain specific components of vitamin A. The tretinoin attaches to a receptor site, which provides information to the cell, telling it to behave in a more healthy manner. In this regard, tretinoin can play a vital role in changing the way skin cells are formed and shaped, not just exfoliating. If a skin cell has a healthier form and shape, it can do its job of natural exfoliation.

Helping skin to grow in a healthier manner by using Retin-A, Micro Retin-A, Renova, or any other tretinoin product can have extremely positive effects on both sun-damaged and acne-prone skin by literally changing how skin cells are formed and how they are shed, which makes skin feel smoother and helps unclog pores. But what about wrinkles? According to a 1996 study from the University of Pennsylvania School of Medicine's department of dermatology, "Tretinoin has been shown to stimulate synthesis of collagen in photo-aged human and hairless mouse skin. It has been suggested that this partial reversal of photodamaged skin by tretinoin is a consequence of low-grade inflammation. [But this test demonstrated that the] tretinoin-induced zone of new collagen was twice the depth of that induced by [other] irritant vehicles [which included glycolic acid]."

Regardless of these positive effects, tretinoin products will be useless if you do not wear a sunscreen as well. Not a wrinkle cream in the world, even one approved by the FDA, can have positive results if you don't use an effective sunscreen.

For now, tretinoin products aren't cheap. Renova costs about $60 for a 40-gram tube (a one- to two-month supply), and that doesn't include the cost of a visit to your doctor. The good news is that prices for tretinoin products will be changing now that the patent for Retin-A has expired. This allows other pharmaceutical drug manufacturers to make their own tretinoin products. Lots of them are already in the process of doing just that, which should make pricing more competitive and attractive for the consumer.

The big question is, are AHA and BHA products a replacement for tretinoin? It depends on whom you talk to. Some "experts" recommend using AHA products and a tretinoin product like Retin-A or Renova, while others say tretinoin can be used all by itself. Although AHA and tretinoin products have somewhat similar results, they do not work in a similar fashion. Tretinoin affects actual cell growth, while AHAs and BHA simply help the skin to shed dead skin cells. BHA also helps unclog pores by exfoliating skin inside the pores.

Given the evidence that tretinoin can help produce collagen and unclog pores, plastic surgeons and dermatologists alike tend to prescribe it. However, with AHAs the results are immediate; it can take two years to see an increase in collagen production when using tretinoin, and the potential for irritation is fairly high. AHAs can be much less irritating.

Many physicians recommend both tretinoin and AHAs, applying AHA in the morning and tretinoin at night. How BHA figures into use for different skin types is not clear. Like BHA, tretinoin can unclog pores, so generally if you are using Retin-A or Renova it isn't necessary to use BHA. Because people react differently to skin-care products, I would suggest experimenting to see which item or items work best for you. There is no reason in the world not to judiciously try out a combination, always remembering sunscreen, to see what has the most benefit for your skin.

Again, what tretinoin, AHA, and BHA products have in common is that once you stop using them, your skin will revert to the way it was before. These products will not produce permanent change. The smooth exterior lasts only as long as you use them. This is one of the major reasons that researchers don't believe AHAs, BHA, Retin-A, or Renova really change the deeper layers of the skin.

If you do choose to get a prescription for Retin-A or Renova or one of the new tretinoin products soon to appear on the market (or if you cross the border into Mexico to get it over the counter), it is important to be careful when using them and/or AHA and BHA products. Review and remember the following list of cautions.

- It is dangerous to tan after you start using Retin-A, Renova, or an AHA or BHA product. As the surface skin peels and becomes somewhat thinner, it becomes more sensitive to sunlight and is therefore more subject to serious sunburn. Also, tanning will negate any positive effects you hope to gain from using these exfoliators. If you are using any of these products, it is essential to wear a sunscreen rated at least SPF 15, with avobenzone (Parsol 1789), titanium dioxide, or zinc oxide, whenever you venture outside. The idea is to keep your sun exposure at a minimum.

- Retin-A, Renova, and AHA and BHA products can irritate the skin. If you use any other irritant on the skin at the same time, you will exacerbate the initial negative side effects of the product. You must eliminate all of the following from your skin-care routine during your first months of using these products (it's probably best for your skin to always avoid these, by the way): washcloths; hot water; cold water; all astringents, toners, fresheners, clarifying lotions, refining lotions, and the like that contain irritants; scrubs; clay facial masks; bar soaps; skin-care products that contain fragrances or strong preservatives; and saunas and steam rooms (used on a regular basis, saunas and steam rooms can cause spider veins and other problems for the face).
- If you want Retin-A, Renova, or AHA or BHA products to work, you must use them regularly. To sustain the results, you must continue using them on a regular, patterned cycle for the rest of your life. The changes that take place on the skin are not permanent. Once you stop using the product, the skin slowly reverts to its original condition. Using something forever is a tremendous commitment. But according to the majority of women I've interviewed and who have written to me, the difference is positive enough to warrant a long-term relationship.
- If you want to use Retin-A or Renova with an AHA or BHA product, most doctors recommend using AHAs during the day and Retin-A or Renova at night.

See Chapter Six, "Special Battle Plans for Blemishes," for more information about using Retin-A for breakouts (instead of for sun damage).

Skin Vitamins Inside and Out

You can't feed the skin from the outside in. You can't put food on your face and have lunch, and you can't put vitamins on your face and provide nutritional benefit for skin tissue. That is why the FDA regulates how names of vitamins must appear on cosmetics labels. Legally, the chemical name of the vitamin must be used—tocepherol acetate instead of vitamin E, or retinyl palmitate instead of vitamin A. According to the FDA, this is so consumers won't be misled as to what they are putting on their face—a chemical with cosmetic properties and no nutritional or medical value. Regrettably, most women don't pay as much attention to ingredient lists as they do to marketing copy, which is scarcely regulated.

That's not to say there isn't some benefit to be derived from putting vitamins in their chemical form on the skin. In other words, vitamins B, C, and E, among others, are helpful to the skin, not because of their nutritional value but because they can provide some kind of barrier on the skin that prevents dehydration, works as an antioxidant, or helps with some amount of exfoliation. Are they the only or even preferred way to get these benefits? No. Many other cosmetic ingredients do the same things.

Why can't vitamins feed the skin from the outside in? Now it gets complicated. Vitamins are essential, fundamental compounds required for maintenance of life. But vitamins do not work alone. Without a whole litany of other physiological processes (meaning an interactive process with innumerable other factors that include a mixture of other vitamins, enzymes, coenzymes, proteins, amino acids, oxidation, hormones, metabolic cycles, circulation, and so on), vitamins would have no effect. That is why vitamins used topically can't really feed the skin, nourish the skin tissue, or change your metabolism (meaning build collagen). Again, that doesn't mean vitamins in skin-care products don't have a function, but they don't do what you might be hoping they will do for your skin.

To complicate matters a little further, there are fat-soluble and water-soluble vitamins. Fat-soluble vitamins are stored in body fat and may therefore accumulate in quantities that can be toxic; these include vitamins A, D, E, and K. Most water-soluble vitamins, such as the B-complex vitamins and vitamin C, are rapidly eliminated in the urine and thus rarely cause toxicity, even when ingested in excessive amounts. Even if vitamins could feed the skin, you wouldn't want to risk building up too much of the fat-soluble vitamins in skin tissue, but because topical vitamins aren't utilized that way, they can't negatively impact the skin in that manner.

What makes the cosmetic value of an ingredient like vitamin A differ from the pharmaceutical or medical value of a drug like Retin-A, a vitamin A derivative? Retin-A is retinoic acid, and its resemblance to vitamin A is so distant as to be several generations removed. Derivation tells you only an ingredient's source; it doesn't tell you anything else. Retinoic acid is extracted via a very precise procedure that renders it compatible to only certain points on a skin cell. This is comparable to needing one correct-sized screw (out of a million possible screws to choose from) to tighten one specific hinge (out of a million possible hinges). Breaking down a food or vitamin into the appropriate molecular elements to perform a physiologically altering task is not the realm of cosmetics, and given the way cosmetics are regulated, you absolutely would not want that to be otherwise.

What about taking the new oral vitamins for skin care being sold by many cosmetics companies, particularly in-home sales companies like Mary Kay? As long as you don't megadose, taking vitamin supplements is just fine for the entire body, and that includes hair and skin. Can you take certain vitamins hoping they will target just your hair to make it grow fuller and thicker or just your skin to erase wrinkles or acne? Sadly, no. If you are deficient in a particular vitamin (though deficiency is a rare occurrence in most Western countries), supplementing your diet is great for many, many reasons. There is plenty of evidence that the American diet, built around processed and fast foods, is inadequate in fresh fruits and vegetables, and may indeed be lacking nutritionally. But unless you have a true vitamin deficiency, the excess vitamins you take will either be stored in fat cells, a potential problem, or excreted when you go to the bathroom. Remember, vitamins don't work alone. So when you hear or read cosmetic babble suggesting vitamin A or folic acid is the most important vitamin for skin, remember that vitamins don't work alone. They need other vitamins to do their job, and too much of this good thing can be toxic (vitamin A is one of those fat-soluble vitamins).

And don't assume for one second that vitamins can prevent sun damage or replace sunscreen. It isn't possible. Vitamin supplements also can't replace a healthy diet. Perhaps this is the most distressing aspect of the entire vitamin industry. **The benefit a person receives from consuming a whole food cannot be duplicated in a pill. While the list of vitamins, minerals, and other bionutrients in a vitamin supplement may look impressive, they are only a small part of what you would actually get from eating a balanced diet.** Say you take a vitamin C supplement. Not a bad thing to do, but if you think for one second that the pill replaces eating an orange or tomato (tomatoes are high in vitamin C) you are truly cheating your health. An orange or tomato contains a complicated mix of vitamins, minerals, fibers, sugars, amino acids, and, as research in this area continues, probably lots more things we don't yet know about. Eating the orange or the tomato or other whole foods is what can make us healthy and beautiful, not the supplements or exotic herbs from the Far East that offer only a small part of what the body needs to be OK.

Regarding the issue of vitamins and skin, in all my research I have yet to come across one published study indicating that vitamins or minerals can change one wrinkle or affect acne. Consult any of the various issues on vitamin supplements done by *Consumer Reports* if you don't believe me. Their debunking of the vitamin industry is exemplary, and will be insightful for anyone interested in better health.

Retinol

A cosmetic ingredient called retinol has, I've noticed, had a recent resurgence. Retinol is a vitamin A derivative, but it is hardly new. In fact, it has been around for some time. Retinol gained immense popularity shortly after Retin-A (tretinoin, or retinoic acid) made headlines as a prescription wrinkle cream back in 1987. Retin-A is a derivative of vitamin A. So is retinol. It wasn't a big stretch for cosmetics companies to try to convince the consumer that a product containing retinol could produce the same effects as Retin-A. Headlines everywhere had made most people aware of vitamin A, and in no time there was a flurry of knock-off Retin-A sound-alike products containing retinol or retinyl palmitate (another vitamin A derivative).

As it turns out, new, though limited, evidence indicates that retinol in rather large quantities can benefit the skin in the same ways Retin-A does. But it takes a lot more retinol than is presently being used in any cosmetic. According to a study by Dr. John Voorhees et al., from the University of Michigan, Ann Arbor, department of dermatology, Retinol must be present in at least a 20% concentration in order for a product to mimic tretinoin. The question is why anyone should even bother with retinol when there is so much evidence that tretinoin, in the form of Retin-A, Renova, and others, offers such good, and proven, results.

Vitamin C

Vitamin C is another popular skin-care ingredient these days. The sensation over Cellex-C, which uses a form of vitamin C called L-ascorbic acid, I've commented on in issues of my newsletter and in *Don't Go to the Cosmetics Counter Without Me,* as well as in the first chapter of this book. The reason this issue deserves so much attention has a lot to do with the cosmetics industry getting carried away with the subject and spawning a horde of vitamin C products. To sum up, the commotion about vitamin C as an anti-aging ingredient is not only exaggerated, it borders on preposterous. L-ascorbic acid turns out to be a very good antioxidant, but an exceptionally unstable one. When exposed to air, sun, or heat, it decomposes. Longevity is definitely an issue for these types of products. **The only research available about vitamin C indicates that it can help prevent some amount of sunburn. Preventing sunburn is great, but the effect of that takes years to show up on the face. Plus, preventing sunburn is only one part of what it takes to prevent the sun's rays from damaging the skin. Sunburn is caused by UVB radiation. Skin cancer and wrinkles are caused by UVA radiation. So while some forms of vitamin C may help reduce sunburn, they won't stop wrinkling or reduce the need for sunscreens with UVA-blocking ingredients like titanium dioxide, avobenzone, and zinc oxide.**

L-ascorbic acid and other forms of vitamin C are decent antioxidants, and it is well established that antioxidants are beneficial in enhancing the effects of other sunscreen agents, helping to reduce sun damage. But is L-ascorbic acid the be-all and end-all of antioxidants? No. L-ascorbic acid is only one of an entire new breed of antioxidant ingredients showing up on the skin-care scene. Many other antioxidants are as good as or even more impressive than L-ascorbic acid for increased sun protection, and many are far less unstable, including selenium, vitamin E, superoxide dismutase, and beta glucan, to name a few.

The entire arena of antioxidants is new, and there is nothing definitive to warrant the cost or tumult. They won't get rid of wrinkles or replace sunscreen, so calm down! They can offer increased sun protection, which is important, but that's it. Of course, that doesn't stop the companies promoting these products from making claims about building collagen and feeding the skin from the outside in, despite the fact that they have no studies supporting either contention.

Vitamin K and Spider Veins

You may have run into advertisements or heard cosmetics salespeople discussing the effectiveness of Vitamin K creams and lotions for reducing or eliminating surfaced spider veins (technically referred to as telangiectasias). These creams can't change spider veins, but let me explain why some people erroneously think they can. The vitamin K in these products is considered a cosmetic ingredient, not a pharmaceutical or drug. As a cosmetic, it is not necessary for companies to prove their claims about what it can do. All of the information I've seen about this ingredient's effectiveness comes from companies that sell these products. One medical expert in particular, a Dr. Melvin Elson, who sells creams that contain vitamin K, makes a lot of claims about treatment of spider veins. His company, Cosmeceutical Research Institute, is the only source of information suggesting this stuff works. There are no published studies or peer-review studies that add up to results you can even remotely count on.

According to Dr. Craig Feied, M.D., director of the American Vein Institute and associate clinical professor of emergency medicine at George Washington University, vitamin K is associated with veins and blood because it is a prominent factor in the blood's ability to clot. If you take too much vitamin K orally, it can cause blood clots (which can lead to death). Blood clots can choke off the blood flow through a vein or capillary and make it disappear. However, shutting down a vein or a surfaced capillary (spider vein) this way can be risky business. Applying vitamin K to the surface of the skin does nothing, and that's good. If vitamin K could penetrate the surface of the skin to affect the blood flow in spider veins, it could also affect the blood flow in healthy veins. If you're already using a vitamin K product, don't worry; in order for vitamin K to form blood clots to shut down a vein or capillary, it must first be digested and then metabolized in the liver, where proteins are formed. These special proteins are what causes the blood to clot. It isn't the vitamin K that has the effect of shutting down veins, but a by-product that is created after digestion.

If you are interested in doing something that truly eliminates tiny surfaced spider veins from the face, the Photoderm laser is considered one of the most effective and safest ways to go about it. Treatment of very tiny spider veins via Photoderm is an outstanding procedure. Photoderm zaps the tiny spider vein and literally makes the blood boil, which closes down the vein and the surrounding surfaced spider veins. The sensation is about the same as being poked by a tiny needle. If you have a fear of needles, Photoderm is a blessing. It is best for tiny spider veins because it treats only the surface of the skin, where the problem exists. Photoderm can't get deep enough to cause damage or problems for veins you don't want it to affect.

Getting rid of existing spider veins on the face is one issue, but preventing them is even more important. Sunburn, heat (prolonged exposure to saunas, Jacuzzis, or just cooking for long periods over a hot stove), pressure on the face (from severely blowing your nose or rough massages), injury, and repeated local irritation and inflammation from irritating skin-care ingredients can all increase the occurrence of spider veins. Avoid these things and you can prevent their formation as well as reduce their appearance.

Antioxidants

Many women nowadays are fairly certain that free-radical damage is bad for the skin, and they are right. It is bad for the skin. It is also well known that oxygen and UV rays (not pollution and smog, as you may have heard from cosmetics salespeople) are the main catalysts of free-radical damage. Theoretically, free-radical damage can cause deterioration of the skin's support structures, decreasing elasticity and resilience. What plays a part in slowing down free-radical damage is the presence of antioxidants in the diet, and, possibly, the topical application of antioxidants in skin-care products. Antioxidants are ingredients such as vitamins A, C, and E; superoxide dismutase; flavonoids; beta carotene; glutathione; selenium; and zinc. Technically there are thousands (yes, thousands) of viable antioxidant compounds in the plant world, of which we have discovered a mere handful.

Despite the proliferation of skin-care products containing antioxidants, according to many researchers, including Dr. Jeffrey Blumberg, chief of antioxidants research at Tufts University, "There is no conclusive scientific evidence that antioxidants really prevent wrinkles, nor is there any information about how much antioxidant(s) or exactly which one(s) has to be present in a product to have an effect," if any noticeable effect is even possible. Agreeing with Dr. Blumberg are such skin-care experts as Retin-A inventor Dr. Albert Kligman, from the University of Pennsylvania, and Dr. Jim Bollinger, from Galderma Laboratories, who both state emphatically that "everything we know about antioxidants is theoretical, and there is no proof they can do anything to stop wrinkling."

Even if antioxidants did work on the skin to prevent free-radical damage, the results would hardly be immediate. Free-radical damage in the human body takes years and years before any noticeable deterioration can be detected. You can't slap the stuff on and immediately notice your wrinkles disappearing.

Despite this lack of hard evidence, fashion magazines have heralded the elimination of free-radical damage as the fountain of youth for the '90s. The excitement around antioxidants is understandable. According to many skin experts (both legitimate experts and those endorsing specific products), all aspects of aging, including wrinkling, are caused by free-radical damage. Vitamin companies and cosmetics companies alike want you to believe their antioxidant products can eliminate it. The evidence is fairly convincing that free-radical damage is an insidious "natural" process that causes the body to break down. What isn't known is whether you can really stop free-radical damage inside and outside of a human being from taking place.

Explaining free-radical damage is like trying to explain how television works. No matter how many times I'm told how transmission and reception happen, all I know is that I can watch television whenever I turn on the set, and nothing else makes sense. Nevertheless, here's a simplified explanation of free-radical damage.

Free-radical damage has to do with oxygen and ultraviolet radiation. Oxygen molecules (O_2) are generally stable, but when they become unstable, due primarily to the presence of ultraviolet radiation and other unspecified molecules (there's a lot about free-radical damage we don't know yet), the unstable oxygen molecules grab other molecules as a way to become stabilized. What happens then is that those other molecules also become unstable and grab more molecules to become stabilized. This chain reaction can go on indefinitely and there seems to be primarily one way to stop it, but I'll get to that later in this section.

A good, but extremely simplified, example of how free-radical damage takes place involves paint. When paint is shut off from air (oxygen) and sunlight in a sealed container, it remains liquid. When it is exposed to air, however, it hardens. What takes place is that an unstable oxygen molecule gets into the exposed paint and interacts with specific parts of the paint's molecules, changing their form. The paint molecules become unstable, creating free radicals, which in turn grab all the other molecules, resulting in solid paint. Actually, referring to this process as damaging can be misleading. Free-radical damage is a major life function, in plants as well as the human body. Immune systems, metabolism, cells communicating with each other, and collagen production (as well as destruction) are all affected both positively and negatively by the presence of free-radical damage.

So what does that have to do with aging? No one is exactly sure. When the free-radical reaction continues unrestrained, it can cause systems to break down. Instead of building collagen or other components of skin, free-radical damage destroys it, and it has a similarly bad effect on all other aspects of human physiology. How can you control free-radical damage? The answer to that question will make some person or corporation very wealthy.

One thing thought to stop free-radical damage from going too far is the presence of free-radical scavengers. As silly as that sounds, they really do exist, and they stop, or, a better term, "eat" free radicals. These scavengers are better known as antioxidants. Antioxidants keep air (specifically, unstable oxygen molecules) from interacting with other molecules and causing them to become unstable and start the free-radical chain reaction. The only problem with this theory is that free-radical damage is constant and extensive. How could you ever use enough antioxidants to stop it? How much oxygen or sunlight can you really keep away from all skin cells, or even some skin cells? What if you miss an area when you apply whatever product you bought? How fast do the antioxidants get used up? Do they last 20 minutes, one hour, two hours, or more on the skin? No one has the vaguest idea, and you can't suffocate the body to find out.

In relation to the skin, free-radical damage from sun exposure is a lifelong process that starts at birth and continues until death. Targeting the problem for the short term is pointless. Oxygen and sunlight are all around us every day of our lives. The world of skin care makes it sound like antioxidants are a quick fix, and that is absolutely not true.

Major investigation is being done in this fascinating area of human aging that most unquestionably influences wrinkling. Even though a lot of respected researchers are working on this issue, the research is in its infancy, and suggesting anything else is sheer fantasy. For now, in regard to your present skin-care routine, check the back of your moisturizer and see if it contains any free-radical scavengers (antioxidants) such as superoxide dismutase, vitamin C, vitamin E, or cysteine (among others), and make sure they are close to the top of the ingredient list and not at the end. Almost every company makes moisturizers that contain antioxidants, so they aren't hard to find. You won't see any difference in your skin, but if free-radical damage, and thus the destruction of the skin's structure, can be slowed, or if sun damage can be reduced, the antioxidants should help. It's a long shot, but many scientists think that if there is a fountain of youth, this could be it. For now, it's all theoretical, and no one can give you any definitive amounts or specific ingredients to look for despite the cosmetics industry's attempt to do so. As Dr. Blumberg puts it, "Cosmetics companies are not known for doing the work it takes to prove anything."

Oxygen for the Skin

Here is the most pathetic but clear-cut demonstration of how insane the world of cosmetics truly is. After selling us products to ward off oxygen's effects on the skin (antioxidant means anti-oxygen), the beauty industry then sells us products that claim to provide oxygen to the skin. Doesn't the beauty industry have anything better to do? (No, it doesn't, especially if there is an interested consumer willing to make a purchase.)

Many cosmetic products contain antioxidants, ingredients that keep oxygen off the face, such as vitamin C, superoxide dismutase, and vitamin E. On the other hand, the cosmetics industry also sells products that contain hydrogen peroxide (H_2O_3) or some other oxygen-releasing ingredient, which supposedly delivers an oxygen molecule when it comes into contact with skin. It is logical to wonder if the extra oxygen would just trigger free-radical damage and cause more problems for the skin. And if you were also using products that contained antioxidants, wouldn't they "scavenge" up the free-radical oxygen? There is no real answer to this question because it is so hypothetical and unfeasible as to be little more than sheer science fiction. If any of that were possible, meaning if you could put oxygen in a cosmetic and deliver it to the skin, the amount of oxygen trapped inside a cosmetic wouldn't be enough to provide one puff of air to even one skin cell, let alone the entire face. Likewise, the amount of antioxidant any cosmetic may contain has no measurable effect on free-radical damage.

Why the concern about supplying oxygen to the skin? Oxygen depletion is one of the things that happens to older skin, regardless of whether it has been affected by sun damage or any other health issue. Why or how that happens is a complete unknown, and delivering extra oxygen to the skin doesn't reverse it. After all, there is plenty of oxygen in our environment. The earth's atmosphere is 21% oxygen; the oceans, lakes, and rivers are about 88% oxygen. Oxygen is a constituent of most rocks and minerals, and 46.7% (by weight) of the solid crust of the earth. Oxygen makes up 60% of the human body, and is in every cell and organ (which further explains why using antioxidants is probably futile). It is a constituent of all living tissues; almost all plants and animals, including all humans, require oxygen to maintain life. However, oxygen is utilized by the body almost exclusively through respiration. Oxygen on the surface may affect the very top layer of skin, but so what? How much extra oxygen does skin need? Again, no one knows. Can it be absorbed? No. Plus, none of this answers the question about more free-radical damage.

Unquestionably, there is no shortage of oxygen anywhere in our world, but that doesn't stop the cosmetics industry. If anything, it fuels new fads for women who are desperately seeking beauty products to waste their money on.

Speaking of oxygen, the beauty industry is promoting a senseless regime involving hyperbaric oxygen booths. Spas and salons are offering them as a beauty treatment. Hyperbaric refers to a way of producing higher than normal atmospheric pressure. Increasing oxygen in a closed environment is one way to increase atmospheric pressure. (Ironically, too much oxygen is bad for the skin. Pure oxygen kills, and any amount of oxygen triggers free-radical damage.) Why would you want this increased oxygen around you? Because you've been convinced that the reason your skin isn't looking so good is due to a lack of oxygen. How did your skin come to be oxygen-deprived in an oxygen-filled world? Smoking or the skin's natural aging may be to blame. Changing that isn't possible unless you stop smoking or stop aging.

How did this caprice of oxygen booths get started? Oxygen booths are utilized medically to heal leg ulcers. This information was translated somehow to skin care. Assuming your face could benefit from an oxygen booth the way an ulcerated wound does, you would need to live in there. Leg ulcers are a temporary condition, but skin aging is ongoing, a "wound" that doesn't go away. The notion that oxygen treatments affect aging, wrinkles, or any other skin malady is a joke. Nary a study exists anywhere.

Pointing to oxygen as the way to prevent skin from aging would be almost laughable if so many women weren't falling for this hoax. How the skin ages is very complicated and involves an almost limitless range of physiological occurrences. There isn't any one cause that can be addressed with a cosmetic to erase or minimize the inevitable. Skin, all by itself, ages in at least 50 identifiable ways, so adding some oxygen to the equation solves, at best, only one-fiftieth of the problem—not enough to make a difference, even if it could. Besides, if extra oxygen were the answer, we would all simply live in oxygen tents, and no one would wrinkle. **It isn't just oxygen depletion, or free-radical damage, collagen destruction, reduced cell turnover, abnormal cell formation, decreased fat content, intercellular deficiency, genetically predetermined cell shutdown, and so on, that affects the way skin ages—it is all of these things combined.** What we know for sure is that the sun is the biggest culprit in causing the wrinkles associated with aging, and that is easily handled by using a good sunscreen. Bottom line: We needn't spend more than $10 to $15 to really make a difference in how our skin looks as we age.

Pycnogenol, Algae, and Beta Glucan

As the list of new miracle skin-care ingredients grows, the task of combating the misleading information is becoming repetitious. How many times can I explain that the claims don't match the research, not even a little? Yet it is essential to let you know when you need to pay attention and when you should turn a deaf ear. Pycnogenol, algae, and beta glucan are definitely a case of the latter. Pycnogenol, which is actually another name for beta glucan, and algae are good skin-care ingredients and may have some antioxidant effect, but I would not substitute them for other antioxidants and they don't in the least replace the need for a sunscreen. The following letter is typical of the inquiries I receive about this issue almost daily.

Excerpt from Cosmetics Counter Update

Dear Paula,

I recently read some information about the "latest and greatest" ingredient in anti-aging and anti-wrinkling, called pycnogenol (beta glucan). After reading about it in a magazine, I searched on the Internet and found additional information and products to order. I decided to jump in and try it. It was endorsed by a dermatologist and other scientific sources. I have yet to see a difference in my skin. In fact, nothing has changed.

That's why I am writing to you, the expert in what works and what's hype in the world of cosmetic and facial products. The two products I found for sale were Pycnogenol Ultra Moisturizing Gel by Martin Health Care Products (888-867-9673) and Pycnogenol distributed by Healthy Source (505-856-5004).

Can these products really do what they say: are they anti-aging and anti-wrinkling? If so, does pycnogenol take the place of all the AHA products on the market, or can it be used in conjunction with an AHA product? I look forward to hearing from you before placing my next order for these new wonder products. Thank you in advance for any information you may provide.

Connie

Dear Connie,

I am familiar with the studies regarding pycnogenol (a plant-derived substance), and I am not convinced. I don't think it is a bad ingredient, and it does seem to be a good antioxidant, but that is neither spectacular nor unique. There are thousands of antioxidants in the plant and animal worlds, and many are being used in cosmetics. "Antioxidant" is merely the buzzword of the moment in the cosmetics industry, which means everyone has to have their own super-duper antioxidant. Pycnogenol is just one of many. Cellex-C (which uses a form of vitamin C), Avon (which uses its own form of vitamin C), and Estee

Lauder Day Wear (which uses superoxide dismutase) are among the many companies and products vying to offer women the benefits of antioxidants.

I have been looking into this topic from day one, and there is no evidence, and I mean none, that indicates topical antioxidants can change, prevent, or stop wrinkling. All the commotion is generated because the theory behind antioxidants and some lab work done in this area are compelling, at least when it comes to preventing sun damage. That is why they sound so good, but translating what you can prove in a petri dish or on animal skin to human skin is a monumental leap.

I have interviewed some of the top cosmetic chemists and dermatologists researching cosmetics, and all of them said the same thing about pycnogenol (beta glucan): "It won't hurt your skin, but the hoopla around it is absurd and will be replaced by the next super-antioxidant to come along, and that still won't mean anything for the skin."

Even if antioxidants work, their effect isn't anything you will see overnight or even over months. They are still, in theory, a preventive measure. However, one area where antioxidants are proving to be helpful is in sunscreens, where they can boost the effectiveness of the blocking agents. Now, that's good news. Meanwhile, the entire topic of antioxidants has a lot of controversy and yet-to-be-answered questions. Pycnogenol or beta glucan is not the answer to these questions.

Glycerin: A Classic!

While many cosmetics lines boast all sorts of exotic ingredients, from plant extracts to vitamins, proteins, essential oils, and other exotic and scientific creations, it turns out plain old glycerin, long known as a humectant, may be a best friend for someone with dry skin. For some time it was thought that too much glycerin in a moisturizer could pull water out of the skin instead of into the skin. That theory now seems to be completely unfounded. What appears to be true is that glycerin shores up the skin's natural protection by filling in the area known as the intercellular layer and by attracting just the right amount of water to maintain the skin's homeostasis. The intercellular layer is, in essence, the mortar or natural barrier of the skin. Keeping the intercellular layer intact keeps bacteria out, moisture in, and the skin's surface smooth. There is also research indicating that the presence of glycerin in the intercellular layer helps other skin lipids do their jobs better.

Ceramide, Hyaluronic Acid, Cholesterol, and . . .

Ceramide is good stuff. So are hyaluronic acid, cholesterol, fatty acids and triglycerides (jojoba oil, jojoba wax, apricot oil, canola oil, coconut oil, shea butter, corn oil, safflower oil, soybean oil, olive oil, and sesame oil, among many others), glycosphingolipids, linoleic acid (linseed oil), glycosaminoglycans, glycerin, and mucopolysaccharide. What all these skin-care ingredients share is their presence in the intercellular structure between the skin cells. When any of these ingredients (along with a horde of other related ingredients) are used in skin-care products, they appear to help stabilize and maintain this complex, intercellular skin matrix that is so easily depleted by sun damage, irritating skin-care products, dry climates, indoor heat, smoking, and inherent aging factors. None of these very good water-binding agents can permanently affect or change skin, but they are great at temporarily keeping depleted skin from feeling dry and uncomfortable. More important, all of these ingredients, and lots more, can help support the intercellular area of the skin by keeping it intact. This support helps prevent surface irritation from penetrating deeper into the skin, helps keep bacteria out, and aids the skin's immune/healing system.

Is any one of these ingredients the be-all and end-all for your skin? Hardly. All of them perform similarly. Limiting yourself to a single ingredient, such as ceramide or vitamin C, or a single concept, such as "natural" or "purifying," as the answer to your skin-care needs, is the way to do the greatest disservice to your skin.

Triglycerides, Palmitates, Myristates, and . . .

Standard to most *all* cosmetics, both so-called natural ones and not so natural ones, are soft, supple, waxlike, emollient, thickening agents that read like a science journal with long indiscernible names. These pliable skin-softening agents have many functions. Not only do they have an affinity for skin, effortlessly smoothing over the surface and readily merging with the natural structures of the skin, they also provide the very feel and texture of the cosmetics we use. If a cosmetic has an elegant, smooth, feel; or looks like a light, gel-like lotion; or has a soft, translucent appearance; or has a thick, creamy, white texture, it is the mix of these thickening, emollient ingredients producing those finishes.

The assortment of names for these technical-sounding ingredients is nothing less than astounding. There are more of them than you can imagine. They range from cetearyl alcohol, to isopropyl myristate, myristic acid, palmitic acid, peg 60 hydrogenated castor oil, glyceryl linoleate, cyclomethicone, dimethicone, hexyl laurate, isohexadecane, methyl glucose sesquioleate, decyl oleate, stearic acid, and thousands more. These unsung heroes of moisturizers, sunscreens, cleansers, foundations, eyeshadows, and blushes the world over are the mainstay of cosmetic formulations. What all these ingredients share in common is their molecular resemblance to the natural lipids (sebum/oil) and intercellular substances found in skin. An issue for dry skin is the very lack of these lipids and intercellular substances. Cosmetics with innumerable formulary recipes are invaluable sources to fill in what the skin lacks. This is what prevents dry skin, makes rough skin feel smooth, soothes irritated skin, and replenishes what skin loses from irritation, cleansing products, and sun damage. Although these indispensable ingredients are relatively indecipherable, to a cosmetic formulation they are as important as, or even more important than, any natural-sounding ingredient could ever be.

While these thickening, emollient ingredients work great for a wide range of skin types, they may cause problems for someone with either oily, combination, or acne-prone skin. Because all of these ingredients to one degree or another mimic the skin's own oil production, adding more to your own naturally abundant oil supply will only make things worse. This is also true for natural-sounding ingredients like jojoba oil, shea butter, cocoa butter, safflower oil, lanolin, olive oil, and so on. This is one of the primary reasons why someone with oily, combination, or acne-prone skin should avoid any and all moisturizers. When you have your own moisturizer (the oil produced by the oil gland) flowing freely onto your skin, it makes no sense to apply someone else's fabricated version to your skin.

Melaleuca/Tea Tree Oil

In the limitless procession of miracle skin-care ingredients, melaleuca (tea tree oil) takes a backseat to none. In-home sales companies have sprung up selling everything from tea tree oil shampoos and conditioners to tea tree oil cleansers, anti-acne lotions, anti-wrinkle creams, and, believe it or not, dog shampoo. According to the companies that sell these products, this little oil can do it all, from changing the appearance of wrinkles to clearing up acne, healing the skin, and, well, just about anything else you want. As is usually true with skin-care ingredients claiming to do everything and be perfect for everyone, there is some element of truth behind the hype. Melaleuca, the volatile oil of a tree indigenous to Australia, demonstrates some analgesic (pain- and inflammation-relieving) and antiseptic (disinfecting) properties. That's not bad, though it is hardly worth running out and investing in.

On closer look, the supposedly melaleuca-based products being sold by these lines contain very little melaleuca (it's almost always one of the last ingredients), and not all the products contain it. Does the skin need a plant-based disinfectant and analgesic? Well, it can be beneficial, but it doesn't take the place of a lot of other important ingredients like sunscreen, exfoliants, and other nonirritating ingredients. There are lots of other good anti-inflammatory and antiseptic skin-care ingredients (so-called natural ones too), that don't have skin-care product lines built around them. Besides, several of the melaleuca products I've reviewed contain other ingredients I wouldn't recommend.

It is also important to note that there is little to no independent research or information about melaleuca. All the positive declarations are solely from the companies selling the stuff. Their brochures quote studies that are neither published nor substantiated. They sound impressive, but as is true with any spurious scientific study, missing are statistics, double-blind data, comparison details (what the product was tested against), and evidence of how the study was conducted.

Beware any company that hangs its hat on one skin-care ingredient or theory. Whether it be melaleuca, ceramide, pycnogenol, vitamins, beta glucan, retinol, alpha hydroxy acids, antioxidants, or what have you, it means the company won't react to new research as it becomes available. If a company's raison d'être is based on one ingredient, like melaleuca, but new research shows a different ingredient is more helpful for the skin, it can't exactly respond by changing its company name and marketing strategy.

We are still learning about how best to protect our skin from the sun, what types of antioxidants exist in our world and how they work (new ones are being discovered every day), the need for exfoliation, how the intercellular structure protects the skin, and how cleaning affects the skin, so basing your skin care on one ingredient is reckless and foolhardy. You need objective information to take good care of your skin.

Enzymes

Whether in the form of papaya or in a substance such as papain (a proteinase derived from unripe papaya), enzymes have been used for quite some time as exfoliants—not as good as AHAs, but exfoliants nonetheless. The new enzymes being put in skin-care potions are supposed to stimulate your skin's own biological processes that have slowed down because of age or sun damage.

Enzymes are proteins that function as biological catalysts. They accelerate chemical reactions in a cell, reactions that would proceed minimally or not at all if enzymes weren't there. Most enzymes—and a lot of different enzymes affect skin cells—are rather finicky about how they interact. Sometimes it takes several enzymes to produce a chemical reaction. Some enzymes depend on the presence of smaller enzymes, called coenzymes, in order to function. What that all boils down to is that it is pretty complicated to stimulate enzyme activity in the skin. One little enzyme in a skin-care product won't turn on your skin's ability to create, say, collagen or elastin. It's a nice idea, but the theory is much more impressive than the effect, if any, on the skin.

Furthermore, even if enzymes were effective in skin-care products, they are an exceedingly unstable ingredient. Enzymes deteriorate quickly depending on the pH of the product, the presence of other enzymes, and decreases or increases in temperature. Most likely, in any enzyme product you buy, the enzyme has long since deteriorated even before you have a chance to open the product.

Hormone Creams?

(Most of the following information was obtained from interviews with Dr. Claude Hughes, research professor and attending physician in obstetrics and gynecology at Duke University; Dr. Cathy Kapica, Ph.D., professor of nutrition and clinical dietetics at Chicago Medical School; Dr. Nia Terezakis, clinical professor of dermatology at Tulane University; and Dr. Ronald Chez, professor of obstetrics and gynecology at the University of South Florida; and from an article entitled "Phytoestrogens: Friends or Foes?" that appeared in the May 1996 issue of *Environmental Health Perspectives.*)

Thankfully, most cosmetic ingredients are completely benign. I do worry about irritating skin-care products, the lack of sun protection, and how marketing hype about plants and vitamins takes attention away from products that can really be of help. It is this last issue that has me very concerned about a controversial barrage of skin-care products hitting the market that purportedly contain plant estrogen and/or plant progesterone. Tofu extract is reputedly the source of the plant estrogen, and wild yam extract is the source of the plant progesterone. Skin-care products that contain estrogen and progesterone are directly aimed at female baby boomers who are seeking solutions to the side effects of menopause. When the subject of menopause is on the table, the subsequent discussion usually centers around hormone replacement therapy (HRT).

HRT is a medical (prescription-only) solution to warding off most of the serious and not so serious side effects of menopause, including heart attack, bone deterioration (osteoporosis), hot flashes, vaginal dryness, and changes in skin texture. Usually the hormone prescribed to women is not progesterone but estrogen. Estrogen replacement therapy (ERT) is incredibly successful at reducing the side effects of menopause. Unfortunately, there are problems associated with ERT, especially estrogen-positive cancers, and until you find the right dose, you can experience mood swings and agitation. It takes patience, as well as a very understanding doctor, to get the dosage straight.

Despite ERT's well-known success, it has also been getting some bad press lately, in part because of the increased risk of breast cancer, but also because of the way it is produced (from aborted fetuses from horses that are kept constantly pregnant, or from synthetic sources). Besides, there is mounting evidence that a diet high in foods that contain plant estrogen can have effects similar to ERT. Why bother with the former when the latter can be effective? That is a very good question!

It isn't surprising that alternative, nonprescription sources of estrogen would appeal to a wide audience of women enamored with "natural" products. Plus, there is enticing anecdotal information suggesting that Asian women, who have diets high in soy (an estrogen-laden food), experience low rates of estrogen-positive cancers (particularly breast cancer) and their menopausal symptoms are reduced (but not eliminated).

According to the research I've seen and the experts I've interviewed, there is indeed reason to believe that a diet consisting of foods high in estrogen, such as tofu, kudzu (a root from Japan but also grown in the United States), dates, pomegranates, and flax seed (and probably lots more we don't yet know about), can prevent some of the side effects of menopause and potentially reduce some risks of estrogen-related cancers, but this is all strictly theory—encouraging, but there is simply not enough research to make a definitive statement one way or the other.

The current understanding regarding plant estrogen is that it may work by interfering with the body's own estrogen, preventing it from being out of balance. Plant estrogen may fool the body into thinking it has the right balance of this hormone. If the body has too much estrogen, the plant estrogen may prevent the body from utilizing it (thereby preventing estrogen-related cancers); if the body has too little estrogen (as during the stages of menopause), plant estrogen may make the body think it has more, reducing some of the more uncomfortable side effects. In essence, a woman's estrogen level needs to be in balance in order for things to go right internally and externally. Too little or too much and you can have problems. It's like any other physical issue. Insulin is a hormone secreted by the pancreas. If too little insulin is present, you have diabetes; too much, and you go into insulin shock. The same is true for estrogen: too much or too little can cause havoc with the body (and the emotions).

Given this information, those of us entering midlife should be interested in plant estrogen, in regard to both diet and estrogen replacement therapy. But rather than focusing on diet, many companies interested in serving (preying on) baby boomers and their seemingly unlimited checkbooks are marketing "natural" estrogen supplements as well as "natural" progesterone supplements. Why take a progesterone supplement? Many of the researchers I spoke to wondered the same thing.

There is actually some research that indicates progesterone can increase the risk of breast cancer and deplete calcium from the bones. Though there may be some small benefit to taking plant progesterone to reduce menopausal symptoms and reduce the risk of endometrial cancer, this is a high-risk, roundabout way to get results that could be much better achieved by eating foods that contain estrogen.

One source of plant progesterone that is getting a lot of attention is wild yams from Mexico. Voilà! Wild yam creams and pill supplements are now thriving in multilevel marketing lines and health food stores. But clearly, taking plant supplements of progesterone is not as beneficial as taking estrogen. If a woman wanted to try some kind of alternative plant hormone supplement, she would be far better off with concentrations of soy, kudzu, or other plant sources of estrogen. Still, there are many reasons why plant hormones, especially the wild yam stuff, can be problematic for female consumers.

As many researchers and gynecologists have pointed out to me, just because diet may play a significant part in menopausal symptoms, that doesn't mean the American diet can duplicate the Asian diet. There is little information about how much and for how long a woman must consume estrogen-laden foods in order to reduce or eliminate the effects of menopause. Women who choose to use plant estrogen instead of medical sources of ERT could be putting themselves at risk for heart attack and osteoporosis, because we just don't know if plant and animal estrogens really do perform in the same ways, particularly in regard to these more serious health issues. In other words, adding estrogen-bearing foods or supplements to your diet won't necessarily prevent breast cancer, heart attack, or osteoporosis. (Especially because the typical American's diet is high in animal protein, combined with a low rate of physical activity and exercise, which can have an adverse or negating effect on menopausal symptoms.)

Another potential problem is that if plant estrogen in a cream form could be absorbed through skin and act like the body's naturally produced estrogen, it could suppress fertility, reducing a woman's ability to get pregnant. And if a man used this kind of product, it might produce secondary female characteristics like enlarged breast tissue. If a child or teen started using these creams, animal studies suggest they could cause an earlier than normal onset of the menstrual cycle, which is linked with a higher risk of estrogen-positive cancers.

The true crux of the matter, when it comes to cosmetics, is just what kind of yam or soy extracts are being used in these "hormone" creams. It is one thing to say a product contains plant hormones; it's another thing altogether whether it really does. I suspect the wild yam creams do not contain one drop of progesterone and the soy creams do not contain one drop of estrogen. You have to process food in a very specific and controlled way in order to extract the progesterone or estrogen and get it into a product (or pill) intact. The likelihood of that being the case in a cosmetic is at best a long shot. The wild yam extract can be anything, but is probably just wild yam juice, processed and preserved to be mixed into the cream, without any kind of hormone whatsoever. You can't rub crushed plants on your skin and get any of the dietary plant hormone benefit. Plus, when it comes to progesterone, why would you want to?

I strongly suggest that a woman who is at risk for serious menopausal symptoms or estrogen-positive cancers should not wander into this arena without consulting a doctor first. These cosmetic hormone creams most likely pose little risk or benefit, but if they delay the use of other hormonal treatments, that can be dangerous.

In terms of your skin, prescription ERT creams can make the skin feel smoother and softer, not because of what they do topically but because of what they do systemically. Estrogen, in a chemically appropriate form, works internally (even when it is absorbed by the skin), where your body's estrogen does its thing. More to the point, because the cosmetics and natural-supplement industries are not regulated, there is no way to really know what you are getting, and leaving your health up to marketing schemes is not a wise direction to go.

On a personal note: Having spent some time over the past year researching plant estrogen, I have changed some of my eating habits as a result. Some of that is because I wanted to lose weight and made a conscious lifestyle change, eating less fat and little to no animal protein (animal protein leaches calcium out of the bones and contains a lot of fat), but it is also because of the growing evidence about the benefits of plant estrogen and vitamins and minerals in general. I now eat a lot of soy products, including tofu, soy milk, and soy-based prepared foods. Nevertheless, I would never consider using a cream, lotion, or supplement that had any possibility of containing a plant hormone. As one researcher explained it to me, "The American public loves getting things in supplements or extracts, yet every nutritionist and biochemist knows there is no way you can replace the complexity and perfect balance of a plant. It just isn't possible. You may think taking a vitamin C supplement can take the place of oranges or tomatoes, but the almost limitless number of other plant chemicals and minerals present in these foods can not be re-created in a pill or tea." Nor can it be stuck in a cream. Nature just isn't that simple. Consumers cheat themselves when they think that what comes in a pill is somehow better than what comes in whole foods. More to the point, extracts and supplements are so unregulated as to be almost scary, leaving consumers in the dark as to what they are actually taking.

The Last of the Ingredient Gimmicks

Just when I think I've tackled every possible issue or marketing angle the cosmetics industry has created, such as the insanity surrounding fad ingredients; the benefit, or lack thereof, of natural ingredients; and the entire realm of what is and isn't real or possible in the world of skin care and makeup, I realize the cosmetics industry has dozens more. Royal bee jelly, yeast extract, a rare vitamin, minerals from the Dead Sea or from a spa in Iceland or Europe, volcanic mud, placenta extract, a variety of animal organ extracts, and lord knows what else get thrown into the mix as bait for hooking impressionable consumers. After a while I just want to cry out, "I can't take it anymore. Go ahead, buy it all, see if I care!" Most of the time I'm above this type of mental weariness. (If you had a desk like mine, littered with reams of cosmetics advertising and propaganda, you would lose it occasionally too.) I tell myself to get a grip, sigh loudly, and hope that women will steer clear of such pointless, ineffectual gimmicks once they have the information it takes to make rational consumer decisions. Needless to say, none of those ingredients mentioned above has any effect or benefit for the skin. Volcanic mud is mud, nothing more and nothing less; minerals are too big to be absorbed into the skin and most can be irritants (soaking in the Dead Sea can burn and cause skin rashes for some); royal bee jelly is great food for bees but has no purpose for skin; and the animal organ extracts are completely futile.

Skin Patches for Wrinkles

I recently saw an ad for some new products, called Methodo Medique Complete, that were developed by an Italian physician named Dr. Romano Cali. Dr. Cali is supposed to be a renowned plastic surgeon who has created beauty patches that deliver special benefits quickly into the skin and derive their healing powers from botanical extracts and other natural ingredients. Isn't it astonishing how many healing plants, herbs, and vegetables there are in the world? The package of three patches costs $99.95, plus $10.75 for shipping. Are they worth it? That's always the question, and in this case, it's a $110 (and change) question. They definitely seem to be a bit of a bother. You're supposed to peel off the patch and then apply it to the skin under the eye, over the cheek, or any other place a wrinkle dares to show up, for 30 to 45 minutes or longer, preferably overnight.

Not only is Methodo Medique Complete greasy and messy, it is also an incredible waste of time and money. Healing power of botanicals? Helps combat the ravages of time? So extraordinary it has received worldwide patents? I want to scream. In fact, sometimes I just let out a (mental) flurry of curses at these companies and the marketing people who write their ads. For $99.95 you receive precut pieces of material shaped to go over the cheek area, eyes, and lips. What magic formula are these strips covered with? Nothing more than Vaseline. That's right, Vaseline (petrolatum), plus wax, plant extracts (which can be skin irritants), and plant oil. And each box contains only four treatments. I can practically assure everyone who orders this junk that they will be grossly shocked and disappointed. I don't know about you, but if this Dr. Cali exists, I'd like to string him up by his stethoscope.

Facing Up to Facials

I suspect there is more pressure lately to spend money on facials than ever before. The rapid proliferation of day spas, which seem to be showing up in every hair salon and mall from Manhattan to Los Angeles, is probably what has brought this form of beauty treatment back into the spotlight. For the record, I have never been a big proponent of facials because there is truly very little a licensed aesthetician can provide that regular use of good skin-care products can't duplicate, and do better.

(Separate from my sentiments about facials, let me emphasize the need to consult only a licensed aesthetician. Although "licensed" doesn't tell you anything about the capability of the aesthetician, it does mean the person has been trained in sanitation and application techniques and, more to the point, has been tested on those procedures and is certified to be able to accomplish those tasks. Of course, while that is just the beginning of what you should expect in the care of your skin, it is essential to know that your skin will be handled in as safe and hygienic a manner as possible.)

Given the popularity and effectiveness of high-concentration alpha hydroxy acid peels and the occasional or regular need to remove stubborn blackheads and deep-rooted blemishes, facials can indeed play an important role in a person's skin-care needs. AHA peels at concentrations of 20% to 35% with a pH of 3.5 are extremely effective at providing a temporarily smooth appearance to the skin. That is within the ability of a good facialist, and the results can be very satisfying. But be extremely cautious. This is, at best, a controversial salon treatment. Many cosmetic surgeons, dermatologists, and the FDA consider AHA peels unsafe when done by someone without medical training. That is an extremely rational concern, especially considering the wide disparity in training and licensing, and there are plenty of doctors who charge exorbitant prices for AHA peels but have an assistant or an aesthetician in their office perform the service instead.

When it comes to acne, a reliable aesthetician can definitely soften the skin and safely remove blackheads and blemishes without scarring. In these cases there is every reason in the world to get a facial every six weeks to every other month. But please don't expect any of this to permanently stop breakouts. If anything, facialists can get carried away with applying creams and masks, and rubbing and wiping at the skin, which can cause blemishes and irritation. Keep in mind that the skin-care products being sold by facialists and spas are not any more effective or better formulated than those sold anywhere else.

Along with the viable and relaxing facial treatments out there, a whole host of facial masks and procedures that pass as premium skin care are really nothing more than a waste of time and money. Two of the more ridiculous treatments are "detoxifying" masks and machines that purportedly drain lymph. Let's address these one at a time. First, repeat after me: masks cannot pull toxins out of the skin. We don't even know what toxins reside in the skin. Are artificial sweeteners toxins? (Is anyone willing to give up Equal?) What about Diet Coke? Pesticides? Car exhaust? Preservatives in packaged foods? Even if we could identify which toxins are causing what damage, how do you get them out without harming the cells? And assuming you could detox the skin, a bigger question, at least in terms of common sense and how you spend your money, is what good it does if you live in a world where untold toxins inundate the environment. It would be much like fasting for a day, only to eat large, gourmet meals for the next three weeks. That would get you nowhere fast. These masks may feel good, but the benefits for the skin and your budget are nonexistent.

In regard to those bogus machines, you can't drain lymph and you wouldn't want to, even if you could. Draining the lymph glands from the outside in (which isn't possible, but again, assuming for the moment it is) would be like draining hormones or blood from the outside in. How would the machine know what to suck out? The lymph system carries our body's immune defenses. Lymph runs through the body the way blood does in veins and capillaries. You wouldn't want someone draining your blood or hormones (without lots of proof that it was safe and worthwhile), and the same goes for the lymph.

Interesting side note: Has a facialist ever told you that it is normal to break out after getting a facial? Well, it may be typical, but it isn't normal. Many facials involve the use of heavy creams or lotions, regardless of your skin type, and overmassaging is also common. Overmassaging causes the skin to become inflamed and irritated, and the creams and lotions can clog pores. Inflammation, irritation, and skin-care products that contain pore-clogging ingredients are a surefire way to provoke an eruption of breakouts.

Facial Masks

I have never been a big proponent of facial masks, but I've never been against them either. When facial masks don't contain irritating ingredients (and some fit that bill), they are just fine for the skin. Nonirritating facial masks can be a pampering, sometimes soothing, mostly optional, and usually unnecessary skin-care step. Why am I so ambivalent about this popular group of skin-care products? Because things we do intermittently to our face have much less impact than what we do every day. Facial masks are meant to be used only once a week or once a month. The benign masks have little impact on the health of the skin.

They provide no sun protection, little moisturization (at least not any more than can be provided by a moisturizer), and, if they are soothing, they are no more so than a toner.

Lots of facial masks, if not the majority, are little more than clay. Although there is much ado about the quality of clay from various parts of the world, conjuring images of volcanic ash, or minerals derived from exotic waters, the truth is that clay is clay, and its value for the skin is negligible. Clay has some ability to absorb oil, and when the mask is removed it takes a layer of skin with it, which can make your face feel smoother—temporarily. But that doesn't compare in the least with regular use of AHAs, BHA, Retin-A, or Renova.

When facial masks don't contain clay, they often contain a plasticlike hairspray ingredient that places a Saran-wrap layer over the face. These peel-off masks, when they don't contain other irritants, can be fun. Like the clay masks, they take off a layer of skin when they are removed but, as with the clay masks, the benefit is at best insignificant and very short-term.

Some facial masks contain AHAs or BHA. Although those ingredients definitely benefit the skin, they work best when used daily, not once a week or once a month. Some facial masks contain sulfur, particularly masks that are part of a skin-care routine for acne. Sulfur can have some benefit as a disinfectant for breakouts. However, sulfur is a fairly strong, unnecessary way to disinfect the skin, especially when you leave it sitting on your face for a period of time in a facial mask. There are gentler ways to disinfect the skin. Anyway, when breakouts are the problem, killing the bacteria that cause the eruptions needs to be done daily or even twice a day, depending on the severity of the problem. Sulfur masks are applied too sporadically to be effective in preventing breakouts.

If you are shaking your head at my comments, you may be thinking, "But facial masks feel so good." As long as facial masks don't contain irritants, they do feel good, and your face can feel nice and temporarily smoother after they are removed because they take off the top layer of skin. You can mimic this effect by placing a layer of glue on the back of your hand, letting it dry, and then peeling it off. The back of your hand will feel incredibly smooth, at least for a short period of time. That's fine, but there is no long- or short-term benefit. There may even be a problem if peeling off these masks also removes some of your skin's intercellular protection.

If you are going to use a facial mask, and you have normal to dry skin, I suggest using only those that are lightweight and soothing—no peeling agents or clay needed. For someone with oily skin, the only mask I recommend is plain milk of magnesia (no mint or cherry flavors), just like you buy at the drugstore for an upset stomach. Milk of magnesia is just liquid magnesium. Magnesium, like clay, is an earth mineral, but, unlike clay, magnesium has some disinfecting and anti-inflammatory properties and can absorb more oil for its molecular weight than clay can.

Facial Exercises

Recently, a friend sent me a book all about facial exercises for working off wrinkles. The book was published in 1884. Can you imagine? This inane concept of facial exercises has been around for quite some time. Why are facial exercises so idiotic? Because while sun damage causes the network of fine wrinkles on the face, the deeply furrowed lines (laugh lines, the lines between the brows, and the lines on the brow) are caused mostly by using face muscles too much. Skin loses elasticity from too much smiling, being pulled, and gravity. The facial muscles move downward from overuse as well as gravity. Between gravity and use, the skin stretches and the muscles of the face slip down and forward. All of the facial exercises in the world won't move a muscle back to where it belongs. If building up a muscle could help, it would bulge in the wrong place; it wouldn't lift the skin back and up where it belonged. If anything, facial exercises promote more stretching and overuse, by contorting the skin with unnatural movements. Facial exercises didn't work back in 1884, and they don't work now.

What about sleeping on your back to prevent wrinkles? It turns out to be not such a bad idea, if you can figure out how to sleep with your face straight up. Any stretching and pulling sags the skin. Sleeping on your face can bunch up skin all night, which can promote more wrinkling. Sleeping on your back may prevent that.

Natural Is as Natural Does

Forrest Gump might have made just such a statement about natural ingredients, and the puzzling question would still remain: exactly what do natural ingredients do and exactly what is a natural ingredient? I know this repeats some of the material in the first chapter, but it deserves reiteration as a way to combat the tremendous amount of incessant misleading information that exists concerning "natural" ingredients.

It would be great if natural cosmetic ingredients worked the same way in cosmetics as they do in food, but that just isn't the case. A bunch of herbs seasoning a pot of spaghetti sauce isn't remotely the same as the herbs used in a moisturizer or toner. First and foremost, there are a lot of great natural ingredients, but they are no more effective than so-called synthetic ingredients. **Say a natural ingredient works as a disinfectant; that doesn't make it better than a synthetically derived disinfectant. In fact, because natural ingredients have a larger range of limitations, synthetic ingredients are often safer and more**

reliable for the skin. As Dr. Blumberg from Tufts University has pointed out most eloquently, "Just because it is in nature doesn't mean it's good for the skin."

Among the reasons to be wary of natural ingredients (aside from the lack of a regulated definition, as I mentioned in Chapter One) is that their manufacturers do not make their research available to the Cosmetic Ingredient Review (CIR) panel of the Cosmetic, Toiletry, and Fragrance Association (CTFA). This association is the cosmetics industry's attempt at self-regulation. The efforts of this group are interesting, but the cosmetics industry doesn't always cooperate. According to an article in the June 1997 issue of *Drug & Cosmetic Industry* magazine, CIR panel members were "frustrated by a lack of specific information to allow them to characterize [natural] ingredients in a manner specific enough to determine safety [or benefit]." The panel further noted that "botanicals are frequently poorly defined, subject to seasonal variations or variations due to different species sources and varying extraction procedures." Specifically lacking is sufficient information regarding composition, usage concentrations, and possible contaminants, which raises serious doubts about the safety or use of botanicals. And that's the industry's point of view. Imagine what all this looks like from my vantage point or to scientists from other disciplines.

While plants sound great, pure and natural and all that, and while sesame oil and licorice extract sound far better than capric/caprylic triglyceride and glycyrrhetinic acid, they aren't better, or worse. Each has its pros and cons, and it would be a delusion to assume otherwise.

CHAPTER THREE

Sun Sense

Just the Facts

Because sun exposure is responsible for most of the aging, discoloration, sagging, deep wrinkles, basal cell carcinoma (skin cancer), and general deep and surface tissue damage for women (and men) of all skin types and ethnic backgrounds, it deserves a chapter to itself. Spending time discussing skin care without a thorough understanding of the serious consequences of sun exposure would be like discussing fashion and never talking about clothing.

Wearing sunscreen is vital. If you would never leave the house without clothes, likewise, you should never leave the house without sun protection. Sun defense is a 365-days-a-year commitment. **You can drown your skin in all the wrinkle creams, repair lotions, and antioxidant serums you can find and it won't make one teeny bit of difference, but if you put on good reliable sun protection every single day of your life you can truly prevent wrinkles and skin aging.**

When it comes to your skin, consider the following information as part of your owner's manual.

The sun causes most of the aging seen on the skin.

The sun causes most of the brown patches on white skin, and the ashy discolorations on women of color.

The sun's damage is cumulative. The wrinkles you see today at 40 were started from the sun exposure you got before the age of five.

The sun's cumulative damage cannot be permanently removed or undone with skin-care products.

There is no such thing as a safe suntan. All unprotected sun exposure is bad for the skin.

Sun damage begins within the first few minutes of sun exposure. Repeatedly walking to the car and then to the office or school without sun protection causes most of the wrinkles and discolorations you will eventually see on your skin.

The sun's UVB rays cause sunburn and some skin cancers; the UVA rays cause wrinkling and skin cancer.

Only certain ingredients protect the skin adequately from UVA radiation. Most sunscreens prevent sunburn by protecting skin from UVB radiation, but unless they contain either avobenzone (Parsol 1789), titanium dioxide, or zinc oxide, they do not block enough UVA radiation to mitigate the risk of skin cancer.

Sunscreen is crucial for sun protection. Every day of your life, as long as there is daylight, there is a risk of sun damage.

It takes only a few *minutes* in the sun on a daily basis to cause skin damage.

Expensive sunscreens are a waste of money! Sunscreen ingredients are regulated by the FDA, and it determines the SPF ratings. Regardless of the price tag, if the product doesn't contain avobenzone, titanium dioxide, or zinc oxide, it is worthless for adequate UVA protection.

Sunscreens must be applied generously to all exposed parts of the body every day of your life, at least if you want to reduce the risk of skin cancer and wrinkles!

Apply sunscreen 20 minutes before you go outside to give the active ingredients a chance to be absorbed and get in place to do their thing.

Hats with brims protect you from only about 50% of the sun's rays. Another 50% of the sun's rays bounce back off reflective surfaces such as cement, water, and sand.

Windows do not protect from sun damage. Windows block UVB radiation (the sunburning rays), but they do not block UVA radiation (skin cancer and wrinkle-causing rays).

Your eyes can be damaged by sun exposure, so sunglasses are necessary to protect the eyes from sun-related injury.

Now for more explanation and some repetition. The sun causes most of the aging you see on your face. Aside from wrinkling, most brown or ashy discolorations on the skin are caused by the sun. For people with whiter skin tones, the brown spots and brown patching occur on the parts of the body that have been exposed repeatedly to the sun over the years. For people of color, the ashy, darkened, uneven skin tones are often caused by sun exposure. All skin types, all skin colors, and all ethnic backgrounds are affected negatively by unprotected sun exposure. Yes, white skin wrinkles sooner than darker skin and lighter skin definitely is more susceptible to skin cancer, but all skin types wrinkle, discolor, and age with sun exposure.

Some words of warning: Sunscreen ingredients can be irritating no matter what the product's label says. The way these ingredients work can cause a reaction on the skin. Even the ingredients titanium dioxide and zinc oxide, which are almost completely benign and nonirritating, are occlusive sun-blocking agents, and as a result can clog pores or feel greasy on the skin. It is important to experiment until you find the combination of ingredients that works best for your skin type.

How long do sunscreens last? Should you throw them away after a year or two if you haven't used them up? Sunscreens don't last forever, on your skin or in the bottle. The FDA considers sunscreens to be over-the-counter (OTC) drugs, meaning they are subject to much more stringent guidelines and regulations than cosmetics. According to the FDA's OTC regulations, sunscreens should be stamped with an expiration date. From the time a sunscreen is packaged, it has about a two-year period of efficacy. Unfortunately, the cosmetics industry is sort of loosey-goosey with this one, and not all products are identified with an expiration date. That's a risk for the consumer, because there is no telling how long that product has been sitting around at the warehouse or on the shelf. Look and ask for sunscreens with an expiration date whenever possible, and avoid sunscreens that don't have one.

The Backside Test of Aging

As I've said before, one of the biggest beauty myths is the idea that dry skin causes wrinkles. Lately that's been embellished with new myths about wrinkles being associated with a lack of cellular renewal or antioxidants in the skin. Nothing could be further from the truth. Neither those things nor any of the other buzzwords going around the world of cosmetics are associated with wrinkling. According to every expert I've spoken to in the fields of dermatology, oncology, and cosmetic chemistry, 95% of wrinkling is a direct result of sun exposure! That's it!

You can prove this for yourself with something I call the backside test of aging. I've talked before about this indisputable, clear-cut evidence of wrinkling's direct relationship to sun damage, and it is as valid today as it was years ago when Dr. Kligman, the inventor of Retin-A, first described the phenomenon. If you are over the age of 40, preferably not more than 20 pounds overweight (fat helps plump up skin and smooth out wrinkles), you need only compare the skin on your face, hands, or the other parts of your body that are consistently exposed to the sun, with your backside. (If you don't meet the qualifications for this test, you can sneak a peek at women in the locker room at your exercise club and do the test surreptitiously.) Most people who have never, or rarely, exposed their bare backside to the sun will see a radical difference between it and those parts of the body that have been exposed to the sun. What you will notice on the face and hands is crepey skin, some loss of elasticity, lines, furrows, some skin discoloration (usually darkening, redness, or ashiness), and signs of new freckling. However, the skin on your bottom will be smooth, evenly toned (no freckling or discoloration), and elastic (unless there has been a fluctuation in weight, in which case the backside may be out of shape and saggy), without lines, "crow's-feet," crepiness, or any sign of wrinkles. These differences become more enhanced the older you are and the more sun exposure you've experienced.

How does the cosmetics industry account for this difference in skin texture and appearance when it comes to wrinkle products? Why don't the backside and the tummy (if you don't wear bikinis) need wrinkle creams like the face does? The cosmetics industry doesn't have an explanation; they just ignore this fact, and so does the consumer. Out of sight, out of mind, I imagine. You aren't faced with this contradiction about what causes skin wrinkling if you don't see it right there in front of you on a daily basis.

The Greatest Sunscreen Story Ever Told

If you take to heart only one section of this book, make it this one. What makes the following information so vital is not only the prevention of wrinkles, but the prevention of skin cancer. We're talking serious skin care. In the spring of 1997, the world of sunscreens changed forever in the United States, but you may not have noticed. The cosmetics industry doesn't want you to know, at least not until they've sold all of their old sunscreens. Before I explain these changes and what this all means, let me go over some facts and review the previous situation for sunscreens sold in the United States.

Perhaps the most important fact is that sunscreens are tightly regulated by the FDA as over-the-counter drugs, not as cosmetics. And as you know by now, cosmetics don't have to prove their claims, or their efficacy for that matter, while over-the-counter drugs have to prove both efficacy and safety. The FDA also allows only specific claims to be made for specific ingredients. That means if a product is labeled as SPF 15, whether it's Chanel or Coppertone, it must utilize one or more of the limited number of approved sunscreen ingredients, in very specific concentrations, allowed to warrant such a rating.

In the United States, the typical SPF 15 formulation provided very nice protection from ultraviolet B (UVB) radiation, which unquestionably prevented sunburn and deep tanning. Anyone who applied a sunscreen correctly (I explain that below) knew they wouldn't get burned and could stay in the sun with no painful side effects. Despite this remarkable protection, as well as the notably increased use of sunscreens, skin cancer rates did not decline. If anything, they increased. It is well known that sun exposure and skin cancer are inseparably linked, but why weren't sunscreens doing their part to reduce the problem?

To the dismay of dermatologists, oncologists, and researchers, it eventually became clear that UVB radiation is not the culprit in many types of skin cancers. Rather, ultraviolet A (UVA) radiation is the primary cause of skin cancer. Because sunscreens were so successful at preventing sunburn (protecting against UVB radiation), they allowed people to stay out in the sun for even longer periods of time, absorbing more cancer-causing UVA radiation. It turned out that the typical sunscreen formulation protected against only about 20% of

UVA radiation and 80% of UVB radiation. Keeping a large percentage of the UVB rays off the skin was great, but evidently not enough for the long-term health of the skin. It is easy to see why cancer rates were going up, not down.

What changed in sunscreens in the United States in 1997 had already been implemented in Europe, Canada, and Australia. In those parts of the world, three specific active sunscreen ingredients—avobenzone, titanium dioxide, and zinc oxide—were used and accepted as providing much greater protection against UVA radiation. The FDA has now accepted the research and safety data proving these ingredients are indeed effective at blocking about 80% of UVA radiation.

What does this mean for you, the consumer? If you are looking for a sunscreen—and everyone absolutely must wear a sunscreen—you now need to pay attention to more than just the SPF. The SPF is still important, but it's only part of the story. Regardless of what sunscreen products you buy, whether tints, foundations, oil-free sunscreens, sprays, or lotions, they must be rated at least SPF 15 and they must contain titanium dioxide, avobenzone (Parsol 1789), or zinc oxide on the active ingredient list, either alone or in combination with other sunscreen agents. (In Canada avobenzone may be listed as butyl methoxydibenzoylmethane.)

What About SPF?

A sunscreen's SPF (sun protection factor) rating is still incredibly important, but it is no longer the only guide when buying sunscreens. All the SPF number lets you know is how long you can stay in the sun without burning while wearing that product. For example, let's say you're like me and you can stay in the sun for about 15 minutes before your skin starts to turn pink. Applying a sunscreen rated SPF 15 (both the new formulations with zinc oxide, titanium dioxide, or avobenzone, or those without) will allow you to stay in the sun 15 times longer (three and three-quarters hours: 15 times 15 minutes) without getting pink. In other words, the SPF number, 15 in this case, multiplied by the amount of time you can normally stay in the sun without getting pink, tells how long you can stay in the sun after you've applied the sunscreen. If you normally can stay in the sun 25 minutes without getting pink, applying an SPF 15 sunscreen would let you stay in the sun six and one-quarter hours (15 times 25 equals 375 minutes) without burning.

But, as we now know, the SPF rating refers only to protection from UVB radiation. It gives you no information about protection from UVA radiation, which causes skin cancer and, most likely, wrinkles. If that SPF 15, SPF 30, or SPF 45 sunscreen doesn't contain avobenzone, titanium dioxide, or zinc oxide, you are receiving minimal protection from UVA radiation—only about 20%.

Foundations with SPF

As many of you already know, wearing a foundation with a high SPF is an excellent idea, particularly for women with oily skin who don't want to wear any more layers of skin-care products than they absolutely have to and for women who are just tired of wearing layers and layers of skin-care products and makeup. Luckily, about a dozen foundations and tinted moisturizers with good SPF numbers containing titanium dioxide (one of the new FDA-approved ingredients to protect against UVA damage) with excellent color choices and textures are available. The one negative about using a foundation with sunscreen is you need to apply it generously; thin, sheer applications don't work for any type of sunscreen.

Also, if you wear a foundation with SPF you might forget to use a sunscreen on your hands, neck, throat, chest, or any other area of your body that is exposed to the sun on a daily basis. Those brown "age spots" and crepey skin texture are related to sun damage. Like wrinkling on the face, wrinkling on the rest of the body can't be prevented or stopped without daily use of sunscreen, and that means reapplying your sunscreen every time you wash your hands and putting the sunscreen on exposed parts of your body day in and day out.

Waterproof Sunscreens

Aside from SPF ratings and UVA ingredients, there is a major difference among sunscreens when it comes to claims about being waterproof. If you are swimming or sweating, you absolutely want to use a sunscreen that's labeled as waterproof. Waterproof sunscreens are formulated quite differently from regular sunscreens. Waterproof sunscreens utilize acrylate technology in their formulations, which can hold up remarkably well for a period of time under water. Acrylate-type ingredients are, like hair spray, holding agents. These plasticizing ingredients form a film over the skin and they can take a great deal of wear and tear with water before the sunscreen protection is rinsed away. Generally, waterproof sunscreens can hold on for about 90 minutes of swimming or exercising before they are no longer effective. Some sunscreen products make claims of being able to last longer, and these should be able to live up to their claims. To be safe, it never hurts to reapply sunscreen when you are done swimming or exercising if you are still going to be outside.

During the day, for normal wear, I do not recommend the daily application of waterproof sunscreens. The acrylate-type ingredients that help keep sunscreens on when swimming or sweating also make them somewhat tacky or sticky under makeup. For regular application, when you aren't exercising outside or taking a dip, a regular sunscreen with SPF and good UVA protection is the best choice.

Shopping for Sunscreens

I've been in and out of every department store imaginable, every makeup boutique and drugstore. I've called in-home sales companies and infomercial companies. Why? To find sunscreens that contain the newly FDA-approved active ingredients that protect skin from UVA radiation as well as UVB radiation. To recap, it is no longer good enough (or safe enough) to buy a sunscreen based only on its SPF rating. It is now essential to buy sunscreens that not only are at least SPF 15 but also contain titanium dioxide, zinc oxide, or avobenzone as one of the active ingredients. When those ingredients are present either alone or with other sunscreen agents, you are guaranteed of getting equal protection from UVA and UVB radiation. UVB radiation causes sunburn, but UVA radiation is even more insidious and causes skin cancer and skin damage.

Please understand that labeling on sunscreens can be misleading. If the label says "protects from UVA and UVB radiation" but the active ingredients don't include titanium dioxide, zinc oxide, or avobenzone, the sunscreen will not provide adequate protection from skin cancer and wrinkling-causing rays, despite the claim. The reason products can say this even when they don't contain the pertinent ingredients I've mentioned is because of a technicality. Most sunscreen formulations at best block only about 20% of the UVA rays and about 80% of the UVB rays. You get some UVA protection with most sunscreen formulations, but not enough to protect you from skin damage, cancer, and wrinkles. So when the product states "protects from UVA and UVB rays," it isn't exactly lying even though it doesn't contain avobenzone, titanium dioxide, or zinc oxide, but it isn't telling the whole truth either.

I know the following list seems relatively small, but as the cosmetics industry catches up with this new information and reformulates their sunscreens (which they surely will) I will keep you updated on which ones do the best job in my newsletter, *Cosmetics Counter Update.*

Recommended Sunscreens (with titanium dioxide, zinc oxide, or avobenzone)

Avon Age Block SPF 15 *($12.50 for 1.7 ounces)*

Bain de Soleil All Day Extended Protection SPF 15 *($8.50 for 4 ounces)*

Bain de Soleil All Day Extended Protection SPF 30 *($8.50 for 4 ounces)*

Basis Face the Day Lotion SPF 15 *($6.55 for 4 ounces)*

Bobbi Brown Essentials SPF 15 *($38 for 1.7 ounces)*

Clarins Creme Solaire Bronzage Securite SPF 15 *($18.50 for 4.4 ounces)*

Clarins SunBlock Stick SPF 15 *($16.50 for 1.7 ounces)*

Clinique City Block SPF 15 *($13.50 for 1.4 ounces)*

Clinique Special Defense Sun Block SPF 25 *($13.50 for 3 ounces)*

Elizabeth Arden Sunwear Daily Face Protector SPF 15 *($18.50 for 1 ounce)*

Estee Lauder Face Block SPF 25 *($19.50 for 1.7 ounces)*

Estee Lauder Verite Sheer Sunscreen SPF 15 *($25 for 1.7 ounces)*

Garden Botanika Waterproof SunBlock SPF 20 *($8.50 for 4 ounces)*

Hawaiian Tropic 15 Plus SunBlock *($5.99 for 5 ounces)*

Johnson & Johnson Purpose Dual Treatment Moisturizer *($9.87 for 4 ounces)*

Neutrogena Sensitive Skin SunBlock SPF 17 *($9 for 4 ounces)*

Origins Silent Treatment SPF 15 *($15 for 1.7 ounces)*

Paula's Choice Essential Moisturizing Sunscreen SPF 15 *($9.95 for 6 ounces)*

Paula's Choice Essential Nongreasy Sunscreen SPF 15 *($9.95 for 6 ounces)*

Philosophy The Naked Truth SPF 15 *($30 for 4 ounces)*

Physicians Formula Sun Shield for Faces Sensitive Skin Formula SPF 15 *($6.11 for 2 ounces)*

Shade UVA Guard SPF 15 *($9.99 for 4 ounces)*

Recommended Tinted Sunscreens (with titanium dioxide, zinc oxide, or avobenzone)

Lancome Immanance SPF 15 *($27)*

Lancome Immanance Mat SPF 15 *($27)*

Shiseido Vital Perfection Protective Tinted Moisturizer SPF 10 *($26)*

Recommended Foundations with Sunscreen (with titanium dioxide, zinc oxide, or avobenzone)

Clinique Almost Makeup SPF 15 *($25)*

Clinique City Base Compact Foundation SPF 15 *($20)*

Clinique Sensitive Skin Foundation *($18.50)*

DermaBlend Active Cover Creme Foundation SPF 15 *($18.50)*

Estee Lauder Double Wear Makeup SPF 10 *($27.50)*

Estee Lauder Enlighten Skin-Enhancing Makeup with SPF 10 *($27.50)*

Maybelline Natural Defense Makeup with SPF 15 *($5.26)*

Physicians Formula Le Velvet SPF 15 Foundation *($5.50)*

Physicians Formula Le Velvet Liquid Cream Makeup SPF 15 *($5.95)*

Physicians Formula Sun Shield Foundation SPF 15 *($5.50)*
Revlon New Complexion One-Step Makeup SPF 15 *($8.78)*
Shiseido Advanced Performance Compact Foundation SPF 10 *($30)*

What About All-in-One Products?

Lots of women want to pare down the number of skin-care products they use (which is a good thing to do for both the skin and the budget), so it makes sense to combine steps. Some women don't realize that sunscreens already come in an excellent moisturizing base, which means you won't require any other moisturizer during the day. (Of course, it makes no sense to use a sunscreen at night because the active agents in the sunscreen are best used only in the sun.) By the way, sunscreen can and should be used around the eyes, which also cuts out a step.

For women with oily skin, there are a handful of sunscreens that leave a matte or smooth, dry finish on the skin, but not many. Using a foundation with a good SPF reduces the number of products you need to apply.

Many women who use AHA or BHA products and diligently apply sunscreen would love to combine those steps as well. Wouldn't it be nice if these two product types could be formulated together so you would need only one product, not two? Theoretically, it is absolutely possible to combine an AHA or BHA product with a sunscreen, but I've yet to see a formula that integrates the two in a way that optimizes the effectiveness of their very different active ingredients. As this book goes to press, I've reviewed every single AHA- or BHA-with-sunscreen-type product, and there isn't one with a high enough concentration or a low enough pH for either the AHA or the BHA to be an effective exfoliant. Furthermore, none of these so-called all-in-one products uses the new FDA-approved sunscreen ingredients that prevent UVA damage. Until things change, there are no all-in-one products available that aren't a burn for both sun protection and exfoliation.

It Really Makes Me Mad

Perhaps one of the most irresponsible, reckless, and unethical marketing positions the cosmetics industry takes is selling skin-care routines that don't include sunscreen. Almost without exception, cosmetics line after cosmetics line sells an endless array of cleansers, toners, anti-wrinkle serums, eye creams, throat creams, face creams, and facial masks but never mentions the indispensable need for regular, consistent use of a sunscreen. Almost every line does have "sun-care" products, but they are often promoted separately from the "daily care" routines. I've personally spoken to hundreds and hundreds of cosmetics salespeople about their products and repeatedly found a gross lack of information about sun protection. I'm always told how important moisturizers, eye creams, serums, toners, cleansers, and eye makeup removers are, but not about the daily value of sunscreen.

Most of us think sun damage occurs from baking in the sun and getting a deep, dark tan. That is only part of the picture. Sun damage begins the moment you walk out of the house, any time during the day, whether it is sunny or cloudy (at least 40% to 50% of the sun's rays penetrate a cloud cover). It may take 20 minutes for some of us to get burned, an hour or two for some of us to start tanning, but the damage associated with wrinkling and skin cancer begins the moment your skin sees sunshine. It is the repeated sun exposure, several minutes a day, 365 days a year, *even when sitting near a sunny window (UVA radiation comes through windows),* that adds up to a great deal of damage both aesthetically and physically. Regrettably, windows do not protect you from sun damage. UVB rays (the ones that cause sunburn) don't filter through a window, but UVA rays do, and those are the ones that cause skin cancer and wrinkles.

According to the Skin Cancer Foundation and the American Academy of Dermatology, that means daily use of a sunscreen with a minimum rating of SPF 15 (with avobenzone, titanium dioxide, or zinc oxide, of course, for UVA protection) is a must. Without a good sunscreen you cannot prevent, stop, or change wrinkles and there is no way you can properly manage your skin-care needs.

Sun Protection for Different Skin Types

In Chapter Five, "Skin-Care Planning," and Chapter Six, "Special Battle Plans for Blemishes," I discuss how to work sun protection into many different types of skin-care routines. There are indeed many ways to get good sun protection, regardless of your other skin-care needs. It would be unconscionable to discuss any skin-care routines, skin-care problems, or skin-care concerns and not include, first and foremost, sun protection. If you've been intrigued by a new miracle skin-care line, but a sunscreen is not mentioned in their ranting, they clearly do not take skin care seriously or ethically and you would be wasting your money and hurting your skin (unless you took the time to find a good sunscreen from another line).

Perhaps the trickiest part of sunscreen application as part of a daily skin-care routine is finding one that doesn't cause problems for someone with normal to oily skin, acne-prone skin, or sensitive skin. Active sunscreen agents including avobenzone, benzophone, padimate-o, octyl methoxycinnamate, oxybenzone, and many others can cause irritation on the skin, creating patches of dryness, itching, rashlike breakouts, redness, and swelling. Because these other sunscreen agents can be potentially irritating, many dermatologists feel that titanium dioxide is the best sunscreen ingredient since it is so completely benign on the skin and almost fully blocks both UVA and UVB radiation. I wish the subject could end here and I could unequivocally recommend titanium dioxide as the only sunscreen ingredient to look for, but that isn't the case. As safe and effective as titanium dioxide is, it can be occlusive, and then can block and clog pores.

The issue for any ingredient causing breakouts is threefold: how occlusive it is, meaning how much it blocks oil flow out of the pores; how irritating it is on the skin, including whether it causes rashlike breakouts; and how much the ingredient duplicates what the pore produces, adding more fuel to the fire. Titanium dioxide poses the first problem for skin. Are you guaranteed to break out if you use a sunscreen with titanium dioxide? Absolutely not, but it is a possibility. Everyone's skin reacts differently to any and all cosmetic ingredients. One other issue with a sunscreen that uses only titanium dioxide as the active ingredient: cosmetically, these products tend to have a thick, white appearance and can feel heavy on the skin. That can be a problem for all skin types. In response to that shortcoming, many sunscreen products include titanium dioxide among other sunscreen agents. That reduces the amount of potentially irritating ingredients and reduces some amount of titanium dioxide's occlusive tendency.

What to do? It takes experimentation to find what type of sunscreen works best on your skin. There is no one formula that will work for everyone. As long as the product contains in part titanium dioxide, avobenzone, or zinc oxide and is at least an SPF 15 (though 8 to 10 may be fine for casual daily wear when you are minimally exposed to the sun), you will be doing just fine.

Suntan vs. Self-Tanners

And the winner is—self-tanners! Every season, remind yourself that suntanning is something you must avoid at all costs. You all know the hazards, so there is no reason to belabor the point, other than to remind you of a few basics, such as the fact that hats with brims protect the face from only about 50% of the sun's rays. The other 50% of the sun's rays bounce back up off cement, water, and sand, causing sun damage reflected from the ground up. Apply sunscreen 20 minutes before you go outside to give the active ingredients a chance to be absorbed and get in place to do their thing. If you've been perspiring or swimming, which is likely in hot weather, be sure to reapply sunscreen every one and a half hours. Do not buy expensive sunscreens; they are no more effective than inexpensive ones, and it is essential to generously apply sunscreen when sitting out in the sun. How generous are you going to be when applying a $30 SPF 15 versus a $6 SPF 15? And all sunscreens should contain either titanium dioxide, zinc oxide, or avobenzone (Parsol 1789) to protect from UVA (skin cancer–causing ultraviolet radiation).

Self-tanners are the only way to get a tan that is safe for the skin. All self-tanners are created equal in that they all use the same ingredient, dihydroxyacetone, to chemically turn the skin brown. Some products contain a greater concentration of dihydroxyacetone than others, which determines how fast the skin will change color. The key is the application, which is always tricky. It takes experimenting to figure out how much to use, how dark to go, what areas to go over lightly (like knees and elbows), what areas to avoid (like palms of hands and armpits), and where to start and stop the application (do you stop at your ankles or continue down to your toes?). All of these are questions you need to answer for yourself, depending on your own personal preferences and blending techniques.

My suggestion is to use a self-tanner that is labeled either "light" or "medium" and not "dark." This way you can build the color slowly, so in case you make a mistake or don't like the way it looks, you can alter the course without looking streaked, smudged, or mottled. Companies that make self-tanners promising to turn the skin instantly dark, so you can instantly see exactly how much and where you've applied it, never explain what you can do if you make a mistake. Once the skin changes color, it doesn't wash off, and I have no idea what you do about the palms of your hands, which will also turn instantly tan. However, some women feel that using a fast-darkening self-tanner is preferred because it changes the skin's color immediately, thereby making mistakes apparent immediately so they can easily be corrected. I have not been able to perfect that technique, but I understand how that could be advantageous. The choice is yours.

There are techniques I've seen recommended (and ones I've recommended as well), such as exfoliate first, apply the self-tanner over a moisturizer to help spread the product evenly, and use a spray to spread a thin layer, or use a cream so you can control spreading, or apply in sections to assure evenness so you can remember where you have and haven't put it and how much you've applied. All of these are valid application techniques, but none offers a guarantee, which is why experimenting and going slow is the best option of all. The following list is a way to help prevent fake tans from looking fake.

Note: If you choose to buy a self-tanner, whether it contains a sunscreen or not, please be aware that brown skin does not offer any protection from the sun. All of the rules for wearing sunscreens apply to these products too. In Chapter Eight, "Makeup Application Step by Step," I discuss how to use makeup to enhance the color you get from a self-tanner.

Self-Tanning Guidelines

1. Before you get started on your whole body, experiment with a small section of your body first to see how your skin responds to the self-tanner and your application technique. You can choose a part of your body few people are likely to see.
2. When you're ready, take a quick shower first to make sure the skin is clean. A long shower or bath can make the skin swell and become engorged with water, making application less smooth.
3. Use a liquid cleanser like Nivea Shower and Bath or Caress Body Wash rather than bar soap. This will help keep a soap film from building up on the skin.
4. While in the shower, do exfoliate the skin with a washcloth or loofah, but don't overdo it. Too much scrubbing can rough up the skin, and that won't help smooth things out.
5. Be sure your skin is absolutely dry before you begin any application.
6. If you have dry skin, apply a tiny amount of a lightweight moisturizer (Nutraderm or Lubriderm works just fine) evenly over the entire body. Self-tanners work better if applied over a smooth, even surface. If your skin isn't dry, this step isn't necessary. It is best, especially for your face, to use no other skin-care products before or after the self-tanner. Skin-care products such as AHAs, BHA, Retin-A, disinfectants, or sunscreens can affect the self-tanner's action on your skin.
7. Allow at least an hour to apply self-tanner to the body and face. An hour gives it time to be absorbed and to dry.
8. Have a game plan that includes which parts of the body you want to work on, and where you do and don't want color; then proceed systematically. It is important to have a clear idea of where you do and don't want to have color. You have to make decisions about whether you want your ears, tops of feet, toes, hips, abdomen, ankles, eyelids, or the underside of your arms to be tan. As a rule, apply color only to those parts of your body that would normally get tan. Keep in mind that some body parts look odd with color; for example, it can look weird to have tan armpits.
9. Starting with your face, do your forehead, cheeks, nose, and chin. Then proceed to your neck, chest, shoulders, arms, and so on. Use only enough of the self-tanner, the smallest amount, to cover one area at a time.
10. Do each section completely and thoroughly before moving on to the next. If you want color on your back, enlist the help of a friend to get hard-to-reach areas so you don't miss a spot.

11. The self-tanner can collect anyplace on the body where there are creases, like the neck, or where there is rough skin, like the knees and elbows, and cause excess pigment to be created. Either go over those areas very lightly or use a paper towel to dab off the excess.
12. Wait at least 20 minutes before you get dressed so you don't transfer any self-tanner to your clothing.
13. To maintain the color, gently exfoliate every day, and reapply self-tanner every three or four days depending on the look you're going after. This all takes experimenting to see what works for you and what doesn't, so be patient.
14. I recommend applying self-tanner before you go to bed as opposed to during the day. This way you have plenty of time, and if any residue is left it won't affect your clothing (you can wear an old T-shirt to sleep in). More important, it is best to leave the skin alone after applying a self-tanner. Doing it at night, when you don't have to apply makeup or a sunscreen, prevents other cosmetic ingredients from inhibiting the self-tanner's effectiveness.

Tanning Machines

According to the FDA, the FTC (Federal Trade Commission), the American Academy of Dermatology, and the Skin Cancer Foundation, tanning machines are nothing more than skin cancer machines and should be made illegal. They radiate the most damaging effects of the sun only inches away from your body, and, worse, they are available day after day, month after month, in areas of the country where you would not normally see the sun on a daily basis, exposing body parts that are usually covered. Not only do they put the skin at serious risk for skin cancer, in all likelihood they age the skin faster than normal sun exposure would because of the intensity and proximity of the radiating light source.

Shockingly, I have received pamphlets and brochures from tanning-machine companies and from salon managers who own these machines explaining how safe these machines really are because of the type of radiation they emit. It makes me want to scream, or cry, or both. None of it is true or substantiated by anyone other than those promoting the use of tanning machines. Please, if you heed no other information this book provides, protect your skin from sun damage, both artificial and natural. There are lots of ways to look and be beautiful, but this isn't one of them.

Skin Cancer and Sun Damage

According to the Centers for Disease Control and Prevention (CDC) and the American Academy of Dermatology (AAD), one million new cases of skin cancer are diagnosed each year. That gives skin cancer the ignoble distinction of being the most common form of cancer in the United States. As reported by Dr. Darrell S. Rigel from the New York University School of Medicine, the chance that an American will develop melanoma in his or her lifetime is 1 in 84. Those aren't the kind of odds you want to gamble on, at least not when it comes to losing portions of your skin. Most skin cancers fall into three categories: basal cell carcinomas, squamous cell carcinomas, and melanomas. Basal cell carcinomas are caused by repeated, unprotected sun exposure. Scientists believe that exposure to UVA and some UVB radiation triggers mutations in the replicating skin cells, causing their genetic coding to go haywire. The cells forget how to maintain the normal cell turnover process because of the radiation damage. Fortunately, nonmelanoma skin cancers are relatively easy to treat if detected in time, and are rarely fatal. Malignant melanomas are much more dangerous, but their connection with ultraviolet radiation exposure is not well understood.

Fair-skinned people are particularly susceptible, but the highest rates of skin cancer in the world are found in Queensland, Australia. The predominantly light-skinned people there are exposed to very high UVA radiation levels, probably due to the depleted ozone layer in that area of the world. (The ozone in the earth's atmosphere helps provide protection from the sun's radiation and heat.)

There are some early, telltale signs of skin cancer you should be aware of. Early detection of skin cancer can save your skin and your life. If you perceive a change in your skin that you are not sure about, talk to your doctor; even a minor difference in a mole or a freckle, or a blemish that doesn't look "normal," can be an indication of skin cancer.

The Five Most Typical Characteristics of Skin Cancer (Basal Cell Carcinoma)

1. **An open sore, any size, that bleeds, oozes, or crusts and remains open for three or more weeks. A persistent nonhealing sore is one of the most common signs of early skin cancer.**
2. **A reddish patch or irritated area that doesn't go away and doesn't respond to cortisone creams or moisturizers. Sometimes these patches crust over or flake off, but they never go away completely.**
3. **A smooth growth with a distinct rolled border and an indented center. It can look like a small blemish or wound, but tends to grow and doesn't heal.**
4. **A shiny bump or nodule with a slick, smooth surface that can be pink,**

red, white, black, brown, or purple in color. It can look like a mole, but the texture and shine are what makes it different.

5. A white patch of skin that has a smooth, scarlike texture. The area of white skin can have a taut, clear appearance that stands out from the appearance of the surrounding skin.

The American Academy of Dermatology has a list of the "ABCDs" of identifying skin cancer, as follows:

A—Asymmetry: one half of the lesion or suspect area is unlike the other half.

B—Border: there is an irregular, scalloped, or poorly circumscribed border around a suspected skin lesion or mole.

C—Color: color varies from one area to another, with shades of tan, brown, black, white, red, or blue.

D—Diameter: the area is generally larger than 6mm (diameter of a pencil eraser).

After-Sun Care

I worry about the concept of "after-sun care." It sounds as if you can undo all the sun damage you incurred during the day. I admit it's a great marketing concept, but it is risky business for someone to buy into the notion that skin can be repaired following unprotected sun exposure. If you leave your skin defenseless and exposed to the sun's rays, and then slather some lotion, toner, or serum on afterward, you cannot miraculously or even in a minor way heal, eliminate, correct, or cancel the devastating injury (and all sun exposure over time is devastating) to your skin. The skin does want to heal on its own, but what we do to it in the name of skin care can get in the way of the skin's own immune/healing response.

Slathering too much moisturizer on after a long day outside, or just in general, can prevent the skin from doing what it does on its own naturally, namely healing. Too much moisturizer can turn off the skin's natural ability to heal. Most skin is best left alone or, at most, given a lightweight, thin layer of moisturizer, especially after sun exposure.

What about taking care of sunburn? Well, why are you getting sunburned in the first place? Why would you ever leave your house any time of the day or year without a good sunscreen on (one rated at least SPF 15 that contains either avobenzone, titanium dioxide, or zinc oxide as the active ingredient)? OK, that's enough guilt—just don't do it again, and now take care of your burn wisely. It is essential to treat sunburns the same way you would treat a burn injury from any heat source. Unquestionably, whenever the skin is burned you first need to cool it off to prevent the skin tissue from either retaining the heat or continuing to react negatively. Trapping the heat in the skin by covering it with a thick, waxy, or heavy lotion or cream will literally continue to fry the skin even after the heat source has been removed. Likewise, it promotes swelling, redness, and pain.

Some of you may remember the days when you got burned in the kitchen and your grandmother or mother would slather butter on it. Absolutely nothing could have been worse for the skin. Butter, like any emollient moisturizer, places a relatively occlusive layer over the skin, encapsulating the heat and preventing it from leaving the skin. It does nothing to reduce the swelling or redness.

All burns need to be cooled to dissipate the heat simmering in the lower layers of skin and to reduce the resulting inflammation. If you have a sunburn over most of your body, I advise a cool to slightly cold bath (not ice-cold: ice applied directly on the skin is too severe and can burn the skin in other ways). If you do want to use a moisturizer or soothing agent, I recommend a light layer of aloe vera, but not for the reasons the cosmetics industry tells you to use the stuff. Using aloe vera helps cool the skin and prevents trapping the heat with creams and emollient moisturizers.

If your burn is serious or extremely painful, do not hesitate to find the nearest hospital emergency room. Heat trauma from sunburn can be a serious threat to your health.

Why Aloe Vera May Work on Sunburns

What we are now learning about moisturizers is that they can be overdone, hampering the skin's healing process. Lots of people attribute to the aloe plant miraculous abilities to help the skin to heal. Aloe juice is 99.5% water and 0.5% minerals and amino acids. There is no real evidence that those minerals and amino acids help the skin in any significant way, although they may provide a slight anti-inflammatory benefit. However, enough anecdotal evidence about aloe vera exists to make its reputation hard to ignore. It turns out that aloe's reputation may have less to do with what it does for the skin than with the things it helps you keep off the skin. In other words, if you apply pure aloe to a sunburn or other injury site, you won't apply anything else. In essence, you are just cooling off the skin and leaving it alone to do its own thing. Once the aloe juice dries, and because it is mostly water that happens fairly quickly, the skin can heal quite nicely on its own.

Buying Sunglasses

I love wearing sunglasses. I think they are one of the most sexy, sultry, and instantly attractive, as well as utilitarian and practical, fashion accessories a woman can own. It is for this reason alone I regret living in Seattle. There just aren't many opportunities to wear sunglasses. (The rumors are true: it does rain here all the time, and in the winter there is no sun at all. Thank goodness for Starbucks.) Yet, whether you buy inexpensive sunglasses like the stunning $20 pair I found in Palm Springs or top-of-the-line shades like the $250 Chanel number I couldn't swallow buying (not only did they not look that good, but I lose my sunglasses all the time, and knowing I could easily lose a $250 anything is more than I can tolerate), they are a waste of money if they don't protect your eyes from ultraviolet radiation.

Eyes exposed to sunlight are at risk for cataracts, sunburn (the eyeball itself can get sunburned), irritation, skin cancer of the eyelid, and dry eyes. As it turns out, most sunglasses do protect well from the sun, but there is no easy way to know which ones do and which ones don't. Some sunglasses come with labels indicating UV radiation protection, but there are no regulations or standards in this field. It doesn't hurt to buy sunglasses with a UV protection label, but there are some things you need to check out to make sure you purchase a pair that does more than just look good.

I strongly recommend buying sunglasses that hug the face and have wide rims and earpieces. This way, you shield the eyes from any sunlight coming in from above, below, or around the sides, as well as protect more of the delicate skin around the eyes from sun damage.

The American Optometry Association has a few extremely helpful guidelines for finding the best protection. First, be sure that the lens tint is uniform, not darker in one area than another. Next, hold the glasses at arm's length. Look through them from this distance at a straight line—say, the edge of a bookcase or wall. Then slowly move the glasses across the straight line. If the straight edge distorts, sways, curves, or moves, the lenses have imperfections and you should not buy them.

The most important test (aside from fit) is to see if the glasses block enough sunlight. Try the sunglasses on in front of a mirror. If you can see your eyes easily through the lenses, they probably aren't dark enough. In this regard, the darker, the better. This does not apply to lenses that darken when exposed to sunlight, but if you're looking at this kind, check them in a mirror outside in daylight to see if they become dark enough to block enough of the sun's rays.

Tinted sunglasses have an impact on sun exposure aside from their impact on the face. Red- and yellow-tinted lenses can cut haze, but may not adequately protect from sun exposure. Check them in daylight or consult an ophthalmologist. Gray, green, and brown tints are known for providing good viewing as well as good sun protection. Black and blue tints can be too dark, impairing good vision.

CHAPTER FOUR

Understanding Skin Type

Forget Skin Type

I know, I know: you turned to this chapter to get some solid information about your skin type, and the first thing I tell you to do is forget about skin type—but that is the key to making good decisions about your skin-care needs. Some women are quite aware of their skin type; for other women it's a complete mystery, an elusive conundrum of changes and setbacks that never settles down into one specific direction. Regardless of how sophisticated some companies are in approaching the issue—with computers and questionnaires to help you discover what is going on with your skin, or seemingly knowledgeable salespeople looking at your face and evaluating what you need—their final determination of skin type is usually inaccurate. **That's not to say understanding skin type isn't important, because it is, but not in the way the cosmetics industry approaches it or the way we've been indoctrinated to think about it.**

What I'm really saying is to forget about skin type as the cosmetics industry has defined it. The rigid categories you find at cosmetics counters and the information about what your skin needs as analyzed by a salesperson are often wrong or at best incomplete. Skin type in terms of the standard normal, oily, combination, or dry types is one of the most misleading and misused beauty concepts around, but it is usually where we begin making decisions about our skin-care routine.

The primary difficulty in understanding your skin type is recognizing that outside factors can and do influence what you see and feel on your face. You can't know what to do for your skin type until you know why your skin behaves the way it does. There can be no rational discussion of your skin-care needs until you evaluate what you may be doing that affects your skin's health (such as smoking, exercising too little or not at all, exposing yourself to the sun without adequate protection, or using hormone replacement therapy), what kind of environment you live in (someone living in cool, moist Seattle has radically different skin-care concerns from someone coping with the hot, dry air of Phoenix or Los Angeles), what you're doing to clean your face (too many or the wrong skin-care products can wreak havoc), what products (moisturizers, scrubs, AHAs, BHA, masks, and so on) you are using, whether you have a skin disorder such as rosacea or psoriasis, and whether you have a physical health concern that can affect the skin such as a thyroid disorder.

All those complex, integrated circumstances, combined with your skin's genetic predisposition for certain traits (oily versus dry), contribute to what is taking place on and in your skin. To complicate matters a little further, skin type is not static. **What you see today may not be what you see tomorrow, next week, month to month, and season to season.** Judging skin type from one moment in time (such as when you are shopping at a cosmetics counter and the salesperson says you have dry, oily, or combination skin) doesn't give you enough information to create an effective skin-care routine.

Let's forget, for a moment, your genetically inherited skin type or physical health, and talk about your present skin-care routine. The products you use can affect the skin's oiliness, dryness, and sensitivity; may trigger allergies, redness, surfaced capillaries, or changes in skin texture; and can aggravate breakouts. The way your face feels right now can be a result (although not solely) of the way you clean your face. Your skin-care routine could be creating the very problems you're trying to eliminate.

For example, if you wash every day with a bar soap (which is drying), followed by a toner (which may also be drying) and several moisturizers (which can be greasy and potentially can block pores), you can create a severe combination skin condition and cause breakouts. Or if you wipe off your makeup with a cold cream (even expensive ones can be greasy), then follow up with a toner (which might also be greasy or contain irritants), you should not be surprised if you develop breakouts and dull-looking skin. If you have fairly normal skin but you use an alcohol-based AHA toner, plus a scrub, an AHA moisturizer, and a clay mask, your skin may end up looking very dry, irritated, and subject to rashlike pimples. Typing skin without taking into consideration the products you use relies on an assumption that the skin is the way it is all by itself, regardless of what you do to it, and that is rarely the case. **Before you can know what your skin type really is, you have to start at square one to discover what your skin type is not, and find out what is causing the conditions you see on the surface.**

Another problem is the assumption that once you've been typed, your skin will be the same forever, or at least until you grow older, but that's rarely the case. The face can be affected by emotions, weather conditions, hormonal levels, menstrual cycles, stress, physical changes, weight fluctuations, and whatever else life brings. All these things can directly affect your skin. If your skin-care routine focuses on skin type alone, it can become obsolete the moment the season changes, or you lose your job (or get increased responsibilities), or you decide to change boyfriends.

If you go to the cosmetics counter and the salesperson determines your skin type, she can base that judgment only on what your skin feels and looks like at that moment. If you make a decision about what products you should use based only on that information, you will be making a big mistake.

To complicate things even more, in any given period of time a woman may have many skin types! Over the years, even when using gentle, irritant-free products, I've experienced irritated skin patches at the same time I had oily skin, or acne flare-ups along with dry skin around my eyes. Present that list to cosmetics salespeople and they go wild, because the products they sell cannot address those variances. **It is not unusual for women to have a little bit of each skin type going on simultaneously or overlapping each other. An overview of how your skin behaves and changes is necessary to assess what your skin needs.**

The biggest problem with identifying skin type is the way the cosmetics industry handles that information. As far as the cosmetics industry is concerned, every woman can and should have normal skin. Yet the very idea of normal skin is a slippery, precarious issue. Like the rest of our bodies, skin is in a constant state of change. Even women with perfect complexions go through phases of having oily, dry, or blemish-prone skin; what is certain is that all women age, and it is the rare individual who does not have sun-damaged skin. In reality, no one is likely to have normal skin for very long, no matter what she does. Those of us who struggle with oily skin, breakouts, dry skin, sensitive skin, or sun damage know that normal skin is at best fleeting. **If determining your skin type helps control your skin problems better, that's great, but chasing after normal skin can set you up on an endless skin-care buying spree, running around in circles trying everything and finding nothing that works for very long.**

In any case, determining skin type is highly subjective. Many women have really wonderful skin but refuse to accept it. They are distressed by the smallest blemish or wrinkle, or the slightest sensation of dry skin. I can't tell you how many women I've met who get one blemish and run to the dermatologist complaining about acne. Or the women who see a line or two around their eyes and immediately buy the most expensive anti-wrinkle creams they can find in the hope of warding off the worst-imagined nightmare. Overreacting to what you see in the mirror makes for more mistakes in cosmetics purchases than almost any other aspect of skin type. **This is one of those times when being realistic is the most important part of your skin-care routine.**

Identifying your skin type is made even more difficult by the omnipresent combination-skin complaint. Almost everyone at some time or another, if not all the time, has combination skin. This is not surprising; it happens to be the way the skin functions. The nose, chin, center of the forehead, and center of the cheek areas have more oil glands than other parts of the face. It is not surprising that those areas tend to be oilier and break out more frequently than the other areas of the face. Problems occur when you buy extra products for combination skin, because many ingredients that are appropriate for the T-zone (the area along the center of the forehead and down the nose, where most of the oil glands on the face are located) won't help the cheeks or jaw. Some products claim they can regulate themselves over each area; this is a complete impossibility. The ingredients that can absorb oil can promote dryness, and the ingredients that moisturize dry skin can cause breakouts. **You may need different products to deal with the differences in skin type on the face, because you should treat different areas of the skin differently.**

The most frustrating aspect of skin type is the fact that it's often used (by cosmetics salespeople and by the cosmetics industry in their ads) to instill a sense of immediate need. Once your skin is classified as a "type" and it isn't normal, or if it stops being normal (this ploy is usually aimed at the 30-something crowd, with the salesperson saying something like "You had better do what you can do now to make sure it stays the way it is"), a sense of desperation can set in. I've seen it happen a thousand times as I've listened to or been subjected personally to a salesperson's rebuke over skin-care mistakes that are destroying my skin. **What destroys skin is unprotected sun exposure, smoking, and using irritating skin-care products. Not using the right skin-care products (other than a good sunscreen) may cause problems, but it does not damage skin in the long run, and that includes not using a moisturizer.**

Determining skin type doesn't answer questions of need that may not be apparent on the skin's surface. Sun damage is not evident when you are young, but sun protection is imperative for all skin types. Dry skin and oily skin that are present at the same time along with some redness may be an early sign of rosacea, a condition that cannot be treated with cosmetics. Your skin may be breaking out, but those blemishes on the surface took a few weeks to get there. Breakouts begin in the pores, and may involve sebum (oil), cellular debris (dead skin cells), dead hair shafts, and/or bacteria. It takes consistent long-term planning to handle each aspect of the blemish problem, and treating only what you see (as in zapping zits or spot treatment) can make matters worse. Large patches of flaky, dry, red skin may be caused by psoriasis, and cosmetics can make this condition worse. Dry patches of scored skin could be caused by an allergic reaction or by eczema.

Get the picture? What you see on the surface of the skin does not always indicate the type of skin-care products you should buy, or even if you need a skin-care product at all. To summarize:

1. **Your real skin type can be camouflaged by the skin-care products you are now using.**
2. **Skin type changes with emotions, weather conditions, hormonal levels, menstrual cycles, smoking, heat (including a sauna or Jacuzzi), and sun**

exposure. Recognize these changes when they happen and adapt your skin-care routine accordingly.

3. Skin can be more than one skin type, because of an oily T-zone, skin rashes (dermatitis), or areas that tend to break out.
4. The idea of identifying your skin type so that you can make it "normal" is not realistic.
5. Skin type is highly subjective; what may look like normal skin to one person may seem oily or wrinkled to another.
6. Combination skin does not require special products, but it does require treating each area differently.
7. Skin type should not be a reason to beat up your ego or spend lots of money.
8. Skin type isn't the only thing to define need, because some problems are not immediately apparent on the surface of the skin, such as sun damage, breakouts, and rosacea.

Skin Type Has Nothing to Do with Your Age

Older skin is different from younger skin. That is indisputable. Yet it is a mistake to buy skin-care products based on a nebulous age category. Treating older or younger skin with products supposedly aimed at dealing with those attributes is inappropriate because not everyone with "older" or "younger" skin has the same needs. An older person may have acne, blackheads, eczema, rosacea, sensitive skin, or oily skin, while a younger person may have dry, freckled, obviously sun-damaged skin. Products designed for older skin are almost always too emollient and occlusive, and those designed for younger skin are almost always too drying. Both extremes can cause problems when the issue becomes age as opposed to the condition of your skin.

Treating older skin or younger skin with an age-related unified skin-care routine is a trap lots of women fall into, particularly older women. I understand the anxiety caused when a woman notices her skin is looking older (which is more about sun damage than age), but buying skin-care products in hopes of stopping that damage (as opposed to alleviating it and preventing more damage with sunscreen) is a waste of money. Skin-care routines should be based on the current condition of your skin along with protection from sun damage, and that may not have anything to do with your age.

Describing the aging process of the skin is complicated. There are over 50 identifiable factors that affect skin aging. Researchers generally agree that the visible signs of aging on the surface of the skin—deep wrinkles, lines, discolorations, skin texture—are only one aspect of a multilevel composite of events.

Surprisingly, leathery, crepey skin and brown "age" spots are directly caused by sun exposure, while sagging is a result of facial muscles shifting down and forward along with gravity's pull on the skin. None of those factors is genetically predetermined. What does seem to be genetically predetermined are a vast range of occurrences in the skin that can cause it to look older. This explains why the anti-aging trade is hitting us over the head with so many different products.

Looking at the issue objectively can help us better understand what is happening to our skin and what can and can't be done for it. Gaining insight into why wrinkle products make the claims they do and why it is most unlikely that they can actually live up to those claims will ultimately benefit our skin and our budget. For example, while we know that collagen and elastin, the support structures of the skin, break down and flatten as a result of repeated sun exposure, they also become less pliant and more hardened with age, so the skin becomes less elastic. Some products claim to only build collagen or only improve elastin. That is much like building a house with only cross beams and no support beams. One without the other is useless, because the house won't stay erect.

But, for the sake of argument, let's say these products can build more collagen or elastin. If elastin gets less elastic as we get older, what good is it? **Changes in collagen and elastin are only a small part of what makes the skin age. Just rebuilding elastin or collagen or any other single part of the skin isn't enough to halt or reverse the skin's intricate, puzzling aging process.**

A notable characteristic of older skin versus younger skin is that younger skin has more fat cells in the dermis than older skin. That is one reason older skin looks more transparent and thinner than younger skin, and why someone 30 pounds or more overweight tends to have fewer wrinkles. Furthermore, for some unknown reason, the skin keeps growing and expanding as we age, despite the fact that the supporting fat tissues of the lower layers of skin are decreasing. That is why the skin begins to sag: too much skin is being produced, but there aren't enough bones (remember, bone also deteriorates with age) and fat to shore it up. Simultaneously, the facial muscles lose their shape and firmness, giving the face a drooping appearance.

Certain components of the skin also become depleted with age. The water-retaining and texture-enhancing elements in the intercellular structure, such as ceramides, hyaluronic acids, polysaccharides, glycerin, and many others, are exhausted and used up. Older skin is also more subject to allergic reactions and sensitivities than younger skin, which suggests older skin is less capable of defending itself against irritants because of a weakening immune system.

On a deeper molecular level, the DNA and RNA genetic coding of the skin cells turn off and the cells stop reproducing as abundantly or in the same way as they did when we were younger. This preprogrammed change makes cells become abnormally shaped, which further changes the texture of the skin and prevents the cells from retaining water. This is why older skin tends to be drier than younger skin. DNA breakdown seems to happen for a variety of reasons: it is genetically predetermined, a result of sun damage, and a result of toxins built up in the skin cells over a period of time.

You have probably connected the dots and noticed that many of these factors of aging are targeted by corresponding cosmetic ingredients that claim to counteract the effect of their depletion. Collagen, elastin, ceramide, hyaluronic acid, polysaccharide, DNA, RNA, and other skin components are popular in wrinkle creams. (DNA and RNA are the biggest jokes in this group of ingredients because not only do you not want to mess around with the cell's genetic coding, you can't. If you could, you would have the cure for cancer.)

Putting collagen and elastin in a skin-care product is cute, but they can't bond to the collagen and elastin in your skin, although they can work as moisturizing ingredients. Ingredients like ceramides and hyaluronic acids do work to help support the intercellular structure of the skin, but they don't make the skin produce more ceramides and hyaluronic acids, nor will they prevent their continuing depletion. (Good old glycerin is also abundant in the layers between the skin cells, and it's just as reliable in helping the skin to feel better, but the cosmetics industry doesn't talk much about glycerin because it is too commonplace to sound distinctive.) Unfortunately, the cosmetics industry loves to use phrases, such as "replaces what skin has lost," that lead you to believe these kinds of ingredients can affect skin structure. The point of all of this is that growing old cannot be reversed with a skin-care routine or a handful of specific skin ingredients (but the progression can be stopped or slowed with adequate sun protection).

Is It Good for Sensitive Skin?

Hopefully by now you are sensitive (pun intended) to the fact that the cosmetics industry doesn't always tell you the truth. They are particularly unforthcoming on the issue of allergic reactions and unfavorable skin reactions. Allergic reactions and skin sensitivities are not technically the same thing, but they can feel the same on your skin. Regardless of the physiologically precise definition, we have all used some type of cosmetic, only to have part of our face or body burn, tingle, swell, flake, redden, itch, blister, break out, or just feel bad. How could this happen? Given how many products we use and the diversity of ingredients, I'm shocked it doesn't happen more frequently.

Fragrance and preservatives are often thought to be the major culprits when our skin goes a little crazy from a cosmetic. Preservatives are impossible to avoid:

how many of us want to use a moldy, contaminated skin-care or makeup product? This is what would happen to an unpreserved cosmetic. However, you can and should stay away from cosmetics, particularly skin-care products, that contain fragrance. It is simple enough to avoid products with fragrance, perfume, or parfum on the ingredient list. But ingredient lists aren't always that easy.[1]

The cosmetics industry knows that most women emotionally and psychologically prefer cosmetics that smell nice, even if they say they want to avoid fragrance. But if a cosmetics company produces products without fragrance, you will instead get the scent of the ingredients, which are not in the least as appealing as a sweet added fragrance. In order to kill two marketing birds with one cosmetic stone, rather than listing fragrance or perfume on the label, they list its components, usually as essential oils. As lovely as essential oils sound, they are almost all fragrant, volatile oils that can prove quite irritating and sensitizing to sensitive (or even not so sensitive) skin. **So while your eyes don't see the word "fragrance" on the list, and you may approvingly think wintergreen oil, lemon oil, cardamon oil, ylang-ylang oil, or other oils sound pleasant and healthy, your skin may respond disapprovingly.**

There are more factors that can trigger allergic or sensitizing skin reactions than I can even begin to list. Plant extracts (if you suffer from hay fever, plants are the last thing you want in abundance in skin-care products); stimulating and drying ingredients like sodium lauryl sulfate, SD alcohol, mints, menthol, camphor, eucalyptus, and citruses; and lanolin, vitamin E, chamomile, and some sunscreen agents are among the many more-common ingredients that can cause problems. And while most women fret over "oils" in their cosmetics, all of the thickening agents used in everything from blushes to oil-free moisturizers (yes, even "oil-free" is meaningless) can clog pores and spawn blemishes.

---

[1] I have not included specific warnings for preservatives I have mentioned in the past, such as quaternium-15, 2-bromo-2-nitropane-1,3-diol, and phenoxyethanol. At one time research seemed to show that these ingredients posed a higher potential for irritation than other preservatives. More recent data, however, strongly disputes that conclusion. After discussing this matter with several cosmetic chemists, I have concluded that all preservatives can be a problem for many different types of skin, so it would be unfair to pinpoint one specific preservative as a problem. If you are concerned, you can easily avoid any of these ingredients; however, as several cosmetic chemists warned me, a reliable preservative system is essential for any skin-care product because microbial contamination of a product causes more problems for the eyes, lips, and skin than the risk of a reaction to a preservative.

On a related matter, some of you may be familiar with research that warns against using cosmetics that contain triethanolamine or TEA-lauryl sulfate along with formaldehyde-releasing preservatives such as imidazolidinyl urea, quaternium-15, 2-bromo-2-nitropane-1,3-diol, or dmdm hydantoin. There is evidence that suggests these combinations can form nitrosamines in a cosmetic, creating a potential carcinogen. There is substantial disagreement among the cosmetic chemists I spoke to as to how significant a problem this is for the skin (or even if it is a problem). They suggested that going out of the house without a sunscreen or sitting in a bar exposed to secondhand cigarette smoke poses more risk to the skin than any combination of skin-care ingredients ever could, but the decision is up to you. You can read the ingredient listings to discern which ones meet your specific concerns.

Over and above the issue of skin-care ingredients, women tend to use too many different products (less is best for the skin, but more is better for cosmetics sales) while ignoring the huge lists of ingredients on the labels. I can't stress this one enough: the less of everything you put on your face or body, the better, and that goes for all skin types but especially for those with sensitive skin.

Is there one line of cosmetics that's best for sensitive skin? It would be great if there were, but it just doesn't exist. Skin reactions are amazingly random and dissimilar. What you're allergic to has little to do with what someone else reacts to, and then there's the intricacy of ingredients being combined on the face. The culprit may not be the product you think caused the problem. You may think a new moisturizer made your eyes swell, but it could turn out that the nail polish you were wearing in combination with the new moisturizer triggered the problem.

Everyone Has Sensitive Skin

Most of us have sensitive/irritated skin. Regardless of your primary skin type, ethnic background, or age, minor or major irritating skin conditions can be present, even those you can't feel. The skin can burn, chafe, or crack, and you may have patchy areas of dry, flaky skin related to weather conditions, hormonal changes, the skin-care products you use, or sun exposure. Skin can also break out in small bumps that look like a diaper rash. Skin can itch, swell, blotch, redden, and develop allergic reactions to cosmetics, animals, dust, or pollen. If that isn't enough, just think about the number of cosmetics most women use daily. The average woman uses at least 12 different skin-care, makeup, and hair-care products a day, with each one, on average, containing about 15 different ingredients. That means her skin is exposed to anywhere from 100 to 180 different cosmetic ingredients on any given day. The fact that any of us have skin left is a testimony to the skin's resiliency and the talent of cosmetic chemists. Whether we like it or not, most of us have sensitive skin to one degree or another.

Your skin is the protective armor that keeps the elements and other invaders from entering the body. We protect most of our anatomy with clothing, but our faces are left painfully exposed to everything. It's no wonder the skin on our faces acts up now and then. Sensitive skin is probably the most "normal" type of skin around.

Everyone has the potential to develop sensitive skin, so the precautions for sensitive skin should be heeded by women of every skin type. What are the precautions? There is really only one, and it goes for all skin types: **Treat your skin as gently as you possibly can. Whether you think of your face as oily, dry, or mature, you still need to be gentle with your skin and avoid those things that cause irritation.**

The operative word is gentle. Preventing skin irritation, regardless of skin type, is the course of action I recommend throughout this book. Of course, some skin types can and should try to tolerate certain potentially irritating ingredients, such as a topical disinfectant (2.5% benzoyl peroxide, for instance) for someone with acne, or a BHA solution (a salicylic acid exfoliant) for someone with blackheads, or AHAs (an alpha hydroxy acid product to exfoliate) or Retin-A or Renova (to improve cell formation) for someone with sun-damaged skin. Other than those departures from the gentleness rule, if something is irritating it can be detrimental for all skin types. If it is bad for sensitive skin, it is probably bad for oily skin, acned skin, combination skin, dry skin, or mature skin. As you begin to integrate this gentleness philosophy into your skin-care routine, you will slowly solve many skin problems you may have been experiencing.

Excerpt from Cosmetics Counter Update

Dear Paula,

I can't even imagine how much money you've saved me, not to mention the grief I used to go through buying the wrong products. I would now like your thoughts concerning what I have noticed about Asian skin. I have noticed that Asian skin does not seem to wrinkle as much (or as fast) as Caucasian [skin]. I am of Chinese heritage and spent [my] first 18 years in Southeast Asia, where it is sunny all year round. Admittedly, most Asians wear hats, do not sunbathe, and pretty much stay out of the sun, particularly the midday sun. Nonetheless, they do not use sunscreens. I don't go out of my way to avoid the sun, but I don't sunbathe or spend great amounts of time outdoors. Do you know whether Asian skin [types] tend to wrinkle at a different rate from Caucasian [skin types]?

P.C., via e-mail

Dear P.C.,

Your take on Asian skin is accurate. In the past, Asians for the most part have stayed out of the sun, giving no value to the golden brown color of tanned skin. But Asians who don't stay out of the sun (many Japanese love going on holiday to Hawaii now) are doomed to the same fate as anyone else who gets sun exposure-wrinkles and possibly skin cancer. Even African-American women (especially those with lighter skin) will wrinkle if they don't use sunblock, and many cosmetics lines for women of color are starting to raise these women's awareness by including SPF 15 products in their lines. Obviously, whiter skin runs the risk of faster and more serious damage, but wrinkles are wrinkles, and when they start showing up between age 30 and 40, most women start wishing they hadn't spent so much time in the sun. If sunscreen isn't something you can make part of your daily skin-care ritual, avoiding the sun as much as possible is the next best thing, and it really makes a difference.

Learning to Be Gentle

If there is one thing the skin doesn't like in any way, shape, or form, it's irritation. Irritation takes a toll on all skin types. Although many things can cause irritation, the skin tends to react the same regardless of the source. The skin can handle only so much irritation, which isn't much, before it reacts adversely. What can happen is an assortment of problems that are hard to combat: redness, dry patches, blemishes, rashes, cracks along the side of the nose and corners of the mouth and eyes, flakiness, increased skin sensitivity, other skin disorders, and a reduction in the skin's immune/healing response.

Note: It is generally believed that irritation is not responsible for wrinkles and premature aging of the skin. Some dermatologists suggest, however, that repeatedly using irritating ingredients on the skin can suppress the skin's immune/healing response, making the wrinkling process worse. Many products that are advertised as making skin look instantly younger when placed over the lines on the face contain irritating ingredients (such as alcohol) that swell the skin temporarily. With repeated use, they could actually make the skin more wrinkled.

What physically takes place when the skin is irritated? The skin's nerve endings immediately become overstimulated, which causes them to activate whatever they are attached to. The nerves on the face are attached to the skin, hair follicles, oil glands, capillaries, and underlying structure of the skin. If you overstimulate the nerve endings, the oil glands will produce more oil, the skin will flake, and the blood circulation to the small capillaries near the surface of the skin will increase and possibly cause spiderlike veins to appear. If surface capillaries are already present on your face, irritation will make them worse. Irritation will also break down the intercellular substances between the skin cells, diminishing the skin's immune/healing response.

Take this rule at face value: Thou shalt always treat thy skin gently or it will complain loudly that something is wrong. The skin might react to topical irritation immediately, or it may take some time before signs of irritation show up. Possibly the most ominous aspect of irritation is that your skin doesn't have to react at all. Your skin can become irritated and you won't necessarily feel or see anything different. If you use irritating skin-care products, your skin may suffer the negative effects whether or not you can see them taking place on your skin.

It logically follows that learning how to be gentle to your face is one of the most important parts of any skin-care routine. There is no way you can ever begin to hope for soft, smooth skin when your face is being irritated every time you take care of it. Irritation-free skin is the goal.

How to Be Gentle

We do many things to our skin and buy an assortment of skin-care products that can cause serious irritation. It is far easier than you think to eliminate these skin-"care" culprits. With that in mind, here is a list of typical skin-care and makeup ingredients and specific cosmetics products and tools to avoid or use cautiously. The skin can react negatively to all of the following products and ingredients.

Irritating Skin-Care Steps and Products

Abrasive scrubs

Astringents containing irritating ingredients

Toners containing irritating ingredients

Scrub puffs

Cold water/hot water

Facial masks containing irritating ingredients

Loofahs

Bar soaps and bar cleansers

Washcloths

Irritating Ingredients

Acetone

Alcohol or SD alcohol followed by a number (ingredients like cetyl alcohol or stearyl alcohol are standard, benign, waxlike cosmetic thickening agents and are completely nonirritating)

Ammonia

Arnica

Balm mint

Balsam

Bentonite

Benzalkonium chloride

Bergamot

Camphor

Chamomile

Cinnamon
Citrus juices and oils (such as grapefruit or orange)
Clove
Clover blossom
Cocoa butter
Coriander
Cornstarch
Eucalyptus
Fennel
Fennel oil
Fir needle
Geranium
Grapefruit
Horsetail
Lavender
Lemon
Lemongrass
Lime
Marjoram
Melissa
Menthol
Mint
Oak bark
Papaya
Peppermint
Phenol
Sandalwood oil
SD alcohol
Sodium C14-16 olefin sulfate
Sodium lauryl sulfate
TEA-lauryl sulfate
Thyme
Wintergreen

Witch hazel

Ylang-ylang

These ingredients are extremely common; you would be surprised how often they show up in skin-care products for all skin types. Ingredients like camphor, menthol, mint, alcohol, and phenol are sometimes recommended because they are considered to be anti-itch ingredients. The theory works like this: when your skin itches, the nerve endings are sending messages begging you to scratch. If you place these irritating ingredients over the area that itches, the nerve hears the irritation message louder than it hears the itch message and interprets this as a reason to stop itching. That reasoning is fine if minor, sporadic, occasional itching is your problem. If it is not and those ingredients are used in skin-care products meant to be applied every day, they introduce a constantly irritating insult to the skin, causing dryness, rashes, increased oil production, redness, and breakouts. None of those side effects are attractive.

Skin doesn't have to hurt, tingle, or be stimulated even a little to be clean. (If the skin tingles, it is being irritated, not cleaned.) The major rule for all skin types is, if a product or procedure irritates the skin, don't use it or do it again. Pain and cleanliness have nothing to do with each other.

Exception to the rule: If you are initially using AHA, BHA, Retin-A, Renova, Azelaic Acid, or Differin, these can cause some tingling. You may need to cut back, if it is more than a little tingling, or stop altogether, if the tingling persists for more than a few weeks.

Allergic Reactions

In addition to the multiple problems associated with irritation that causes skin to react negatively, it can be both disconcerting and aggravating to have an allergic reaction to the cosmetics you use. Reactions can be subtle, such as a little itching, minor redness and swelling, or small rashlike pimples. They can also involve a full blown flare-up that causes intense but temporary discomfort and an unsightly appearance, or they can trigger a chronic condition requiring medical attention. If you have a tendency to allergic reactions, your skin type can be greatly affected and you will have to pay close attention to what you use. Someone with allergy-prone skin needs to use fewer products with smaller ingredient lists.

I would love to list ingredients that I could guarantee won't cause your skin to have an allergic reaction, but there is no single ingredient or combination of ingredients that can live up to that sweeping claim. Why not? Because everyone is biochemically different. Each of us has a unique chemical makeup, and the endless paradoxical differences in the way our bodies perform account for why we react so differently when exposed to the same thing.

Because of the almost limitless combinations, in all sorts of mixtures and formulations, it is virtually impossible to know if, when, or how anyone's skin will react to any cosmetic. Your only recourse, and this is not the best news, is to keep experimenting until you find what works for you. If you do get a reaction, stop using the product immediately, consult your physician if the reaction is serious or prolonged, return the products that are suspect, and keep track of the ingredients included in products to which you seem to be allergic. Also, just because you've used a cosmetic for a long time doesn't mean you won't develop an allergic reaction to it.

I mention the risk of plants and other potentially sensitizing or allergy-related ingredients throughout this book, and while some, if not all, of these should be avoided, remember that the amount of a suspect ingredient can also determine how a product will affect your skin. The less there is of an ingredient—the further down in the ingredient list it is—the less likely you are to have a reaction to it. Just because the ingredient is suspect or may have a potential for causing skin sensitivities doesn't mean it will always cause problems. Listen to your skin, erring on the side of gentleness, and be cautious. **Moreover, be patient. If you do have an allergic reaction, wait until it subsides before you venture out to try something new or different. Pare down to the absolute basics, usually just cleanser and a touch of moisturizer over very dry areas, try a bit of over-the-counter cortisone cream to reduce irritation, and stay out of the sun.**

It is also important to understand that some potentially irritating ingredients, such as the many preservatives present in cosmetics, are critical to the products' stability, even though they are not good for sensitive or allergy-prone skin. But chemists have literally no other option when it comes to preventing microbes from taking up residence in their products. Fragrances are another known source of skin irritations, and while they are frequently used to mask the unpleasant odor of many cosmetic ingredients, more often they are added to increase sales. Ostensibly most women want their lotions and creams to exude an obvious bouquet. This isn't the fault of the cosmetics companies, although it does reflect a need for consumer education. If you want perfume, use perfume, but choose skin-care products that are fragrance-free to take gentle, soothing care of your skin.

If you have an allergic reaction of any kind to a cosmetic product, stop using it immediately and consult your physician if the problem persists. Do not hesitate to return the product to the place where you purchased it and get your money back. It is not your fault that the product caused problems. Also, returning the product gives the cosmetics company essential information about how their formulas are working.

Skin Disorders and Skin Type

In addition to issues surrounding skin type and skin sensitivities and allergic reactions, a large percentage of the population must deal with medical conditions that can add to skin-care woes. These problems make selecting appropriate skin-care products extremely tricky, yet they are rarely discussed at cosmetics counters. The most common skin disorders are eczema, psoriasis, seborrhea, and rosacea. Early identification goes a long way toward reducing the symptoms of these skin afflictions, and can prevent sufferers from wasting time and money in the cosmetics world. These conditions require a dermatologist's care and cannot be treated at the cosmetics counter or with over-the-counter drugs from the drugstore. Finding skin-care and makeup routines that work with each of these conditions is important, but they must work with the medical treatments available for the specific disorder.

Rosacea

Rosacea is no fun. This stubborn skin disorder is frustrating and extremely difficult to treat. It is thought to afflict at least 10% of the population, and is frequently misdiagnosed by dermatologists and physicians. Rosacea develops over a long period of time, starting with what first seems like a tendency to blush easily, a ruddy complexion, or an extreme sensitivity to cosmetics. This distinctive redness or flushing, which appears in a characteristic butterfly pattern over the nose and cheeks, is the first likely indication of the condition. This distinctive though subtle initial redness is often ignored by women as being just a bothersome skin-color problem and not a skin disorder.

Another problem with identifying rosacea is that pustules and papules (pimples) that resemble acne are often present. That makes rosacea look like acne, and it is often misdiagnosed as a result. Unlike most acne conditions, rosacea is rarely, if ever, accompanied by whiteheads or blackheads. The distinctive flushing and extreme skin sensitivity also differentiate rosacea from acne. The final toll on the face is the presence of flaky patches that may or may not be accompanied by either dry or oily skin, or both at the same time. Rosacea can be extremely confusing for a woman because the dry, flaky skin responds minimally to moisturizers and the acnelike bumps respond minimally, or not at all, to typical acne treatments.

Even more confounding, when rosacea first develops, it may appear, disappear, and then reappear a short time later. This fluctuation also makes diagnosis difficult. Yet, despite its evasive beginnings, the condition rarely reverses itself and almost always becomes worse without treatment. Eventually the skin doesn't return to its normal color and stays persistently red. Other symptoms, such as enlarged blood vessels, flaky patches, oily skin, skin sensitivity, and breakouts, become more and more visible. As rosacea progresses, pimples appear on the face in the form of small, solid red bumps and pus-filled bumps. In more advanced cases of rosacea, a condition called rhinophyma may develop. This is characterized by a bulbous, enlarged red nose and puffy cheeks. It may also involve thick bumps that develop on the lower half of the nose, spreading to the nearby cheek areas. Rhinophyma rarely occurs in women.

For years this disorder was referred to as acne rosacea, which only added to the confusion because rosacea obviously is not acne. Because blemishes can make rosacea look like acne, many doctors misdiagnose it, prescribing everything but the course of treatment that can relieve the symptoms. Only a handful of treatments for rosacea exist, and they are all available by prescription only, including MetroGel, MetroCream, Azelaic Acid, and oral tetracycline. Using the topical MetroCream, MetroGel, or Azelaic Acid with oral tetracycline is the primary mode of treatment. But first, you and your doctor need to know what you are dealing with. Knowing the difference between acne and acne rosacea can make a huge difference in the health of your skin.

Several factors can make rosacea worse. These catalysts include hot liquids, spicy foods, exposure to extreme temperatures (including cooking over a hot stove), alcohol consumption, sunlight, stress, saunas, hot tubs, smoking, rubbing or massaging the skin, irritating cosmetics, and anything else that overstimulates the skin and blood vessels. Rosacea can also be exacerbated by AHAs, BHA, Retin-A, Renova, Differin, benzoyl peroxide, and exfoliants of any kind, including scrubs and washcloths. In terms of skin care, eliminate the use of irritating ingredients and products. The less you do, meaning the fewer products you use and the fewer the ingredients in each, the happier rosacea-afflicted skin is going to be.

Psoriasis

Psoriasis is a chronic recurring disease of the skin, identified by the presence of thickened scaly areas and papules (small, solid, often inflamed bumps that, unlike pimples, do not contain pus or sebum). These bumps are usually slightly elevated above the normal skin surface, sharply distinguishable from normal skin, and red to reddish brown in color. They are usually covered with small whitish silver scales that stick to the cystlike swelling and, if scraped off, may bleed. The extent of the disease varies from a few tiny lesions to generalized involvement of most of the skin. Often the elbows, knees, scalp, and chest are involved. Psoriasis affects over 6 million people in the United States alone, but for most people it tends to be mild and unsightly rather than a serious health concern.

No one really knows exactly what causes psoriasis, although recent studies suggest it may be related to an immune system disorder. To put it simply, psoriasis is the recurring growth of too many skin cells. A normal skin cell matures in 28 to 45 days, while a psoriatic skin cell takes only 3 to 6 days. Both men and women can get psoriasis at any age. Psoriasis appears in several forms. The scaly, papule kind called plaque psoriasis is the most common. Other forms are guttate psoriasis, typified by small dotlike lesions all over the body; pustular psoriasis, with weeping lesions and intense scaling; and erythrodermic psoriasis, characterized by severe sloughing and inflammation of the skin. Psoriasis can range from mild to moderate to severe and disabling. On occasion, some people who have psoriasis experience spontaneous remissions, but no one knows why this happens, and remissions are unpredictable.

Sadly, there is no cure for psoriasis, but there are many different treatments, both topical and systemic, that can clear it for periods of time. Experimenting with a variety of options is essential if you wish to find the treatment that works for you, but all require a doctor's attention.

Of the various therapies available to treat psoriasis, it is generally best to start with those that have the least serious side effects, such as topical steroids (cortisone creams); coal tar creams, lotions, cleansers, or shampoos; and exposure to sunshine. If those methods are not successful, you can proceed to the more serious treatments involving oral medications. More often than not, successful treatment requires a combination of methods.

Natural sunlight can significantly improve, or even clear, psoriasis. Regular daily doses of sunlight taken in short exposures with adequate sun protection are strongly recommended. Sun protection is vital not only to prevent sunburn, which may make psoriasis worse, but also to reduce skin damage from the sun's ultraviolet radiation. This outdoor approach to treating psoriasis is often referred to as climatotherapy. Some people travel to Florida, Hawaii, the Caribbean, or the Dead Sea in Israel (where special clinics offer treatment solariums and supervised medical assistance) to use swimming and natural sunlight as their psoriasis treatment (some people believe immersion in salty, mineral-laden water may also have some unknown benefits). In some countries, medical plans actually cover trips to these types of sunny climates and mineral spas for subscribers with psoriasis.

When you can't get to sunshine, medically supervised administration of UVB lamps may be used to minimize widespread or localized areas of stubborn and unmanageable psoriasis lesions. UVB light is also used when topical treatments have failed, or in combination with topical treatments. The short-term risks of using controlled UVB exposure to treat psoriasis are minimal, and long-term studies of large numbers of patients treated with UVB have not demonstrated an increased risk of skin cancer, suggesting that this treatment may be safer than sunlight. (Sunlight has both UVA and UVB radiation; UVA causes skin cancer, while UVB mainly triggers sunburn.) UVB treatments are considered one of the most effective therapies for moderate to severe psoriasis, with the least amount of risk.

Treating psoriasis with coal tar is a very old and effective remedy. These topical medications are available both over the counter and by prescription; the difference is in the potency and amount of coal tar the medication contains. Coal tar can be combined with other psoriasis medications (e.g., topical steroids) or with sunshine (ultraviolet light). However, coal tar can make the skin more sensitive to ultraviolet light, and extreme caution is advised when combining its use with UV therapy (or exposure to the sun) in order to avoid getting a severe burn or causing skin damage.

Anthralin, another topical prescription medication, has been used to treat psoriasis for over a hundred years. It has few serious side effects but can irritate or burn the normal-appearing skin surrounding psoriasis lesions. Anthralin also stains anything it comes into contact with. It is prescribed in a range of concentrations and there are a variety of regimens for its use, but the negative side effects make it a less than desirable option.

Calcipotriene, a synthetic vitamin D_3 analog, is used to treat mild to moderate psoriasis. It is a prescription medication with few side effects. It is not the same compound as the vitamin D found in commercial vitamin supplements. Calcipotriene is sold in the United States as a topical, odorless, nonstaining ointment and cream under the prescription brand name of Dovonex.

More serious systemic medications such as Methotrexate, Tegison, Accutane, Soriatane, Cyclosporin, and oral steroids are also used to treat psoriasis, but each has pros and cons that need to be researched and discussed at length with your physician.

Discovering whether any of these will work for you, alone or in combination, takes patience and a systematic, ongoing review and evaluation of how your skin is doing. As is true with all chronic skin disorders, success requires diligent adherence to the regimen and a realistic understanding of what you can and can't expect. It is also important to be aware of the consequences of the varying treatment levels. For example, continued long-term use of topical cortisone creams can cause skin thinning, stretch marks, and built-up resistance to the cortisone medication itself, so that it actually becomes an ineffective treatment. Exposure to sunlight without adequate protection (particularly from UVA radiation) can cause skin cancer. Oral steroids can have serious withdrawal effects, including increased bouts of psoriasis. Accutane causes birth defects if a woman becomes pregnant while taking it.

For more information on the current status of available treatment, write to the National Psoriasis Foundation (NPF) at 6600 Southwest 92nd Avenue, Suite 300, Portland, OR 97223; send e-mail to 76135.2746@compuserve.com; or phone (800) 723-9166 (toll-free).

Seborrhea

Seborrhea is a skin disease of the sebaceous (oil) glands, marked by an increased secretion of sebum (oil) or a thickened sebum discharge. It can resemble acne and blackheads. One of the differences between acne and seborrhea is that in seborrhea the increased oil production is often accompanied by a scaly, thickened skin, especially on the scalp, and the oil itself can have a strange viscous texture. However, in seborrhea and sometimes in acne, the sebum (a firm waxlike substance in the pore that liquefies into oil on the surface of the skin) in the sebaceous gland accumulates, causing the gland to become swollen and filled to the brim. When this overproduced sebum is covered by skin, it forms a small, firm mound called a whitehead. When the sebum is exposed to air (not covered by skin) and the duct fills with dead skin cells, the sebum turns dark and the blemish becomes a blackhead. The size of the eruption, the texture of the oil, and the flaky skin are what differentiate seborrhea from acne.

Seborrhea can show up wherever there are lots of oil glands. The scalp, sides of the nose, eyebrows, eyelids, behind the ears, and middle of the chest are the areas most commonly affected. Other areas, such as the navel and the skin folds under the arms, breasts, groin, and buttocks, may also be involved. The swelling, breakouts, and accompanying yellowish, greasy-appearing scales make this skin disorder hard to miss.

Although seborrhea on the scalp can look like dandruff, dandruff and seborrhea are not associated. With dandruff there is excessive scaling that appears in white flakes possibly caused by the presence of a fungus in the hair follicle. With seborrhea, there is excessive yellowing, thickened scaling accompanied by excessive oiliness. Seborrhea can occur at any age, but typically it is seen in infants, when it is called "cradle cap."

Recent evidence suggests that this skin disorder may be intensified or perpetuated by a yeastlike organism in the hair follicle. This organism is normally found on nondiseased skin in low numbers. Feeding off the increased scaling and oil production of seborrhea, this yeast grows and can aggravate the inflammation of the disease. Specific prescription creams and shampoos can be helpful in controlling the condition in some people.

One of the more effective treatments is applying low-strength cortisone cream or hydrocortisone to the affected areas. Frequent use of nonprescription shampoos or topical medications containing coal tar, zinc pyrithione, selenium sulfide, sulfur, and/or salicylic acid may be recommended by a dermatologist. For patients who do not respond to this treatment, there are several other effective medications that a dermatologist can prescribe.

Eczema

I have suffered from eczema for many years. At one point in my life almost 80% of my body was affected, and the resulting itching, sores, irritation, and discomfort were more awful than I can put into words. For years I struggled with medications and a varying assortment of cortisone creams and bar soaps, from Basis to Aveeno, until the day my dermatologist found the right cortisone strength and I started to stay away from topical irritants; then my skin finally settled down.

Eczema, also known as contact dermatitis, atopic dermatitis, irritant dermatitis, allergic dermatitis, and a host of other designations, is without question a difficult skin disease to pinpoint. When you have it, you generally know it by the cracked, abraded, blistered, crusted, weepy, reddened, patchy, dry skin surface, accompanied by persistent, almost unbearable itching and the tendency for everything you touch to make matters worse. A simple act like washing hands, applying eye makeup, or wearing scratchy material can instigate a flare-up that feels interminable.

Almost anything can trigger eczema, and no disturbance at all can precede a bout of oppressive itching and rashes. Wool (clothing to carpets), shampoos, hair dyes, nail polish, jewelry, plants, undergarments (elastic waistband and spandex bras are special villains), deodorant, tight socks, nylons, pet allergies, excessive heat or air conditioning (which increases dry and itchy skin), bathing too often (which leaches moisture out of the skin), harsh or mild soaps, hot water, vigorous rubbing or massaging, chlorinated water, salt water, and even sweat (this triggers my eczema almost instantaneously) are all possible offenders. In the world of cosmetics, lanolin, preservatives, irritants (such as peppermint, menthol, alcohol, camphor, eucalyptus, fragrance, and essential oils), bath salts, bubble bath, scrubs, AHAs, BHA, and loofahs are all potent eczema triggers.

Despite this daunting list, everyone is different, and what irritates your skin might not irritate someone else's. There is no exact science to discovering what causes your skin to react; rather, it is a process of paying attention to what you come into contact with, seeing what makes things better or worse for your skin, and then eliminating or avoiding those things at all costs.

Generally, dry skin is more prone to itching and chapping, so finding a reliable way to deal with dry skin is almost always the starting point for the treatment of eczema. To this end it is important to keep bathing time short, avoid bath salts or bubble baths, use lukewarm to warm water (avoid hot water most of all), and avoid bar soaps of any kind (they all contain potential irritants). Using fragrance-free liquid cleansers that also contain moisturizing agents, and applying moisturizers quickly afterward, can help a lot.

Unquestionably, moisturizers minimize dryness and are a mainstay in treating mild to chronic dermatitis. It is believed that regular and frequent use of moisturizers can reduce the amount of topical steroids needed in the maintenance treatment of eczema. While using a moisturizer twice daily is considered adequate, I keep moisturizer with me at all times to reapply every time I wash my hands. It is important, though, to keep in mind that your moisturizer may be causing eczema flare-ups. Oversaturating eczematous skin can be a problem too, just as it can be for any dry skin condition (see "Stop the Moisturizing Mania" in Chapter Two). The lightest-weight moisturizer you can use to minimize dry skin and eczema will perform the best by helping your skin's own immune/healing response to kick in.

Topical corticosteroid is the drug of choice for treating eczema. It is available in a vast range of strengths and molecular structures that allow for varying skin penetration and potency. The risks associated with prolonged use of a potent corticosteroid may result in skin deterioration and adaptation (that means it stops having an effect on the skin). However, concerns about skin breakdown (which happens with any long-term cortisone use) and adaptation should not limit the use of a good potent steroid. This is the only way to get control of the dermatitis. Once the skin is back to a more normal state, a weaker steroid can be used to maintain results. As much as possible I try to minimize the frequency of cortisone application, but I have also learned there is a point of no return, where if I don't use it my skin becomes an itchy, rashy mess.

The Skin Types

Do all these skin problems mean you can't judge your skin type? Of course not. But you do need to be careful about how you assess your skin type. By understanding the circumstances that can strongly influence what you see and what you can't see on the surface of your skin, you can better make decisions about what kind of skin type(s) you have and what to do about it (or them). I've included several categories in addition to the standard skin-type lists you are used to seeing.

The usual four categories of skin types—dry, oily, mature, and combination—are too general and practically useless for a vast number of women. They never take into account the facts that mature skin is not a type unto itself, that oily skin doesn't necessarily break out, and that there isn't just one type of normal skin, and they ignore skin disorders, allergies, and aged skin. The following list takes into account most skin types and can help you establish a battle plan to take wonderful care of your skin's needs.

Please note that, depending on sun exposure and skin color, wrinkles usually begin to appear between the ages of 32 and 38, become more pronounced and noticeable between 40 and 45, and are formidable from 50 on up. Aside from sun exposure, weight can play a significant factor in the appearance of wrinkles. A woman who is more than 25 pounds overweight can look almost wrinkle-free compared with a woman who is height-weight proportionate, providing both have had the same amount of unprotected sun exposure.

One more note: I use the term "mature" to refer to a woman who may already be showing signs of sun damage, a change in skin texture, and beginning hormonal changes (most noticeable by a change in her menstrual cycle), which can happen at any time over the age of 32. Aged skin (especially sun-damaged skin on someone over the age of 65) refers to skin that has become fragile, thin, and almost translucent.

Basic normal skin. No visible pores; little to no dry skin; few to no breakouts; no excess oil to speak of; no sensitivities or allergies. (Please note that, despite what the cosmetics industry would like you to believe, normal skin does not mean flawless skin.)

Mature normal skin. No visible pores; minimal amount of dry skin; eye puffiness on occasion; no excess oil; minimal presence of whiteheads.

Basic oily skin. Visible pores; visible blackheads; small breakouts mostly occurring on the nose, cheeks, chin, and forehead; usually a buildup of excess oil that gets worse as the day goes on. (Please remember that having oily skin does not prevent or slow down wrinkling. Keeping the sun off the face is what prevents or slows the wrinkling process.)

Severe oily skin. Enlarged pores and blackheads over much of the face but most prominent around the nose, center of the forehead, and cheeks (the T-zone); excess oil present almost immediately after washing face; makeup seems to slide off by the end of the day; intense breakouts can occur during the menstrual cycle or for any reason at all.

Mature oily skin. Visible pores; visible blackheads; a small number of breakouts around the T-zone and eye area; skin around the eyes may be dry and puffy; buildup of excess oil still noticeable by the end of the day; makeup seems not to last; skin color can appear dull.

Acned oily skin. Similar to severe oily skin except that breakouts are more chronic and swollen; blemishes often leave minor scarring or discoloration.

Acned dry skin. This is an unusual skin type, but it does exist. Chronic blemishes; skin is dry, flaky, and taut, with little or no oil present except a slight amount in the T-zone.

Cystic acne. May or may not be accompanied by oily skin; distinguished from the mild acne associated with most oily skin types by the large, deep, and disfiguring lesions on the face.

Basic dry skin. No visible pores; skin tends to flake and peel; dry patches present; lips may feel parched; as the day goes on, the skin tends to feel drier and tighter.

Mature dry skin. No visible pores; skin tends to flake and peel; dry patches are present; lips may feel parched and actually crack; as the day goes by, skin can feel very dry and tight; skin may look dull from lack of natural color.

Very dry skin. No visible pores; skin feels constantly tight and dry, and tends to be sensitive and uncomfortable; flaking may or may not accompany the condition; tightness is hard to eliminate.

Aged dry skin. No visible pores; thin, dry, flaky skin that seems to tear when scratched; pronounced wrinkling; crepiness that moisturizers no longer alleviate.

Aged dry skin with occasional breakouts. No visible pores; thin, dry, flaky skin that seems to tear when scratched; pronounced wrinkling; crepiness that moisturizers no longer alleviate; nose, chin, and eye area may have whiteheads or blackheads.

Oily and dry combination skin. The most classic type of combination skin, in which the T-zone—nose, forehead, and chin—is oily with visible pores and blackheads, while the cheeks, jaw, and eye area are dry and flaky.

Sensitive/allergy-prone oily skin. Skin tends to react to your emotions and to everything you put on it; reaction can be in the form of blemishes, dry patches, redness, irritation, puffy eyes, dry lips, dry skin, and/or rashes, but with a pervasive tendency toward breakouts and oily skin regardless of anything else.

Sensitive/allergy-prone dry skin. Skin tends to react to your emotions and to everything you put on it; reaction can be in the form of blemishes, dry patches, redness, irritation, puffy eyes, dry lips, dry skin, and/or rashes, but with a pervasive tendency toward a constant tight, dry feeling.

Combination skin. The presence of any two or more of the above-mentioned skin types occurring simultaneously or at different times during the day, week, or month.

Rosacea. See earlier description.

Seborrhea. See earlier description.

Psoriasis. See earlier description.

Eczema. See earlier description.

CHAPTER FIVE

Skin-Care Planning

Why Does It Have to Be So Complicated?

As I look over the material and research I've accumulated, from magazine articles, books, and medical journals to interviews with dermatologists, oncologists, and cosmetic chemists and product reviews from hundreds of lines, I am amazed that it's possible to sort through it all. You wouldn't think that cleaning the face, protecting skin from the sun, moisturizing, and fighting blemishes would be so complicated or shrouded in such controversy, but the truth is, it is very complicated.

Despite being such a small part of the whole body, the face has the lion's share of topical problems, far more than what takes place from the neck down. Acne, wrinkles, sagging, sunburn, blackheads, dryness, eczema, psoriasis, seborrhea, swelling, and allergies, not to mention our concepts of beauty, are most evident on the face. There is a lot of money to be made if a cosmetics company can get a consumer to believe that their product(s) will make her more beautiful and do something to tackle one or more of those facial dilemmas. If a company can make the stuff sound utterly unique for the skin, even when it isn't, the sales figures rise astronomically. No wonder the claims are so hard to decipher.

As complicated and emotional as skin care can be, the actual skin-care routines are streamlined and concise. Now that you have an overview of what works and what doesn't, how the cosmetics industry may be hurting your skin, and what the current research is revealing about good skin care, my task is to present all this information in a way that helps you find a good cleansing routine so you can stop wasting money on useless products that may be hurting your skin.

First, let me explain my attitude about skin-care products and your current skin-care routine. If the products you are using work for you, no matter how expensive or inexpensive they are, whether I have rated them as being effective or a waste of money, if you are satisfied with how your skin looks and feels, continue doing exactly what you are doing: there is absolutely no reason in the world to change. I don't want you to use a new routine, mine or anyone else's, unless you are dissatisfied with what you are now doing! Conversely, if the information in my book leads you to wonder about adequate sun protection, the risks of overmoisturizing the skin, not treating blemishes in an effective manner, causing more irritation than necessary (even when the skin doesn't look irritated), or wasting money on overpriced products, then absolutely you should reconsider what you are doing and think about other, more measurable solutions. My ideas and suggestions present options and alternatives. There is no reason to change just for the sake of change. Change needs to be based on a reasonable, factual approach to taking care of your skin.

I hope that what you have previously read and are about to read in this book will shift the way you think about skin care and change the way you spend money on skin-care products. **I feel strongly that my suggestions can save you hundreds, if not thousands, of dollars over the years while helping you take optimum and realistic care of your skin.** Depending on whose products you buy, the skin-care routines I suggest for most skin types cost about $40 for an initial purchase, less for some skin types and slightly more for others. When you do decide to do something different for your skin, these ideas will, for the most part, still be valid. Thousands and thousands of women the world over have been following my advice for almost 20 years now, adjusting what they do as new research becomes available.

I should also mention that my ideas are somewhat radical compared with those of most beauty experts on both sides of the counter. I am known for being a proponent of good, inexpensive skin care that results in beautiful skin but does not take a lot of time or involve a litany of products. I do not want any woman to be preoccupied with taking care of her skin for 15 minutes every morning and evening, and an hourlong weekend ritual for good measure. No one should have to waste her time—we all have better things to do with our lives (I barely have time to eat dinner, let alone time for an elaborate skin-care routine)—especially given that the extra time will not make a difference in the way our skin looks anyway. If I had any evidence that the extra products, extra cleansing, and extra moisturizing made a difference in the way my skin looked or improved my quality of life in any way, I would be the first to find time to make it happen. But there is nothing in an extensive, expensive skin-care routine that makes it any more effective than an uncomplicated one.

The other thing that makes my viewpoint on cleansers, soap, astringents, toners, and facial masks controversial is the products I don't recommend. I am frustrated beyond words at beauty experts and cosmetics lines that continue to recommend products that are irritating, harmful, or useless. Regardless of whether they are recommending natural products, instant youth products, wrinkle creams, or cleansing products, their misinformation puts the consumer's skin at risk. **Using an inadequate sunscreen increases your chances of developing skin cancer, applying blemish products that don't do a good job of disinfection and exfoliation can make breakouts and scarring worse, overmoisturizing can impair the healing process, as can irritating ingredients, and wiping off makeup can sag skin. These problems crop up in cosmetics line after cosmetics line.**

I cringe every time I hear women with oily skin being told to use alcohol-based toners, soaps that are too drying (even worse, alkaline soaps can encourage bacterial growth), scrubs that are too abrasive, facial masks that aggravate the skin, inferior disinfectants, or too many exfoliating products. Incessant recommendations for eye creams, cell-renewal creams, night creams, day creams, throat creams, serums, and moisturizing gels are aimed at women with dry or sun-damaged skin. Yet no one at the cosmetics counters or in fashion magazines informs women about the latest FDA-approved sunscreen ingredients or the risks of overmoisturizing.

It takes only an attitude change to see beauty from an informed vantage point. I'll do my best to continue clarifying why I recommend the things I do and the research that supports my conclusions, so that you, as the consumer, can decide for yourself what is best for you.

The Skin-Care Steps Everyone Should Avoid

Although I'm not one to make sweeping comments, at least not often, I want to go over the primary "don'ts" before I go over the various "dos." The following skin-care steps are just plain bad for the skin and should never be done, regardless of your skin type, age, or needs:

1. **NEVER** wipe off makeup—never, ever. **Whether it's eye makeup or face makeup, wiping pulls at the skin and promotes sagging.**
2. **NEVER** use greasy cleansers. **The greasy residue these cleansers inevitably leave behind can clog pores and inhibit normal exfoliation, and often requires an extra step to be removed.**
3. **NEVER** use drying cleansers. **Whether or not you have oily skin, cleansers should never leave the face feeling tight, dry, or uncomfortable.**
4. **NEVER** use bar soap or bar cleansers. **The ingredients that keep these soaps and cleansers in bar form can clog pores, foster breakouts, and irritate skin. Cleansing agents in these are almost without exception drying and irritating for all skin types.** Plus bar soaps and cleansers usually have high pHs (over 7), which can encourage bacteria growth!
5. **NEVER** use a toner simply because you think you should. **There are reasons to use a toner, but it should not automatically be part of your routine.**
6. **NEVER** use a moisturizer based on the false notion that "everyone needs a moisturizer." **Not everyone needs a moisturizer. You need a moisturizer only if you have dry skin, and then only over those areas that are dry.**
7. **NEVER** use an AHA or BHA product unless you are sure of the concentration and pH level. **If you don't know that, you won't know whether it can help to exfoliate the skin.**

8. **NEVER** use more than one exfoliant, and use it only once or twice a day at most. **The face can handle only so much exfoliation; too much starts breaking down the skin's intercellular structure, fomenting irritation** (even **when you don't feel a tingling sensation, the skin can still be suffering the consequences) and swelling the skin.**
9. **NEVER** use a blemish or acne product unless you understand its part in treating the underlying cause of the problem. **If a product doesn't gently clean, adequately disinfect, effectively exfoliate, or absorb oil without irritating, it is a useless waste of time and money.**
10. **NEVER** rely on the term "oil-free." **Plenty of ingredients that aren't oils or don't sound like they're oils can still clog pores, cause breakouts, and grease up the skin. "Oil-free" doesn't tell you anything about what the product can and can't do for the skin or what it really contains.**

And Let's Go Over the Absolute Basics One More Time

- **Avoid skin-care products that contain irritating ingredients.** They can compound or create countless skin problems.
- Never use **a daytime skin-care routine that doesn't include an adequate sunscreen.** Without this there is no way to prevent wrinkles or skin damage.
- Never **overmoisturize the skin.** A skin-care routine that saturates the skin with emollient moisturizers or more than your skin really needs can hurt the skin. Use the lightest-weight moisturizer necessary to make your skin feel soft and smooth.

Cleaning the Skin

No other aspect of skin care is quite so important as this one. Cleaning the face sets the stage for everything else that will take place on the skin. **Overcleaning or using cleansers that are too drying is a major cause of irritation, dry patches, and redness. Not cleaning the skin well enough can clog pores or leave a residue on the face that can prevent skin cells from sloughing off. Using a cleanser that leaves a greasy film on the face can clog pores and prevent moisturizers from being able to absorb and do their thing. It is essential to get this step right, and that means thoroughly but gently cleaning the face.**

Eye Makeup Removers

Wiping off makeup is damaging to the skin, particularly the skin around the eyes, because pulling and tugging sags it. Skin is made up of an elastic network, and responds much like a rubber band. Regardless of the direction you pull—

up, down, or sideways—if you see the skin move, you are tugging on the skin's elastin[1] fibers and helping the skin to sag sooner than it would otherwise. Repeatedly wiping and pulling at the face, no matter how gently, distends the tissue more than enough to stretch it. Watch closely in the mirror the next time you start wiping off your makeup, particularly eye makeup. Notice that even when you are trying to be gentle the skin is shifting around, which inevitably causes wrinkles and sagging.

Constantly wiping, tugging, and pulling on the skin, particularly in the eye area, stretches out some of the skin's inherent elasticity. Like a rubber band, the skin can take only so much pulling until it won't snap back anymore.

Many skin-care routines involve wiping off eye makeup (and face makeup) and then following up with a water-soluble cleanser. My position is, why bother doing two steps when only one is needed? If everything can be gently washed off, why be inconvenienced with an extra step that may be damaging to the skin?

Most makeup is water soluble, or should be, and because so many of the new water-soluble cleansers use mild ingredients that don't affect the eyes, they can easily remove all of your makeup, including eye makeup. Using water with a water-soluble cleanser that slips over the face and is easily rinsed off decreases friction and minimizes pulling. If you have been used to wiping off makeup, it can take a while to get used to washing it off, but it is the most effective and least damaging way to remove eye makeup.

Of course, water-soluble cleansers don't work on waterproof makeup or waterproof mascara, which is the primary reason I strongly suggest wearing only makeup that is water soluble. Occasional use of waterproof makeup is not a big problem, and in those instances it is fine to wipe that makeup off. What affects the face most is what you do repeatedly to the skin on a daily basis, rather than what you do once in a while.

Depending on the amount of eye makeup you wear and the technique you use to wash the eye area, you may find that tiny traces of eye makeup get left behind. In those circumstances, when you are done cleaning your face, dip a cotton swab in the moisturizer you use around your eyes or in your toner (assuming it is gentle) and softly remove what remains.

One Exception to the Rule

Now that I've carried on about the drawbacks of wiping makeup off the eyes and face, and about the irritation that can be caused by using a washcloth, I

[1] Elastin is a stretchable elastic protein found in skin tissue. It is responsible for the flexible, resilient nature of healthy, non-sun-damaged skin. When skin is damaged by the sun or constant pulling, elastin's orderly arrangement changes to a nonpliable, stiff, or stretched-out mass of fibers. That is what causes the skin to sag.

must mention an exception that overrides this warning. If you are using the new long-wearing, stay-put, ultra-matte foundations and eye makeup, most gentle water-soluble cleansers, no matter how effective or concentrated the detergent cleansing agents are, will have a difficult time cutting through them. (See Chapter Eight, "Makeup Application Step by Step," for additional information on these foundations and their correct application.) To get them completely off, and you do need to get them completely off, you may need to use a washcloth in conjunction with a water-soluble cleanser. I wish it weren't so, but it is. You can also try using a water-soluble cleanser and then thoroughly going over your face with a toner, but you may find that doesn't work quite as well as a washcloth; you'll need to test this for yourself to see which works best. The goal is to always get your makeup off thoroughly every night (leaving any amount of makeup on for that long can cause irritation, breakouts, or dryness) and these new long-wearing foundations bring a tricky twist to the proceedings.

The Water

My adamant recommendation requires attention not only to the right type of cleanser, but to the temperature of the water you use. Water is one of the least irritating things you can use on your skin. Wait, I take that back. There are indeed people with serious atopic dermatitis who find even water irritating to the skin, but that condition should be dealt with by a dermatologist and not by a cosmetic skin-care routine. Although water is the most gentle substance used in cleaning the face, it is gentle only when it is tepid. Hot water can burn and irritate the skin, and cold water will shock and irritate the skin. If the goal is to be gentle (and it always is), then tepid water is essential.

Water is also frictionless, which is a very important reason to use it. When you splash your face with water, your hands glide over the face, keeping you from pulling and tugging at the skin. That means you can remove makeup without stretching the skin tissue. This can prevent irritation and reduce sagging.

Choosing the Best Cleanser

Using the right cleanser makes all the difference in the world because it determines how your skin is going to react to everything else you put on it. Overcleaning your face and drying it out causes problems a moisturizer can't correct. Greasing up your skin with a wipe-off, cold-cream-type cleanser can clog pores and leave a film on the skin, which means all the other products you put on will be sitting on top of that instead of being easily absorbed. Trying to degrease the skin with a drying toner after using this kind of greasy makeup remover can cause irritation and a range of other problems. Using a gentle water-soluble cleanser is the best option for the entire face, and this is true for all skin types.

Most of us are familiar with the three primary categories of cleansers available: wipe-off cleansers (including cold creams and liquid makeup removers), soaps of all kinds (including bar cleansers, which technically are not soap), and water-soluble cleansers (creamy, lotion, or shampoo-type cleansers that rinse off). Obviously my preference is the water-soluble cleansers.

A good water-soluble cleanser is a terrific invention. It is a cross between a shampoo and a cold cream, and it is not a soap. What differentiates a good water-soluble cleanser from a poor one is that it washes off makeup without leaving the face dry (like soaps) or greasy (like cold cream); contains no fragrance (fragrance is an irritant, though these are hard to find), no coloring agents (coloring agents can be irritants, particularly if some cleanser gets in the eye), and no abrasive, scrublike particles; and, most important of all, is gentle to the skin. Some cleansers on the market are labeled water soluble, but in actuality they need to be wiped off with a wet washcloth. If the cleanser must be wiped off with a tissue or washcloth, it is anything but water soluble. Water-soluble cleansers completely do away with the need to wipe off any makeup.

Water-soluble cleansers are not only the most gentle way to clean the face, they are also the most efficient. Everything is done at the sink. Even a heavy makeup wearer can take off all her makeup, including eye makeup, this way. Using a water-soluble cleanser eliminates the need for a separate eye makeup remover or for boxes of tissues to wipe the face with. Imagine splashing your face generously with (tepid) water, then massaging in a water-soluble cleanser evenly over your face, including the eyes, and then rinsing it off with more water, preferably with your hands. Once the face is rinsed, it shouldn't feel greasy or dry.

Using washcloths with water to remove your cleanser is not what I'm referring to when I say a product is water soluble. Water-soluble cleansers should splash off without the aid of a washcloth; if you prefer to use something besides your hands, use a smooth sponge or any smooth cloth. Washcloths are irritating. Many people use smoother cloths on their kitchen counter than they do on their face.

But not all water-soluble cleansers are created equal, and finding a good one can be tricky. Just because a cleanser is labeled water soluble doesn't mean it comes off with water or is gentle. Plenty of cleansers have names that sound great, with words like Milky or Creamy or Foaming or Gel. But many of them leave the face feeling greasy and need to be wiped off, or they rinse off too well, leaving the face feeling dry and irritated. **Also, avoid water-soluble cleansers**

that contain AHAs, BHA, or disinfectants. These can all be irritating to the eye area, and they are rinsed off way before these ingredients have a chance to do anything positive for the skin.

When I first began recommending water-soluble cleansers years ago, there was really only one available. That was Cetaphil Cleanser. It is still available and it is excellent for someone with dry, sensitive skin. But now there are more water-soluble cleansers to choose from than I ever thought possible. Not all of them are really water soluble and many are too drying, but many are very gentle on the skin, remove all the makeup without causing irritation or dryness, do not burn the eyes, and leave no greasy residue.

One thing most water-soluble cleansers have in common, regardless of price, is the same basic ingredient list of water and one or more detergent cleansing agents such as sodium laureth sulfate, ammonium laureth sulfate, cocamide betaine, or sodium cocoamphopropionate, among others. Cleansers designed for dry skin often contain oils and leave a greasy residue. When someone with dry skin uses a cleanser supposedly designed for her skin type, and then follows that with a rich, creamy moisturizer, too many emollients can build up, causing the skin to look dull and preventing cell turnover. Cleansers designed for normal to oily skin can contain one or more standard detergent agents that will dry out the skin, such as sodium lauryl sulfate, TEA-lauryl sulfate, and sodium olefin sulfate (when found in the first ingredients on the label). Drying out the skin is always a problem and often creates the artificial need for a moisturizer, which just greases things back up. This cycle of greasing up dry skin or drying out oily or combination skin causes more skin problems than almost any other facet of skin care.

In my book *Don't Go to the Cosmetics Counter Without Me*, I provide a complete summary of the best water-soluble cleansers for each skin type. Here are a few selections from that list to get you started:

For all skin types where the underlying condition is oily skin, the best water-soluble cleansers are: Alpha Hydrox Foaming Face Wash; Artistry by Amway Clarifying Cleansing Gel for Normal to Oily Skin; Aveda Purifying Gel Cleanser; Avon Purifying Facial Cleansing Gel; Basis Comfortably Clean Face Wash; Black Opal Oil Free Cleansing Gel; Bobbi Brown Face Cleanser and Gel Cleanser; The Body Shop Balancing Cleansing Gel for Normal to Oily Skin; Clinique Wash-Away Gel Cleanser; H_2O Plus Cleansing Gel; Lancome Clarifiance Oil-Free Gel Cleanser; Nivea Visage Hydro-Cleansing Gel; Oil of Olay Sensitive Skin Foaming Face Wash; Orlane Detoxinating Purifying Gel Cleanser; Paula's Choice One Step Face Cleanser for Normal to Oily/Combination Skin.

For all skin types where the underlying condition is dry skin, the best

cleansers are: BeautiControl Chamomile Balancing Cleansing Lotion; Beauty Without Cruelty Herbal Cream Facial Cleanser; The Body Shop Foaming Cleansing Cream for Normal to Dry Skin; Estee Lauder Instant Action Rinse-Off Cleanser; Galderma Cetaphil Cleanser; Hydron Best Defense Gentle Cleansing Creme; Paula's Choice One Step Face Cleanser for Normal to Dry Skin; Pond's One Step Face Cleanser for Normal to Dry Skin; Ultima II Interactives Clean Team Cleanser + Toner Normal/Oily; Yves Rocher Meristem Gentle Cleanser.

Summary: Use only water-soluble cleansers, which rinse off completely when water is splashed on the face, leaving the face with a clean, soft feeling that is neither dry nor greasy. Creamy cleansers, even though they may claim to be water soluble, pull at the skin and can sag it, especially when used with a washcloth. There are many types of water-soluble cleansers on the market, so be careful. A lot of foaming or gel-type cleansers are indeed water soluble, but they may contain ingredients that can be drying or irritating to the face and eyes.

Basic directions: *Wash your hands first and then generously splash the face, including the eyes, with tepid water (not hot or cold). Once the face is soaking wet, take your cleanser and massage it generously all over the face, including the eyelids. Rinse very well. If traces of makeup are left behind, or if you have very oily skin, you may need to repeat this step. Another option is to first cleanse the eye area and rinse, then do the rest of the face separately and rinse again. Do this step twice a day or whenever you need to clean the face, whether or not you are wearing makeup. Using a washcloth might prevent water from being splashed all around the sink, but washcloths can cause irritation, and that's not great for the skin.*

What About Bar Soap?

I never recommend bar soap from the neck up, and suggest avoiding it from the neck down if you have problems with dry skin or breakouts. There are problems with using most bar soaps or bar cleansers no matter what type of skin you have. Actually, I don't have to tell you that, because those of you who have used bar soap—and most of you have—already know it can dry and irritate the skin. Even those of you who feel you can use soap without any problems, keep in mind that the skin can be irritated even without an associated skin reaction, and high-pH soaps can encourage bacteria growth.

Many women believe that the tight sensation they feel after washing with soap means that the face is clean. You know the feeling I'm talking about—where if you open your mouth it pulls the skin around your eyes? The thinking is that the more squeaky-clean your face feels, the better off you are! But that feeling you associate with being clean is nothing more than irritated, dried-out skin. The difficulty with asking someone to break a soap habit is that soap really does clean the skin thoroughly. Unfortunately, it cleans too thoroughly, and that can be irritating! If your skin feels tight for more than two minutes after you wash, you have to run to your moisturizer to prevent it from feeling pulled or taut; if you have oily skin, the oil resurfaces in seconds no matter how clean you felt initially; if you have combination skin, you reinforce that dual condition.

The major reason that soap—all soaps and bar cleansers—can be a problem is because of the ingredients. Almost always the main ingredients in soap are lard or fats (tallowate or some other hard wax that can clog pores is used to keep the bar in its bar form), alkaline cleansing ingredients (sodium cocoate and potassium hydroxide, which are very drying), and/or detergent cleansers (also potentially drying). **Simply put, lard can make you break out, alkaline cleansers and some detergent cleansers can be irritating, and a high pH can foment bacteria; all those consequences can cause breakouts and create dry skin.** According to an article in *Cosmetics & Toiletries* magazine in December 1996, "Studies have shown that washing with a [cleanser that has] a pH 7 [or higher, which is true for most bar soaps and bar cleansers] increases the presence of propionobacteria acne [acne-causing bacteria] significantly when compared to using a cleanser with a pH 5 [more likely in a liquid-form cleanser]."

What about specialty soaps that come in clear bars, have non-soap-sounding names, or contain creams and emollients that appear to have none of the properties of regular soap? All the soaps I've looked at—including Purpose, Aveeno (oatmeal soaps), Pears, Basis, Neutrogena, and Ivory—contain sodium tallowate (can clog pores) and sodium cocoate (strong detergent cleansing agent). So much for specialty soaps being different. Even worse, the soaps designed for oily or acned skin contain even harsher ingredients. Soaps designed for dry and sensitive skin often contain ingredients such as glycerin, petrolatum (mineral oil), or vegetable oil, which might make the face feel somewhat less stiff after you rinse, but won't prevent the irritation caused by the other ingredients.

Don't go by whether the bar soap or cleanser is clear or whether it is labeled as "French milled" (a soap-making process that improves the texture of the soap but has nothing to do with its effectiveness). You need to know what the soap is made of, and you can get that information only from the ingredient list.

Here's a rundown of some basic categories of soaps. Remember, just because a product is advertised as gentle doesn't mean it is.

- *Castile soaps* use olive oil instead of animal fat, but the cleansing agent, sodium hydroxide, is still fairly irritating to the skin.
- *Transparent soaps* like Neutrogena look milder or less drying because of their unclouded, pure appearance, but many contain harsh cleansing ingredients, and the ingredients that give the bar its shape can clog pores.

- *Deodorant soaps* are always irritating for the face and should be used only on other body parts, if at all. The ingredients used to reduce bacteria are too harsh for the delicate skin of the face and they don't stay on the skin long enough to have any real disinfecting effect.
- *Acne soaps* often contain very irritating ingredients in addition to harsh cleansers that, especially when combined with other acne treatments, can super-irritate the skin. There is no reason to overclean the skin. Breakouts have nothing to do with how clean your skin is. Furthermore, if the acne cleanser contains antibacterial agents, their effect is washed down the drain before they can kill one germ.
- *Cosmetic soaps* or bar cleansers are sold at the cosmetics counters for more money than they are worth. Although these are advertised as being gentle or specially formulated, they are no better than or different from what you can buy at the drugstore. The irritating and pore-clogging ingredients are still included regardless of the price or claim.
- *Superfatted soaps* contain extra oils and fats that supposedly make them more gentle for the face. Basis Soap is one of the most popular superfatted specialty soaps. The extra glycerin, petrolatum, or beeswax in these soaps won't prevent irritation and can cause breakouts.
- *Oatmeal soaps* are supposed to be better at absorbing oil and soothing sensitive skin than other soaps or bar cleansers. There are studies demonstrating that oatmeal can have anti-irritant properties. How that translates into a bar cleanser is unknown, but the benefits are probably nonexistent given the amount of time the oatmeal is actually on the skin and the presence of other irritating ingredients.
- *"Natural" soaps* are those that contain vitamins, fruits, vegetables, plants, flowers, herbs, aloe, and specialty oils; these ingredients are gimmicks and serve no purpose on the face. They don't nourish the skin or provide any other health benefits. This is sheer marketing whimsy and nothing more. Plus, the cleansing agents and the ingredients that keep the soap in bar form are the same as in any other bar cleanser.
- *Beauty bars* such as Dove are about 50% sodium cocoyl isethionate (a form of coconut oil); although not as irritating as other cleansing agents found in soaps, it is still potentially irritating and drying, especially in such a high concentration. Dove claims to be moisturizing, and it does contain emollients to help soften the effect of the cleansing agent. If the manufacturers left out the drying and irritating ingredients altogether, they wouldn't need to add emollients to counteract them. Also, the ingredients that help the bar keep its shape can clog pores.

I wish I could recommend one soap over another, but I can't. Soaps and bar cleansers in all forms can still cause irritation and dryness for most skin types, and potentially clog pores. If soap must be part of your personal skin-care regimen, consider using it only at night, and in the morning use one of the water-soluble cleansers I recommend.

What Do Toners Tone?

All toners, no matter what they are called—astringents, fresheners, pore cleansers, clarifying lotions, Sea Breeze, or witch hazel—and no matter who makes them—Borghese, Estee Lauder, or Oil of Olay—are bad for the skin if they contain irritants, and that is true for all skin types. The only toners, astringents, clarifying lotions, fresheners, and pore cleansers you should ever consider using are those that are as irritant-free as possible.

In the past, the primary ingredient in most toners—even many of those designed for dry skin—was usually SD alcohol[2] with a number following it. That's ethanol alcohol—the kind you would never put on a cut or wound, the kind that is a known irritant. In order for an astringent containing alcohol to be an effective disinfectant, it needs to be 60% to 70% pure alcohol. Most astringents are in the 20% range. Even at a 40% level, you would not be getting an effective disinfectant, although you would be getting an effective irritant that kills skin cells and destroys the skin's intercellular layer.

Other irritating ingredients found in toner-type products include acetone (that's nail polish remover), citrus (lemon, grapefruit, and orange juice are incredibly irritating to the skin because of their high acid content), camphor, mint, peppermint, menthol, plant extracts, volatile oils (essential oils, which are nothing more than fragrance additives), and witch hazel. All of these ingredients can hurt the skin because of irritation or skin sensitivity, and should be avoided.

The funny thing—well, maybe not so funny—is that, regardless of the price category, all toners that contain alcohol are astoundingly similar. Water and alcohol, some coloring agents, a few plants, slip agents, and maybe a soothing agent (which won't counteract the irritation from the alcohol, but it's a nice try) are not what I would call exotic. But regardless of the price tag, alcohol irritates the skin, and that is never beneficial.

What do toners, astringents, and the rest of them tone? I have no idea. I'm not sure what the term "tone" means and neither is the cosmetics industry. If it's

---

[2] Do not be confused by cosmetics that contain ingredients that sound like alcohol but are not. For example, cetyl alcohol and alcohol esters are not the type of alcohol I'm warning you about. Remember, the ingredient list will say "SD alcohol" followed by a number. That's the kind to avoid.

about toning skin, what process is that? The term "toner" is a caprice invented by the cosmetics industry and therefore can mean anything they want it to. I have heard that toners do everything from balance the skin and close pores to deep-clean and prepare the skin for other products. They do none of that. In fact, astringents and toners do not close pores; they do not deep-clean pores; and they do not reduce oil production.

If a toner contains irritants, all irritation does to a pore is to temporarily swell it, which can make the pore look smaller for maybe a few minutes. Toners that contain alcohol can remove the surface oil from the skin, but if you've cleansed the skin properly there should be no surface oil left. You can't get inside the pore with a toner to deep-clean it without causing damage; if you could, we would all have spotless, empty pores, so toners surely don't work in that capacity. Most of all, toners do not reduce oil production. Oil production is controlled primarily by hormonal activity. In fact, because irritating ingredients can stimulate nerve endings and because nerve endings are attached to oil glands, toners can increase oil production, which can make pores larger. It is a vicious circle. Astringents and toners can worsen the very problem they are supposedly designed to handle.

So what about the many irritant-free toners on the market? They are fine as an extra cleansing step after removing the cleanser. They won't close pores and they won't deep-clean, but they will leave the face feeling soft and smooth, remove any last traces of makeup or oil, and soothe the skin. For some skin types, they can be the only moisturizer you need to use. That makes irritant-free toners a wonderful cleansing, lightweight moisturizing aid. What is in these products that makes them beneficial to the skin? Well-formulated toners usually are a blend of water, glycerin-type ingredients, soothing agents, water-binding agents, and anti-irritants. Too often, they are accompanied by a fancy price, fragrance (which negates the effects of the anti-irritants), and coloring agents, but there are reasonably priced toners that don't include fragrance or coloring agents. It is hard to find many skin-care products that don't include fragrance or coloring agents, but whenever possible pick those over the ones that do.

In my book *Don't Go to the Cosmetics Counter Without Me*, I provide a complete summary of the best toners for each skin type. Here are a few selections from that list:

For all skin types where the underlying condition is oily or combination skin, the best toners are: Aveda Skin Firming/Toning Agent; The Body Shop Honey Water and Tea Tree Oil Freshener; Lancome Tonique Douceur Non-Alcoholic Freshener for Dry/Sensitive Skin; L'Oreal Plenitude Hydrating Floral Toner; Mary Kay Gentle Action Freshener; Neutrogena Alcohol-Free Toner; Paula's Choice Final Touch Toner for Normal to Oily/Combination Skin.

For all skin types where the underlying condition is dry skin, the best toners are: The Body Shop Hydrating Freshener for Normal to Dry & Dry Skin, and Cucumber Water; Circle of Beauty Skin Refiner Dry Type 4, and Skin Refiner Dehydrated Type 5; Estee Lauder Verite Soothing Spray Toner; Nivea Alcohol Free Moisturizing Facial Toner; Origins Drenching Solution; Paula's Choice Final Touch Toner for Normal to Dry Skin; Physicians Formula Gentle Refreshing Toner for Dry to Very Dry Skin, and Purifying Facial Toner for Normal to Dry Skin.

Summary: Many irritant-free toners are a fine alternative as an extra cleansing step after removing the cleanser. They won't close pores and they won't deep-clean, but they will leave the face feeling soft and smooth, remove any last traces of makeup or oil, and soothe the skin. For some skin types, they can be the only moisturizer you need to use. That makes irritant-free toners a wonderful cleansing/moisturizing aid.

Basic directions: *After cleansing the face, soak a large cotton ball with the toner and gently stroke it over the face and neck.*

Note: The discussion of toners changes dramatically when the subject is how to decrease breakouts. In this case, the only reason to use a toner is if it provides disinfecting properties, eliminating the presence of the bacteria that cause most blemishes to be formed. For more information on this subject, see Chapter Six, "Special Battle Plans for Blemishes."

Exfoliating the Skin

As I've explained in Chapter Two, most skin-care professionals agree that many skin types benefit from exfoliation. During the 1970s the only way to exfoliate the skin was to use toners that contained alcohol and literally burned the skin cells off, leaving more dry skin in their wake. In the '80s the main choices were mechanical scrubs with ingredients such as honey and almond pits, cleansers with scrub particles, facial masks, and more irritating toners. Most of these options worked well enough, but they took a toll on the face and irritation was a typical problem. When it comes to mechanical scrubs, my favorite recommendation was and still is mixing Cetaphil Cleanser with baking soda to create an effective, gentle, and extraordinarily inexpensive scrub. Other mechanical scrubs, with their detergent cleansing agents and wax bases, just can't compare.

Nowadays, with the advent of alpha hydroxy acid, beta hydroxy acid, retinoic acid (found in Retin-A and Renova), Azelaic Acid, and Differin (adapelene), Cetaphil and baking soda are at the bottom of my list as a choice for exfoliating the skin. AHA, BHA, retinoic acid, Azelaic Acid, and Differin all exfoliate the skin chemically instead of physically, which is more thorough and even, with less physical damage to the skin, so the need for mechanical exfoliation has gone by the wayside and I recommend using it only occasionally, if at all.

I provide a complete summary of the best exfoliants for each skin type in my book *Don't Go to the Cosmetics Counter Without Me.* Here are a few selections from that list:

For all skin types where the underlying condition is oily skin, the best alpha hydroxy acid (AHA) products are: Alpha Hydrox Extra Strength Oil-Free Formula 10% AHA; Elizabeth Arden Alpha-Ceramide; M.D. Formulations Facial Lotion with 12% Glycolic Compound; Paula's Choice 8% Alpha Hydroxy Acid Solution.

For all skin types where the underlying condition is dry skin, the best AHA products are: Alpha Hydrox Enhanced Creme All Skin Types 10% AHA, Sensitive Skin Creme 5% AHA, Lotion for Normal to Dry Skin 8% AHA; Avon Anew Perfecting Complex for the Face; M.D. Formulations Smoothing Complex with 10% Glycolic Compound; Murad Advanced Skin Smoothing Lotion; Neostrata Skin Smoothing Cream, and Skin Smoothing Lotion; Pond's Age Defying Complex.

For all skin types with a tendency to breakouts where the underlying concern is dry skin, the best and only beta hydroxy acid (salicylic acid) product available as this book goes to press is: Oil of Olay Age Defying Daily Renewal Cream.

For all skin types with a tendency to breakouts where the underlying concern is oily skin, the best and only beta hydroxy acid (salicylic acid) products are: Almay Time Off Revitalizer Daily Solution, Time Off Daily Solution Pads; and Paula's Choice 1% BHA Solution for All Skin Types. (Please note that the option of using BHA in specific concentrations and pH to treat breakouts and blackheads is quite new and there aren't many alternatives available yet that meet the requirements for effective exfoliation.)

Summary: For oily skin, one of the ways to keep pores from getting clogged is to help skin cells shed as freely as possible so they don't get trapped inside the pore. The more you keep skin cells exfoliating in a normal manner, the less cell debris can fill up the pore and obstruct oil flow out of the pore.

Helping dry skin shed excess dried-up skin cells can make room for plumper, moisture-filled skin cells to come to the surface, which can lend a fresher look to the skin. It also allows moisturizer (the less and lighter, the better) to more easily penetrate the skin because there are fewer dried-up skin cells in the way to block absorption. Exfoliating helps the dead surface skin cells to slough off at a more normal rate to make room for the lower layers of newer skin cells.

If you decide to use a reliable AHA product for sun-damaged skin, or a BHA product for breakouts, or a prescription exfoliant such as Retin-A, Renova, Azelaic Acid, or Differin for either breakouts or sun-damaged skin, the question is, do you still need to use a physical scrub? There is no definitive answer, so you will have to judge for yourself. Most women with normal to dry, sensitive, allergic, mature, or normal skin should use one, and only one, exfoliant and no other. Someone with normal to oily skin with breakouts can use a BHA product, Retin-A, Azelaic Acid, or Differin and may occasionally use a scrub on areas that break out. Stick with Cetaphil Cleanser and baking soda for the most gentle results and listen closely to your skin; irritation is never the goal.

(The only skin types that need to stay away from exfoliating are those with extremely sensitive skin, thin skin, and skin diseases or disorders such as rosacea, eczema, dermatitis, or seborrhea, unless approved by a dermatologist.)

Basic directions: *After cleansing and toning, when the skin is dry, place a small amount of AHA, BHA, Retin-A, Renova, Azelaic Acid, or Differin on your fingertips and smooth over the entire face, avoiding direct contact with the eyes. First-time users who have sensitive skin should apply it once a day (preferably at night). Depending on your skin's tolerance, you may even want to apply it once a day, every other day. If the exfoliant you choose isn't in an emollient base or isn't emollient enough, apply a moisturizer over dry areas. In the morning, apply sunscreen after applying the exfoliant.*

If you started out using the chemical exfoliant once a day or every other day, after four weeks you can start increasing usage to twice a day.

Some dermatologists recommend that after a period of time you alternate treatment for sun-damaged skin by using AHA or Renova (the two best suited for sun-damaged skin). They suggest using it regularly every day for six months and then going one month on and one month off to prevent skin exhaustion.

If you are using an alkaline cleanser such as bar soap (which you shouldn't be, but just in case you are), wait 15 minutes before applying any chemical exfoliant, because the high pH of the cleanser can affect the acidity of the exfoliant.

Sunscreen

Regardless of the time of year, where you live, the color of your skin, or the amount of time you spend in the sun, sunscreen should be an essential part of your morning skin-care routine. It takes only a few minutes in the sun—the time it takes to walk to your car or to your office—for sun damage to begin. Over time this can cause serious wrinkling, even if you don't tan on a regular basis.

There are several ways to fit this vital skin-care step into your daily routine. **Most sunscreens come in a moisturizing base, which means you most likely do not need any additional moisturizer if you have dry skin. A wide variety of sunscreens with moisturizers are available.** As long as the product includes avobenzone, titanium dioxide, or zinc oxide, it is a fine choice. Unfortunately, there are very few sunscreens for someone with oily or combination skin. (See Chapter Three, "Sun Sense," for a list of the sunscreens I like best.)

Basic directions: *Sunscreen is the last thing you apply to the skin during the day. It comes after the cleanser, toner, disinfectant, chemical exfoliant (AHA, BHA, Retin-A, Renova, Azelaic Acid, or Differin), and skin-lightening product (if you use one). If you have very dry skin and feel the moisturizer in your sunscreen is not enough, you can apply a moisturizer over the drier areas and then apply sunscreen over that.*

Moisturizing

If you have dry skin, dry, wrinkled skin, or dry areas (like on the cheeks or around the eyes), you need a moisturizer; otherwise you don't. It's that simple, despite the contortions the cosmetics industry goes through to make moisturizing the skin more complicated and insanely expensive.

Always use the lightest moisturizer capable of making your skin feel soft without feeling greasy or layered. There are more wonderful moisturizers available than bad ones. They contain a vast array of emollients, water-binding ingredients, soothing agents, anti-irritants, and antioxidants, in a dizzying range of permutations with an equally dizzying range of prices. Unfortunately, there is no one formula I can point to as the best one, so don't let the cosmetics industry convince you such a thing exists. It turns out there are hundreds and hundreds of great moisturizers and very few poor ones.

The worst thing about moisturizers is they are often overpriced and erroneously labeled as wrinkle creams, firming lotions, serums, and lord knows what else to make them seem more exotic and miraculous than they really are. While women the world over search for the best wrinkle creams, you can be ahead of the game, taking better care of your skin, by either leaving this step out altogether (because you now know that overmoisturizing the skin is bad) or by using a great but inexpensive moisturizer that can do the job as well as, if not better than, the expensive stuff. Strangely enough, the expensive stuff almost always has too much fragrance (which can cause allergic reactions or irritation), too many plants (and therefore a higher risk of skin reactions), and coloring agents (products sell better if they look pretty, even if the result isn't better for the skin), all of them bad news for the skin.

The only thing that distinguishes a daytime moisturizer from a nighttime moisturizer is the inclusion of sunscreen. All the other claims and descriptions explaining why daytime products are different from nighttime products are bogus. Make sure your daytime moisturizer is rated SPF 15 and contains the active ingredients avobenzone, titanium dioxide, and/or zinc oxide. There are awesome moisturizers with sunscreen available, and more are being created all the time that meet the new FDA guidelines for UVA protection. Don't ignore moisturizers from companies that specialize in sun-care products, such as Coppertone or Bain de Soleil; these types of companies all have good sunscreens in moisturizing bases that are inexpensive and superior for daily use.

At night almost any moisturizer will do, depending on your skin type. Always use the lightest formula possible and only over dry areas. There is no reason to apply moisturizer where the skin isn't dry.

More than 100 excellent moisturizers are listed in my book *Don't Go to the Cosmetics Counter Without Me.* Refer to that summary to see if the moisturizer you are interested in has an acceptable formulation for your skin type. Here are a few of my favorites: Cetaphil Moisturizer; Eucerin Light; L'Oreal Hydra Renewal; Lubriderm Seriously Sensitive Skin Moisturizer; Nutraderm; Paula's Choice Completely Emollient Moisturizer; Revlon Results Line Diminishing Serum.

Basic directions: *During the day follow the directions for applying the sunscreen, because if you have dry skin that's your daytime moisturizer. At night, over clean, dry, or slightly damp skin, sparingly apply the moisturizer over dry areas. Dab it on and let it be absorbed; don't rub it in (rubbing isn't good for the skin). At night, moisturizer is the last thing you apply. If you are using an AHA or BHA product in an emollient base or using Renova, which comes in a moisturizing base (Azelaic Acid and Differin do not come in moisturizing bases), that would be the last thing you apply and probably the only moisturizer your skin needs. If you feel some areas of your face need a little more moisturizer, apply that to the drier areas of the face after you've applied the AHA, BHA, Renova, Retin-A, Azelaic Acid, or Differin.*

What About Eye Creams?

I know this is going to sound shocking, but there is absolutely no reason to use a separate eye cream, lotion, or gel for the skin around the eye. Despite what the cosmetics industry tells you about special ingredients or formulations, most all face products can be used around the eye. Although the eye area is a more delicate, fragile part of the face, the product formulations for eye creams don't differ from the face products.

You might want to use a different product around the eyes if the skin there happens to indeed be different from the rest of the face. For example, my face is normal to oily and doesn't require a moisturizer except occasionally on my cheeks. But the skin around my eyes tends to get dry and wrinkled-looking, and it looks much better after I apply an emollient moisturizer. I use my own Paula's Choice Completely Emollient Moisturizer around my eyes every night and during the day, and also on my cheeks when they're dry. Because my foundation contains sunscreen and I apply foundation over my eye area, I don't need to use a separate sunscreen product around my eyes or cheeks during the day.

Some women don't like the texture of an emollient moisturizer around their eyes, and in those instances a lightweight gel or lotion is just fine. If your foundation or concealer doesn't contain sunscreen, then the daytime moisturizer you use must be rated SPF 15.

How to Handle Skin Problems

The best way to handle a skin problem is to prevent it and then not make it worse. Be sure to get all your makeup off gently but thoroughly every night, and eliminate products that irritate your skin or cause allergic reactions.

Dry Patches

There are many reasons why skin can develop dry patches. Makeup left on overnight, allergic reactions, drying skin-care products, dermatitis, eczema, and heavy moisturizers can all cause dry patches of skin. Avoid drying skin-care products, and use only the lightest-weight moisturizer to handle dry skin areas.

If the dry patches are chronic or itchy, they are probably a topical dermatitis or eczema and may require treatment by a dermatologist. If you've done your best to eliminate whatever is causing the problem and the problem persists, one of the best ways to calm down the appearance of dry patches is with an over-the-counter cortisone cream. Lanacort and Cortaid are 1% hydrocortisone creams meant for short-term use only over dry patches of skin. It is amazing how effective they can be. If the problem lingers, consult a dermatologist, but for many people this is all it takes.

Dry Underneath and Oily on Top

The combination of a layer of dry skin below skin that feels oily or greasy is almost always caused by using the wrong skin-care products. Using a greasy wipe-off cleanser, a toner that is too emollient for your skin type, and an unnecessarily emollient moisturizer can prevent the lower layer of skin from exfoliating, creating a thick, dry, flaky lower layer and a greasy layer on top. Conversely, if you have oily skin, using a drying face cleanser, a toner with irritating or drying ingredients, and then a moisturizer can also create this uncomfortable combination. The condition of dry skin underneath and oily skin on top rarely requires additional skin-care products; instead, take a completely different approach of eliminating rather than adding products. Following my general skin-care recommendations should take care of all this without having to add extra products to your routine. Adding extra products without taking care of the underlying problem would only make things worse.

It is also possible that the dry layer covered by an oily layer could be a result of psoriasis, rosacea, seborrhea, or eczema. Review Chapter Four's sections on those skin disorders before you make a final determination concerning the problems you are experiencing. In those instances you need a dermatologist's help.

Fade Away Brown Spots!

Changes in skin color, called chloasma or melasma, can happen for several reasons. One repercussion of sun damage is areas of skin discoloration known as solar lentigenes, more popularly called liver spots, sun spots, or age spots. They are definitely not associated with the liver, but they have everything to do with unprotected sun exposure. On lighter skin types, solar lentigenes emerge as small brown patches of freckling that grow over time. On women with darker skin tones, they appear as small patches of ashen-gray skin that tend to enlarge over time.

Brown or ashen patches of skin can also occur due to birth control pills, pregnancy, or estrogen replacement therapy. In those instances the discoloration is referred to as pregnancy masking or hormone masking.

Regardless of the source, the issue is the same: site-specific, increased melanin production, or hyperpigmentation. Melanin is the pigment or coloring agent of skin. For some reason, melanin production can get carried away and create brown or ashen areas of skin, especially on the face.

An important factor in terms of selecting treatment is the depth of the discolored pigment within the skin. In most situations the discoloration is superficial. In a few cases, the discoloration lies deep in the dermis. If the pigment is in the epidermis, it can be helped with lightening products, both over-the-counter and prescription.

Understandably, pigment deep in the dermis does not respond well to topical agents. Resurfacing procedures such as chemical peels and laser treatments may help some of these problems, but the results are not consistent and often end up looking worse, particularly for those with darker skin tones.

If the hyperpigmentation is mostly superficial, a lot can be done to lighten the discoloration. Women of all colors can work on hyperpigmentation (especially sun-damage spots and ashy or brown patches of skin) with over-the-counter skin-lightening products that contain between 1% and 2% hydroquinone. Hydroquinone inhibits the production of melanin, which can lighten areas of hyperpigmentation. Hydroquinone does not bleach the skin (calling it a bleaching agent is a misnomer); it only disrupts the synthesis of melanin hyperpigmentation. Many skin-lightening products also contain AHAs and/or BHA, which exfoliate the skin, helping to remove the old built-up layers of melanin. New skin-lightening agents such as kojic acid and song yi acid also help hydroquinone to inhibit melanin hyperproduction.

Some doctors feel that 2% hydroquinone lotions can be more effective when combined with Retin-A or Renova. Higher strengths of hydroquinone (over 2%) are available only from a physician and can possibly reach deeper sources of pigment discoloration. However, higher concentrations of hydroquinone should be approached with caution and require attention from an informed physician. According to an article by Dr. Robert Goldemberg in the February 1997 issue of *Drug & Cosmetic Industry* magazine, the treatment given to some women of color by their dermatologists to reduce hyperpigmentation can actually cause more intense discolorations. Dr. Goldemberg states that studies show "long-term use of hydroquinone at concentrations above 4% can lead to hyperpigmentation."

Depending on the severity of the skin discoloration, you can try an over-the-counter skin-lightening product that utilizes the ingredients mentioned above or you can seek a more potent hydroquinone prescription from a dermatologist. If you choose the latter route, look for a dermatologist who understands the problem of high-concentration hydroquinone products and can perhaps steer you in a different direction, namely, lesser concentrations of hydroquinone along with Retin-A or Renova (tretinoin).

Of course, using skin-lightening products without also using a sunscreen is a waste of time. Sun exposure stimulates melanin production, and that helps maintain the status quo. It is essential to use a good sunscreen with UVA- and UVB-blocking ingredients to prevent the production of more melanin.

My skin-care line has a product called Paula's Choice Remarkable Skin Lightening Lotion. Black Opal, a line of skin-care and makeup products developed for African-American women, also has two skin-lightening products. Both Black Opal skin-lightening products are appropriate for any woman looking to lighten hyperpigmentation spots or areas. Black Opal Advanced Dual Phase Fade Cream is a 2% hydroquinone cream in an emollient moisturizing base. It also contains an anti-irritant, which can be helpful with hydroquinone products. Black Opal Dual Complex Fade Gel is a 2% hydroquinone gel that also contains about 6% AHA and an anti-irritant. This one is best for someone with normal to oily skin, but it can also be worn under a more emollient moisturizer and used by any skin type.

More Than One Skin Type

The cosmetics industry uses the term "combination skin" to denote skin that is dry in some places (usually the cheeks, eyes, and jaw areas), but oily in other places (usually the nose, forehead, and chin). Indeed, many women have this type of combination skin, which isn't surprising because the center of the face has the most oil glands, while the sides and eyes have almost none. Yet as far as I am concerned, and as far as you should be concerned, combination skin refers to the presence of two or more differing skin types on your face. For example, you may have dry skin on your forehead and cheeks, patches of eczema on your chin and jaw, and breakouts or blackheads on your nose and forehead. Another example of combination skin might involve dry areas around the eyes but oily skin with breakouts on the rest of the face. The combinations are almost endless.

Whatever is happening to your skin indicates the direction you should follow. If your cheeks are dry and your forehead is breaking out, do not use the same products on both. It's that simple.

Your skin-care needs may change depending on the time of year or the climate you find yourself in. **Respond to what you see or feel on your face and change what you are doing, always keeping in mind that what you are experiencing might be caused by the skin-care products you are using.** If the latter is the case, adapt accordingly. For example, the cleanser you are using may be fine in a humid, temperate environment, but it may be too drying for an arid, hot climate. It will take some experimentation to find what feels best for your skin in different situations, always paying attention to what works and what doesn't. You can always refer to my book *Don't Go to the Cosmetics Counter Without Me* to see if the product you are using could be causing your skin problems.

Skin-Care Plans for All Skin Types

The following list is a fairly comprehensive compilation of the most effective skin-care routines for different skin types. **Remember, before you choose a routine for your specific skin type, you must determine if what you are seeing or feeling on your skin is being caused by the skin-care products you are presently using.**

In the following list I use the term "mature skin" to refer to skin that has started to show signs of wrinkling. "Older skin" refers to skin that has become thin and fragile. The term "basic normal skin" includes skin that shows no signs of aging or sun damage. "Normal skin" is skin with few or no open pores, no excess oil, no breakouts, and no dryness. Those struggling with blemishes, breakouts, and blackheads should refer to the information and skin-care routines outlined in Chapter Six, "Special Battle Plans for Blemishes."

Exception to the rule: Although it is best to treat only what is happening with your skin, some skin-care problems require consistency even when the problem is not present on the face. If you tend to break out, or have psoriasis, rosacea, or seborrhea, consistency is essential. For breakouts you must use an exfoliant and disinfectant daily in order to see a continuing difference. I explain in Chapter Six, "Special Battle Plans for Blemishes," why you can't spot-treat blemishes. For psoriasis, rosacea, or seborrhea, the same issue of consistent treatment is paramount even when the problem isn't present.

Basic normal skin

A.M.

1. Water-soluble cleanser
2. Toner (optional)
3. Sunscreen in a lightweight or matte base (rated SPF 15 with avobenzone, titanium dioxide, and/or zinc oxide)

P.M.

1. Water-soluble cleanser
2. Toner (optional)
3. Lightweight moisturizer (only over dry patches and around the eyes)

Mature normal skin

A.M.

1. Water-soluble cleanser
2. Toner (optional)
3. AHA product in a moisturizing base and/or Renova (if using both, apply the Renova at night)
4. Sunscreen (rated SPF 15 with avobenzone, titanium dioxide, and/or zinc oxide in a lightweight moisturizing base)

P.M.

1. Water-soluble cleanser
2. Toner (optional)
3. AHA in a moisturizing base and/or Renova (if using both, apply the Renova at night)
4. Moisturizer for dry areas, including the eyes

Basic oily skin

A.M.

1. Water-soluble cleanser
2. Topical disinfectant (if breakouts are present)
3. AHA product in a gel base (if breakouts are present, a BHA product in a gel or liquid base is another option)

4. Sunscreen (preferably in a foundation rated SPF 15 with avobenzone, titanium dioxide, and/or zinc oxide)

P.M.

1. Water-soluble cleanser
2. Toner (optional)
3. AHA product in a gel base (if breakouts are present, a BHA product in a gel or liquid base is another option)
4. Moisturizer (for dry areas only, including the eyes)
5. Facial mask of milk of magnesia (at least twice a week)

Basic dry skin

A.M.

1. Water-soluble cleanser
2. Moisturizing toner
3. AHA product in a moisturizing base, or Renova (if using both, apply Renova at night)
4. Sunscreen in a moisturizing base (rated SPF 15 with avobenzone, titanium dioxide, and/or zinc oxide)

P.M.

1. Water-soluble cleanser
2. Moisturizing toner
3. AHA product in a moisturizing base, or Renova (if using both, apply Renova at night)
4. Moisturizer (if needed, over dry areas and around the eyes)

Basic oily and dry skin

A.M.

1. Water-soluble cleanser
2. Topical disinfectant (if breakouts are present, only over those areas)
3. AHA product in a gel base (if breakouts are present, a BHA product in a gel or liquid base is another option)
4. Moisturizer (for dry areas only, including the eyes)
5. Sunscreen (preferably in a foundation rated SPF 15 with avobenzone, titanium dioxide, and/or zinc oxide)

P.M.

1. Water-soluble cleanser
2. AHA product in a gel base (if breakouts are present, a BHA product in a gel or liquid base is another option)
3. Moisturizer (for dry areas only, including the eyes)
4. Facial mask of milk of magnesia (at least once a week, only over oily areas)

Mature dry skin

A.M.

1. Water-soluble cleanser
2. Moisturizing toner
3. AHA product in a moisturizing base
4. Sunscreen in a moisturizing base (rated SPF 15 with avobenzone, titanium dioxide, and/or zinc oxide)

P.M.

1. Water-soluble cleanser
2. Moisturizing toner
3. Renova
4. Moisturizer (if needed, over dry areas and around the eyes)

Very dry skin

A.M.

1. Water-soluble cleanser
2. Moisturizing toner
3. AHA product in a moisturizing base
4. Sunscreen in a moisturizing base (rated SPF 15 with avobenzone, titanium dioxide, and/or zinc oxide)
5. A more emollient moisturizer (if needed, apply after the sunscreen over the driest areas)

P.M.

1. Water-soluble cleanser
2. Moisturizing toner
3. Renova
4. Moisturizer (if needed, over dry areas and around the eyes)

Older dry skin

A.M.

1. Water-soluble cleanser
2. Moisturizing toner
3. AHA product in a moisturizing base
4. Sunscreen in a moisturizing base (rated SPF 15 with avobenzone, titanium dioxide, and/or zinc oxide)
5. A more emollient moisturizer (if needed, apply after the sunscreen over the driest areas)

P.M.

1. Water-soluble cleanser
2. Moisturizing toner
3. Renova
4. Moisturizer (if needed, over dry patches and around the eyes)

Sensitive/allergy-prone oily skin

A.M.

1. Water-soluble cleanser
2. Over-the-counter cortisone cream (only when irritation or skin reactions occur)
3. Topical disinfectant (over breakouts)
4. Sunscreen (preferably in a foundation rated SPF 15 with titanium dioxide and/or zinc oxide; there are none yet with avobenzone)

P.M.

1. Water-soluble cleanser
2. Over-the-counter cortisone cream (only when irritation or skin reactions occur)
3. Lightweight moisturizer (over dry patches or around the eyes)
4. Facial mask of milk of magnesia (at least once a week, if the skin can handle it)

Sensitive/allergy-prone dry skin

A.M.

1. Water-soluble cleanser
2. Over-the-counter cortisone cream (only when irritation or skin reactions occur)

3. Sunscreen in a lightweight moisturizing base (rated SPF 15, preferably one with titanium dioxide and/or zinc oxide; there are none yet with avobenzone)

P.M.

1. Water-soluble cleanser
2. Over-the-counter cortisone cream (only when irritation or skin reactions occur)
3. Lightweight moisturizer (over dry patches or around the eyes)
4. Facial mask of milk of magnesia (at least once a week, if the skin can handle it)

Combination skin

Treat each area of your face according to what is happening.

Rosacea with oily, flaky skin

A.M.

1. Water-soluble cleanser
2. MetroGel or Azelaic Acid (two prescription-only topical creams designed to treat rosacea)
3. Sunscreen (preferably in a foundation rated SPF 15 with titanium dioxide and/or zinc oxide; there are none yet with avobenzone)

P.M.

1. Water-soluble cleanser
2. MetroGel or Azelaic Acid

Rosacea with dry, flaky skin

A.M.

1. Water-soluble cleanser (Cetaphil Lotion is excellent)
2. MetroGel or Azelaic Acid (two prescription-only topical creams designed to treat rosacea)
3. Sunscreen in a lightweight moisturizing base (rated SPF 15, preferably one with titanium dioxide and/or zinc oxide; there are none yet with avobenzone)

P.M.

1. Water-soluble cleanser
2. MetroCream or Azelaic Acid
3. Emollient moisturizer (for dry areas)

Seborrhea

A.M.

1. Water-soluble cleanser
2. BHA product and/or prescription steroids and coal tar lotions
3. Sunscreen in a lightweight moisturizing base (rated SPF 15, preferably one with titanium dioxide and/or zinc oxide; there are none yet with avobenzone)

P.M.

1. Water-soluble cleanser
2. BHA product and/or prescription steroids and coal tar lotions
3. Emollient moisturizer (for dry areas)

Psoriasis

A.M.

1. Water-soluble cleanser
2. BHA product or prescription steroids, anthralin, or coal tar (all prescribed by a dermatologist)
3. Sunscreen in a lightweight moisturizing base (rated SPF 15, preferably one with titanium dioxide and/or zinc oxide; there are none yet with avobenzone)

P.M.

1. Water-soluble cleanser
2. BHA product or prescription steroids, anthralin, or coal tar (all prescribed by a dermatologist)
3. Emollient moisturizer (for dry areas)

Any skin type with patches of dermatitis, eczema, or rashlike areas

A.M.

Follow the skin-care regime for your skin type. Before applying the appropriate sunscreen, apply an over-the-counter cortisone cream over inflamed areas only. (Lanacort and Cortaid are over-the-counter cortisone creams found at the drugstore.)

P.M.

Follow the skin-care regime for your skin type. Before applying the appropriate nighttime moisturizer, apply an over-the-counter cortisone cream over inflamed areas only. (Lanacort and Cortaid are over-the-counter cortisone creams found at the drugstore.)

Any skin type with brown or ashen skin discolorations

A.M.

Follow the skin-care regime for your skin type. Before applying the appropriate sunscreen, apply a thin layer of a skin-lightening lotion or gel over areas of the face, hands, and body with pigment discolorations. Finally, apply the sunscreen. (Please note that any skin-lightening product can be effective only if a reliable sunscreen is used.)

P.M.

Follow the skin-care regime for your skin type. Before applying the appropriate nighttime moisturizer (optional), apply a thin layer of a skin-lightening lotion over areas of the face, hands, and body with pigment discolorations. Finally, apply a moisturizer if needed.

Severe oily skin with breakouts

See Chapter Six.

Mature oily skin with breakouts

See Chapter Six.

Older dry skin with occasional breakouts

See Chapter Six.

Acned oily skin

See Chapter Six.

Acned dry skin

See Chapter Six.

Cystic acne

See Chapter Six.

CHAPTER SIX

Special Battle Plans for Blemishes

Understanding What Causes a Blemish

There's no way around it: one of the most worrisome and prevalent skin-care problems many of us suffer through at some time in our life is breakouts. Whether it's blackheads, whiteheads, the dreaded "p" word (pimples), or acne, most people have experienced the frustration of dealing with these commonplace skin imperfections. Regardless of your age (teenagers are not the only age group to suffer with breakouts), gender, or skin color, there are certain basics for fighting breakouts that are essential if you are going to have any chance of winning the battle.

In order to create a plan of action—and it does take an organized plan of action—it is essential to let go of the persistent, inaccurate information concerning blemishes and instead learn what can help your skin. You can't choose wisely if you don't know what you're fighting. If you don't understand all your options, focusing on what can work and what can't, you will run around in circles, often making the condition worse than it was to begin with, or finding temporary relief, only to have the problems show up time and time again.

First and foremost, you need to get over three myths about treating breakouts because they not only won't help you prevent or eliminate a blemish, but can cause a whole range of additional skin problems.

The first myth is the notion that you can dry up a blemish. Water is the only thing you can dry up, and a blemish has nothing to do with being wet. Skin cells do contain water, and when you dry up the skin you can cause it to flake, which won't stop breakouts but can lead to irritation and add another predicament to your skin-care woes. Blemishes can be aggravated by oil production, which needs to be reduced and/or absorbed. Absorbing oil on the skin or in the pore is a radically different process from drying up skin.

The second myth is that blemishes are caused by dirty skin. Unfortunately, this mistaken belief causes harsh overcleaning of the face with soaps and strong detergent cleansers. That only increases the risk of irritation and dryness, and doesn't do anything to prevent blemishes. Additionally, the ingredients in bar cleansers and soaps that keep them in their bar form can clog pores and actually cause breakouts. Not a pretty picture.

The third myth is that you can spot-treat blemishes. Sadly, lots of products are based on just this concept. Clearasil is probably the most popular product perpetuating the notion of zapping zits. Once you see a blemish, you can't zap it into oblivion in hopes of changing anything. By the time a blemish shows up on the surface of the skin, it has been at least two to three weeks in the making. It takes time for conditions in the pore to create a blemish. If you don't understand and learn how to deal with that somewhat lengthy process, there is no way for you to successfully tackle recurring breakouts. Dealing with only the blemishes you see means the blemishes that are forming won't be stopped.

Remember, you can't dry up a blemish because it isn't wet; irritating ingredients may stimulate more oil production; and you need to work on the cause of the blemish, not the aftermath.

Of course, there are things you can do to reduce the appearance of a blemish. You can use a mechanical scrub to open the surface of the lesion and help remove what's inside, and you can use a facial mask of milk of magnesia to reduce redness and irritation. But neither of those tactics will prevent other blemishes from being formed.

What truly causes breakouts? There are four major factors that contribute to the formation of blemishes:

1. **Hormonal activity**
2. **Overproduction of oil in the oil gland**
3. **Irregular or excessive shedding of dead skin cells**
4. **Buildup of bacteria in the pore**

Each hair follicle grows from a sebaceous (oil) gland that secretes an oily, firm wax (sebum is the technical name for this oil). This structure that the oil gland and hair follicle share is called the pilosebaceous duct or unit. When things are going well, the sebum smoothly exits the duct through an imperceptible pore and melts on the skin's surface, moisturizing and smoothing your face and body in the most natural, pure, and compatible way possible. When things aren't going well, when the hair follicle/sebaceous gland becomes plugged with sebum and bacteria run amok, a blemish is the outcome.

Surplus sebum is generated by hormone activity. When too much oil is produced, it can become mixed with dead skin cells from the skin's surface as well as poorly sloughed skin cells from the pore's lining and small pieces of hair debris from the follicle. This combination of sebum, dead skin cells, and small pieces of hair can clog the pathway out of the hair follicle/oil gland, creating quite a backup. Now you've got problems.

When your body produces too much sebum/oil, and dead skin cells or hair debris aren't shed normally, they can block the exit from a pore. All this excess solidifies as a soft, white substance. This plug then blocks the pore, causing the walls of the pilosebaceous duct to bulge and the surface to swell. If the surface of the pore is covered by skin, it is called a whitehead (this is not yet a pimple).

If the pore is open, without any skin covering, the top of the plug darkens when exposed to air, causing a blackhead.

Whiteheads or blackheads become pimples when the plug grows too big and the wall of the duct ruptures. *Propionibacterium acnes,* a kind of bacterium that normally lives inside the pore, invades the rupture and, along with the excess sebum, dead skin cells, and hair debris, causes infection. If the rupture takes place deep within the pore instead of closer to the surface of the skin, it forms boil-like infections called cystic acne.

This still leaves some pretty important questions unanswered. What causes the hormones to increase oil production, and can you slow it down? How do the skin cells build up and clog the pore, and how do you stop it from happening? Where did the bacteria that caused the infection come from, and how can you get rid of them? Who can break out or get acne, and why?

Why Me?

Why my skin? Why another blemish or blackhead? Why can't I have smooth, poreless skin? Why me? Believe me, I know this feeling.

Why do you suddenly at the age of 48 have blemishes? Why haven't you outgrown the blemishes and oily skin that have plagued you since you were 14, and at 28 are worse than ever? Why, at 35, do you have incessant blackheads and breakouts that won't go away no matter what you do, and you've done everything? Why do you still have acne when you're 18 and have tried oral antibiotics, Retin-A, sulfur masks, topical antibiotics, and every cosmetic skin-care routine imaginable? Regardless of how old you are, breakouts and oily skin are upsetting, and anyone can be a victim! The main culprit in all these scenarios is hormones, because hormones affect oil production, and hormones can rage out of control at different times of life.

Breaking out is definitely most prevalent in adolescence. Statistics suggest that three out of four teenagers have problems with breakouts and various forms of acne. That isn't surprising when you consider that adolescence is a time of colossal hormonal changes that stimulate sebaceous/oil glands and increase sebum/oil production, which increases the chances for breakouts. But acne can happen at any age. According to the *New England Journal of Medicine*'s publication *HealthNews,* one in five adults between the ages of 25 and 44 experiences acne, and it is estimated that nearly half of all adult women experience mild to moderate acne! Anything that raises hormone levels—stress, the menstrual cycle, pregnancy, birth control pills, or certain medications, such as corticosteroids—can produce blemishes. Androgens and progesterone, male sex hormones present in both males and females, are the main instigators. When hormones gush, blemishes can flare.

There is no question that hormone activity is responsible for oily skin and breakouts. However, hormones alone are not enough to create this annoying skin malady. For some unknown reason(s), something goes wrong in the oil gland, which is activated and made worse by the hormones. These unknown reasons are thought to be related to a genetic predisposition, creating either a defective sebaceous/oil gland, impaired skin and/or oil gland linings that don't shed properly, or the abnormal sebum/oil (too thick or too irritating to the skin). You have to address most, if not all, of these issues in order to reduce the chances of breakouts.

You Can't Zap Zits

Most of us have sought relief from the emotional pain and humiliation that often accompany acne, whether it is one blemish or many, by going to drugstores or cosmetics counters where acne products and skin-care regimes line the shelves. Myriad products promise clear skin, and several pledge to zap zits, dry up blemishes, and drink up oil. The commercials and ads sound fairly convincing, but a closer look reveals that these products can't zap zits or dry up oil (you can't dry up oil), much less stop either from occurring, and the irritation they cause can create more problems than they clear up.

These blemish products claim they are designed for skin that breaks out, offering choices for women with oily, dry, or sensitive skin. But when you read the ingredient lists, where the real information is, you find an array of ingredients that can make breakouts worse and cause problems for sensitive skin. Ingredients that show up repeatedly include alcohol; salicylic acid (also known as BHA, a peeling agent); benzoyl peroxide (a disinfectant); sulfur (a mild antiseptic); boric acid (a toxic antiseptic); and camphor, menthol, eucalyptus, and clove oils. All of these are potential skin irritants. Some of these ingredients do make sense, but which ones?

As I mentioned above, there are things you can do to reduce the redness and swelling, and to eliminate the contents of a blemish. You can use a mechanical scrub such as plain baking soda to open the surface of the lesion to help remove what's inside; you can use a facial mask of milk of magnesia to reduce redness and swelling; you can disinfect the skin to prevent bacteria from aggravating the lesion. But spot-treating only the blemish you see doesn't prevent other blemishes from being formed. It takes consistency (regularly exfoliating, disinfecting, and absorbing oil) to stop breakouts.

The best way to approach blemishes is from a factual basis. If you just pay attention to what you see on the surface without taking into consideration what is taking place underneath, you can't help heal the skin. Finding solutions that address each problem—hormonal activity, oil production, exfoliating the skin (and the pore), and killing the bacteria causing the infection—is the only course of action that makes sense. Focusing on the lesion without keeping the entire picture in mind can result in more breakouts, increased risk of scarring, and additional skin problems like redness, surfaced capillaries, irritation, and dry skin.

What You Can Do

Blemish treatments work by reducing sebum production, speeding up skin-cell turnover, and fighting bacterial infection. The best course of action for blackheads and whiteheads is to **clean the skin gently** (preferably with a water-soluble cleanser that doesn't contain ingredients that can clog pores or irritate the skin) to reduce further irritation and redness and to avoid stimulating more oil production; to **remove dead skin cells** from the skin's surface and inside the pore to help skin shed more normally (that's exfoliation); and to **absorb excess oil** (trying to dry it up can irritate the skin and cause more oil production). If blackheads and whiteheads are accompanied by pimples, you also have to **kill the bacteria** causing the eruption, inflammation, and swelling. The only way to kill bacteria is to disinfect the skin.

You'll need to experiment to discover exactly how to put together these various steps in a combination that works for you. Unfortunately, there isn't one absolutely right way. It is essential to try different options until you find what suits your skin type and your specific condition. If you stay consistent and avoid veering from your special battle plan, you stand a pretty good chance of winning a good part of the war against blemishes and blackheads. But the battle plan must deal with all of a blemish's properties.

There is little, if any, scientific evidence that diet affects acne, although food allergies certainly can, but that depends on what you personally are allergic to. Not everyone has the same food allergies. Likewise, drinking soda pop, smoking cigarettes, popping vitamins, and eating healthy or unhealthy foods will neither help nor hurt acne. Lots of Olympic-caliber athletes have acne-prone skin, and lots of people who smoke, don't exercise, and are overweight have a flawless complexion. However, if certain foods—such as nuts, shellfish (because of their iodine content), milk products, or wheat—seem to make your acne worse, it is best to avoid them one by one to see if it makes a long-term difference in your skin. Incidentally, fluoride in toothpaste can be the source of breakouts around the mouth. If this is a problem for you, transfer to a nonfluoride toothpaste and see if things improve. If indeed you are allergic to fluoride, consult with your dentist about alternative cavity-prevention treatments.

What You Shouldn't Do

What is most frustrating is that many of the blemish products on the market actually make breakouts worse or cause more skin problems than you started out with. Products designed to tackle acne often contain ingredients like alcohol, menthol, peppermint, camphor, and eucalyptus, lemon, or grapefruit oils. All of these ingredients are extremely irritating, and the resulting irritation can further stimulate an already stimulated oil gland.

What makes all these standard, obnoxious blemish ingredients worse is that they don't reduce any of the factors causing breakouts. They can't disinfect, reduce oil production, affect hormonal activity, or help exfoliation. Instead, they kill more skin cells than necessary, which can further clog pores, produce dry skin, cause irritation, and make skin redder. By the way, plants in acne products are also extremely problematic. Pimples are caused by the presence of bacteria in the pore, and plants can be a great food source for these microscopic critters.

A blemish by definition is already irritated, red, and swollen, so it doesn't make any sense to use ingredients that will make it even more irritated, red, and swollen.

Skin-care products with irritating ingredients, such as facial masks, astringents and toners, and facial scrubs (which also contain waxes), are a big no-no. These can all hurt the skin, which can aggravate acne. If a product irritates the skin, if it tingles or burns, it is not helping. And not only does irritation stimulate oil production, promote redness, increase swelling, and dry out the skin, it can also add small rashlike pimples to the breakouts you are already trying to deal with.

Bar soaps and bar cleansers are often recommended for acne, yet all of them contain ingredients that can clog pores. Soaps contain tallow, and bar cleansers contain other heavy, wax-based thickening agents that can clog pores. Shockingly, high-pH soaps and cleansers (a pH of 7) can increase the presence of bacteria in the pore! All this makes matters much worse inside the pore, and that greatly increases the risk of breakouts.

Oversqueezing, picking, digging, scraping, or poking at pimples may be hard to resist, and you may think it speeds healing, but in fact it sets you up for more problems. Bacteria from your hands or from a nonsterile needle or pin can easily get in your skin, leading to more pimples. Creating scabs and constantly reinjuring the lesion increases the likelihood of scarring. There is nothing wrong with gentle squeezing to remove a blemish's contents, but unless you are extremely careful you will create more problems than you started with.

Many women think they can use hot compresses to bring pimples to a head.

Actually, hot compresses severely damage skin by burning it; the heat stimulates oil production, which causes more redness and swelling; and the whole process can also rupture the pore, increasing the possibility of more breakouts. The same is true of steaming the face or using hot water. Hot water burns the skin, stimulates oil production, and causes dryness. Tepid water is what you need to help soothe the skin and calm things down. Use tepid water and a gentle water-soluble cleanser on the face, and do not wipe off makeup. Wiping and rubbing will make the irritation worse, and can also make the skin sag and cause wrinkles.

Finally, do not use moisturizers unless you absolutely have to, and then only where needed. Even if a moisturizer claims it is oil-free, use as little as possible. If your skin feels dry but you are still breaking out and have excess oil, the dryness is probably being caused by the other skin-care products you are using. Throwing moisturizers on top will only make matters worse because you are not doing anything to stop what is causing the dryness. And, regardless of the claims about what they contain, all moisturizers can clog pores.

Be careful that the breakouts you're struggling with aren't a result of hair products getting on the face. Hairspray, mousse, hair gel, and other styling products contain polymers (plasticlike, film-forming ingredients) that can easily clog pores and create something called folliculitis, an infection of the hair follicle. The treatment is the same as for any other type of blemish, but in order to make a difference with this one, you have to get the offending ingredient off the skin.

Oil-Free Is a Bad Joke

But the joke is on us, because "oil-free" is a meaningless claim and may mislead consumers into buying products that can clog pores. There are plenty of ingredients that don't sound like oils but can absolutely aggravate breakouts. **Almost all cosmetics contain waxlike thickening agents that are notorious for clogging pores.** Simple, standard moisturizing ingredients that are great for dry skin can wreak havoc on someone with oily skin or breakouts. Triglycerides, palmitates, stearates, myristates, stearic acid, plant oils (like jojoba oil), plant waxes, shea butter, vitamin E, acrylates, and many other ingredients can all clog pores. These ingredients are used in moisturizers because they duplicate the natural lipids (sebum/oil) in our skin, and that's great. But if you happen to be having problems with the sebum being created in your pores, adding more of the same kind of substance will only make things worse. Despite the problems these ingredients can cause, they show up in lots and lots of so-called "oil-free" products.

Above and beyond the claim of being oil-free, label after label promises that the product is "noncomedogenic" or "nonacnegenic." Most of us have bought products with this assurance, only to find that they did cause breakouts. The terms "noncomedogenic" and "nonacnegenic" have slowly but surely begun to replace "hypoallergenic" on cosmetics labels. Those are all meaningless marketing words, just like "oil-free." The ingredient list is the place to check out whether a product may put your skin at risk.

When to See a Dermatologist

Some women run to see a dermatologist the second they see a blemish. Others put it off well past the time that over-the-counter options have run out but breakouts are still rampant. Though there are many options for dealing successfully with breakouts outside the realm of prescription medications, if your acne is severe or chronic, it may indeed be best to seek medical attention. Dermatologists have in their arsenal a host of options that can more effectively reduce sebum production, create healthy skin-cell turnover, and fight bacterial infection.

However, it is completely acceptable to start with the options available at the drugstore (not the cosmetics counters) or from some specialty lines that pinpoint blemish problems. Many of these are quite similar to what a doctor would prescribe, such as salicylic acid products to exfoliate and benzoyl peroxide products to disinfect. If you select this course of action, it is essential to use only what you now know works and to use it consistently. If after a period of time you find those options don't work or aren't working as well as you would like, you can always make an appointment with a dermatologist.

It is important to mention that dermatologists have many options such as Retin-A, Differin, Azelaic Acid, topical antibiotics, and hormone blockers that basically have no real nonprescription counterpart. Dermatologists also have one option that can be an absolute cure for acne and breakouts. That option is Accutane. Accutane is a powerful, serious oral treatment for acne that can be nothing short of a miracle. Accutane can totally do away with breakouts, blackheads, and whiteheads, and significantly reduce or eliminate oil production, in 85% of the people who take it. Unfortunately, Accutane can also cause serious, frequently fatal birth defects in a fetus if a woman becomes pregnant while taking it. I discuss this issue in more detail later in this chapter.

Fighting Basics for Blemishes

The steps listed below address each of the factors that cause pimples. These are the best options for reducing oil production, the best options for disinfecting the skin, and the best options for improving exfoliation. Finding the combination that works for you is the goal, and then you must focus on hitting all the steps and doing them consistently. I will elaborate on each of the product types I recommend, but the menu approach is necessary because each piece plays a part in dealing with blemishes.

For example, if you choose plan A but find 3% hydrogen peroxide is not effective and you want to try something else, switch to another option for disinfecting blemishes, such as a benzoyl peroxide product or a prescription topical disinfectant. If you decide to try plan C but find Retin-A too irritating, switch to a different prescription exfoliant, such as Differin or Azelaic Acid. Eliminating one of these steps or changing to an ineffective product won't help your skin.

Cleaning the face: Using a water-soluble cleanser gently cleans your skin without stimulating the oil glands, increasing redness, or creating dryness. This step is standard for any skin-care routine because it makes an instant difference in the appearance and feel of the skin, and it is essential for reducing breakouts. Once you stop using drying, irritating, pore-clogging soaps or bar cleansers, and you realize how nice your skin feels when it is no longer dry and irritated, you will never go back to the old way again. Just be certain the water-soluble cleanser you select doesn't contain irritating ingredients and won't dry out the skin. (Check out the water-soluble cleansers recommended in Chapter Five, "Skin-Care Planning," or, for a more complete list, see Chapter Eight of my book *Don't Go to the Cosmetics Counter Without Me.)*

Disinfecting: There aren't many options when it comes to disinfecting the skin. Alcohol (when used in the right concentrations) and sulfur can be good disinfectants, but they are too drying and irritating. Other ingredients that repeatedly show up in products for problem skin, such as lemon, grapefruit, acetone, witch hazel, peppermint, menthol, eucalyptus, and camphor, have no effect at all on bacteria. Currently popular plant-derived disinfectants such as tea tree oil (melaleuca) are not present in high enough concentrations to reliably kill bacteria. For quite some time I have been recommending 3% hydrogen peroxide as a disinfectant, and it is a great starting point in your battle plan. If 3% hydrogen peroxide doesn't prove effective, the next option is benzoyl peroxide at a 2.5% strength, then 5%, and then 10%; to see what works best, begin with the lower strength and work up.

If those products fail, a topical antibiotic or even an oral antibiotic prescribed by a doctor may be the only option left to kill stubborn blemish-causing bacteria, but an oral antibiotic should be a last resort. Oral antibiotics can indeed kill blemish-causing bacteria, but they also kill good bacteria in the body, cause yeast infections, bring about stomach problems, and yellow the teeth. As bothersome and problematic as all those side effects are, the most serious side effect is that your body will adapt to the antibiotic. That means the antibiotic eventually will no longer be effective for fighting acne bacteria or any other bacterial infection you might get. That can pose a dangerous threat to your long-term health.

Exfoliating: Using an 8% alpha hydroxy acid (AHA) product or a 1% to 2% beta hydroxy acid (BHA) product is a crucial over-the-counter starting point for exfoliating the skin. If blemishes are present, I recommend using AHAs or BHA in gel or liquid form, because they are unlikely to contain waxy thickening agents or emollients that can clog pores. If you are seeing a physician, you will probably want to supplement this step with Retin-A, Differin, or Azelaic Acid (though Azelaic Acid is considered a better antibacterial disinfecting agent then an exfoliant). If so, you can use the AHA or BHA product during the day and the Retin-A, Differin, or Azelaic Acid at night. Some dermatologists recommend applying an AHA or BHA product first and then applying Retin-A, Differin, or Azelaic Acid directly over that. The thought is that the AHAs or BHA boosts the effectiveness and penetration of the other products. Again, experiment to see what works best for your skin. (Check out the exfoliants recommended in Chapter Five or, for a more complete list, see Chapter Eight of my book *Don't Go to the Cosmetics Counter Without Me.)*

Also, don't forget good old reliable baking soda as a mechanical exfoliant over breakouts and blemishes. It is not as gentle or as "smooth" an exfoliant as AHA, BHA, Retin-A, Differin, or Azelaic Acid, but many people still find it a handy option for removing dead skin cells and removing the surface of blemishes without damaging the skin.

Absorbing excess oil: While most people think clay masks are the only way to absorb excess oil on the skin, these are my last choice for that purpose. Using milk of magnesia as a facial mask is by far the best way to absorb oil I have ever found or personally used. Milk of magnesia is nothing more than liquid magnesium hydroxide, which is known to soothe skin and reduce irritation, and it has incredible oil-absorbing properties. Magnesium absorbs more oil than clay, and clay has no disinfecting or soothing properties. How often you use the milk of magnesia has to do with how oily your skin is. Some use it every day; others, once a week. Only you and your skin can determine what frequency works best for you.

When all else fails: If your breakouts persist after you've tried these over-the-counter and prescription options for gentle cleansing, disinfecting, exfoliating, and absorbing excess oil, it may be necessary to consider more serious drugs that can affect hormonal production, such as hormone blockers or birth control pills designed to reduce breakouts. Accutane is the last option in this lineup only because of its serious side effects if a woman becomes pregnant while using it (this issue is discussed in more detail later in this chapter).

The following battle plans are presented in order, starting with the most commonly available products with the least potential for side effects such as irritation, and working up to stronger products, some available only by prescription. The first battle plan may be all that is required to heal your skin. As you see how your skin responds, you can experiment with the various options for each category. **The most important element for all these skin-care battle plans is consistency. It takes a minimum of six weeks to six months to see a consistent improvement in your skin.** Remember, spot treatment doesn't work. You have to maintain consistent gentle cleansing, exfoliation, disinfection, and reduced oil production to change the way your skin behaves.

If irritation or skin sensitivity occurs, you may need to cut back on the exfoliant, disinfectant, and/or facial mask you are using. It doesn't mean the skin-care routine isn't or won't eventually work for you, but perhaps your skin can't handle the frequency of application, at least not in the beginning. In that case you may need to reduce how often you apply the AHA, Retin-A, or Differin from twice a day to once a day or every other day, and the same is true with the disinfectant and facial mask.

Battle Plans for Fighting Blemishes

Note: The following plans are not presented in order of use but by types of products needed to gently cleanse (without further clogging pores or increasing the presence of bacteria), exfoliate, and then disinfect. Order of application is described at the end of this chapter, in the section "Special Considerations."

Plan A. Gentle cleanser (Cetaphil, Moisturel Sensitive Skin Cleanser, Pond's Foaming Cleanser & Toner in One, Paula's Choice One-Step Face Cleanser for either normal to oily or normal to dry skin); baking soda over blemishes; 3% hydrogen peroxide used as a disinfectant over blemishes; and milk of magnesia as a facial mask to absorb excess oil.

Plan B. Gentle cleanser; 8% AHA gel or liquid; 2.5% benzoyl peroxide liquid or gel; and milk of magnesia as a facial mask.

Plan C. Gentle cleanser; 1% or 2% BHA gel or liquid; 2.5% benzoyl peroxide liquid or gel; and milk of magnesia as a facial mask.

Plan D. Gentle cleanser; 8% AHA gel or liquid in the morning and Retin-A or Differin at night; 2.5% benzoyl peroxide liquid or gel or 3% hydrogen peroxide; and milk of magnesia as a facial mask.

Plan E. Gentle cleanser; 1% or 2% BHA gel or liquid in the morning and Retin-A or Differin at night; 2.5% benzoyl peroxide liquid or gel or 3% hydrogen peroxide; and milk of magnesia as a facial mask.

Plan F. Gentle cleanser; Differin; 2.5% benzoyl peroxide liquid or gel or 3% hydrogen peroxide; and milk of magnesia as a facial mask.

Plan G. Gentle cleanser; Retin-A, Differin, or Azelaic Acid; a topical prescription antibiotic; and milk of magnesia as a facial mask.

Plan H. Gentle cleanser; Retin-A, Differin, or Azelaic Acid; a topical prescription antibiotic; an oral antibiotic; and milk of magnesia as a facial mask.

Plan I. Gentle cleanser; and hormone blockers or low-dose birth control pills (discussed later in this chapter) to control hormone levels.

Plan J. When all else fails, Accutane can be a consideration. It is a serious prescription drug, with potentially unsafe side effects for pregnant women, but it has a good success rate for curing acne and oily skin. Blemishes do recur for a percentage of those who take Accutane, but that can take years to happen and a second series can nip that in the bud.

Battling Blackheads and Large Pores

Some of the information in this section is identical to that mentioned above, but blackheads and open pores are not exactly the same as pimples and they deserve specific attention. Several of the basic steps are also the same, with only one or two minor differences.

I understand the frustration of battling blackheads. Insidious and glaring, blackheads make skin look mottled and unclean. However, there are only a handful of options for this annoying skin malady, which makes it relatively simple to deal with. Blackheads occur when sebum, dead skin cells, and hair debris get trapped inside the pore and exposed to air. The tendency to have blackheads is determined genetically by hormone levels and the structure of the pore. However, keep in mind that almost any lotion, cream, gel, bar soap, foundation, moisturizer, or cleanser, regardless of claims about not causing breakouts or blackheads, can contain ingredients that clog pores.

If you are susceptible to blackheads, using moisturizers of any kind will perpetuate the problem. Also, mineral oil and petrolatum are not the skin's worst enemy. Trying to avoid those oils as the most heinous of skin-care ingredients can get you and your skin in trouble because you will end up paying attention to the wrong elements in a product. In actuality, although mineral oil and petrolatum are indeed greasy and can make someone with oily skin feel like an oil slick, they don't have the capacity to clog pores! Triglycerides, palmitates, myristates, jojoba, hydrogenated ingredients, and waxes are much more problematic. All of those ingredients liquefy on the surface of the skin but can harden once they are absorbed, and that's what can clog pores. Essential oils may not clog pores because of their viscosity, but they do tend to be irritating and can stimulate oil production.

The bottom line: the primary way to get rid of blackheads is to clean the face gently, so you don't overstimulate oil production; exfoliate the skin and especially the pore lining to unclog the pore; and absorb excess oil. If you have blackheads, the best way to exfoliate is with a 1% or 2% BHA liquid or gel, Retin-A, or Differin. In Chapter Two, "What Works and What Doesn't," I explain at length why BHA can be the best nonprescription choice for treating blackheads and blemishes, at least as far as over-the-counter products are concerned. Milk of magnesia is the best way to absorb excess oil. If pimples are not present, there is no need for topical or oral antibiotics.

Please keep in mind that battling blackheads takes patience. Consistency is essential. It may take weeks or months to get the results you are hoping for.

Removing Blemishes

This isn't a pretty topic, but it is a fact of life and human nature that just leaving a blemish or blackhead alone is almost impossible. Fortunately, gently removing a blackhead or blemish with light-handed squeezing can actually help the skin. Removing the stuff inside a blackhead or especially a pimple relieves the pressure and reduces further damage. Yes, squeezing can be detrimental to the skin, but how you squeeze determines whether you inflict harm. If you oversqueeze, pinch the skin, scrape the skin with your nails, or press too hard, you are absolutely doing more damage than good. Gentle is the operative word and, when done right, squeezing with minimal pressure is the best, if not only, way to clean out a blackhead or blemish.

Although I never recommend steaming the face (heat can overstimulate oil production, cause spider veins to surface, and create irritation), a tepid to slightly warm compress over the face can help soften the blackhead or blemish, making removal easier. First, wash your face with a water-soluble cleanser. Pat the skin dry, then place a slightly warm, wet cloth over your face for approximately 10 to 15 minutes. Once that's done, pat the skin dry again. Using a tissue over each finger to keep you from slipping and tearing the skin, apply even, soft pressure to the sides of the blemish area, gently pressing down and then up around the lesion. Do this once or twice only. If nothing happens, that means the blemish cannot be removed, and continuing will bruise the skin, risk making the infection or lesion worse, and cause scarring. Again, use only gentle pressure, protect your skin by using tissue around your fingers, and do not oversqueeze.

Be sure to use 3% hydrogen peroxide or a 2.5% benzoyl peroxide solution after you're done, and if you wish you can follow up with a facial mask of plain milk of magnesia to soothe the skin and reduce inflammation. Do not remove blackheads or blemishes more than once or twice a week or you can cause too much irritation.

Note: As this book goes to press, I am already receiving hundreds of questions about a new product on the market for blackheads. The gimmick everyone wants to know about is **Biore Pore Perfect Deep Cleansing Strips** *($5.99 for six nose strips).* Biore is being sold in drugstores across the United States. This product is supposed to instantly clean pores. All you do is place a piece of cloth with an incredibly sticky substance on it over your nose, as you might do with a

Band-Aid, wait 15 minutes for it to dry, and then rip it off. Along with some amount of skin, blackheads are supposed to stick to it and come right out of your nose. What does this miracle product contain? A lot of hairspray. The main ingredient is polyquaternium-37, a film-forming hairspray ingredient. It works little better than using regular tape over the nose. (Actually, regular tape may be less damaging to the skin because Biore can leach potentially irritating ingredients into the pores and tape can't.)

What has me most concerned about these so-called Cleansing Strips is they are accompanied by a strong warning not to use them over any area other than the nose and not to use them over inflamed, swollen, sunburned, or excessively dry skin. It also states that if the strip is too painful to remove, you should wet it and then carefully remove it. What a warning!

You may at first be impressed with what comes off your nose. (Well, there is no question: you will be impressed.) Most people do have some oil sitting at the top of their oil glands (most of the face's oil glands are located on the nose), and whether you use these strips or a piece of tape, black dots and some skin will be removed. Is that helpful? Only momentarily, but if you use the Biore product, the plastic-forming agent can get into the pores and possibly cause breakouts and irritation.

Also, despite the warning on the package, most women will try these strips wherever they see breakouts. If I didn't know better, I know I would. The way these strips adhere, they can absolutely injure or tear skin and cause spider veins to surface. They are especially unsafe if you've been using Retin-A, Renova, AHAs, or BHA; having facial peels; or taking Accutane; or if you have naturally thin skin or any skin disorder such as rosacea, psoriasis, or seborrhea.

Biore's brochure claims this product can pull an entire blackhead plug out of the skin. It can't. If you could grab a blackhead out of the skin, your skin would be left with an empty hole (and there is nothing in this product that will close it up), but that's not what happens. Instead, just the very top layer of the blackhead is removed, and then the blackhead returns because the source of the problem was never corrected. Nothing was done to reduce irritation, exfoliate skin cells, and help keep oil flow normal, or close the pore.

You Still Need Sunscreen

There is no way around it: even if you are battling blemishes, you still need to minimize sun damage by using an effective sunscreen. Especially because you should be exfoliating the skin, which can make it more susceptible to the sun's rays.

Unfortunately, the last thing someone with oily skin needs is another product on her skin. Most sunscreens, even those that claim to be oil-free, contain ingredients that can cause blemish flare-ups. The few sunscreens that are indeed lighter-weight tend to be alcohol-based, posing new problems because alcohol can be an irritant. Plus the sunscreen ingredients themselves can cause breakouts, particularly so-called "nonchemical" sunscreens, which contain titanium dioxide. Even though titanium dioxide is a relatively benign ingredient with little to no risk of irritation, it is occlusive and can clog pores. Other types of sunscreen ingredients can cause irritation and result in breakouts. So you're between a rock and a hard place. Yet you still need sunscreen. In my opinion, the best option in this situation is to wear a foundation with a reliable SPF (preferably SPF 15) that uses avobenzone, titanium dioxide, or zinc oxide as one of the active ingredients.

Foundation containing sunscreen is less of a problem than moisturizers when it comes to causing breakouts, regardless of the ingredients. Foundations are designed to stay on top of the skin, rather than being absorbed. I can't give you a 100% guarantee that the foundation won't cause problems, but it reduces the odds. Additionally, it means using one product instead of two, if you were going to wear a foundation anyway. The fewer products you put on your skin, the better, and this is doubly true for someone afflicted with breakouts or oily skin. And please, if you do choose to wear a foundation that contains sunscreen, don't forget that the other parts of your body that are exposed to sun during the day need sunscreen too.

The number of sunscreens that work well for oily skin types has always been limited. Most of the sunscreen formulations on the market are in moisturizing bases or suspended in alcohol. Either way, oily skin loses. The choices were narrowed down even more when the new FDA regulations concerning UVA protection went into effect. Now there are even fewer sunscreens that have a dry, matte finish and contain titanium dioxide, avobenzone, or zinc oxide. I am keeping my eyes open for the best options and will report on the new ones as they become available. In the meantime, **Estee Lauder Advanced Sun Care Sun Block Lotion Spray SPF 15 Body Spray** *($18.50 for 4.2 ounces)* with titanium dioxide can work well on the face and has a dry finish; and my skin-care line, Paula's Choice, offers an **Essential Nongreasy Sunscreen SPF 15** *($9.95 for 6 ounces)*, a dry-finish lotion with avobenzone.

The bottom line: it takes experimentation and diligence to find a comfortable sunscreen for any skin type, but even more so for someone with oily skin and a tendency toward breakouts.

Retin-A for Blemishes

Retin-A, Renova, and Retin-A Micro are indeed worthwhile products for breakouts. The active ingredient in each of these is retinoic acid. Retinoic acid can literally change the way skin cells are formed in the layers of skin as well as in the pore. If skin cells have an abnormal shape, they tend to stick together and shed poorly, getting backed up in the pore. Retinoic acid can literally transform the cells, improving shedding and unclogging pores.

Until the launch of Renova last year, Retin-A hadn't changed formulations for more than 20 years. (Renova is simply Retin-A in a moisturizing base, although the FDA allowed it to make claims of being the first prescription wrinkle cream.) Retin-A came in a variety of strengths in only two basic forms: a gel that contained alcohol, which can further irritate the skin, and a cream that contained isopropyl myristate, which is known for causing breakouts. Yes, it's true: Retin-A has contained a pore-clogging ingredient for years.

Well, apparently Ortho Pharmaceuticals (owned by Johnson & Johnson) finally realized that this is a problem for people who have blemishes. They decided to create a non-alcohol-based version of Retin-A that also did not contain ingredients that could cause breakouts. Yet, as promising as this sounds, don't call your dermatologist for this new version of Retin-A, called Retin-A Micro, just yet. I get the feeling no one at Ortho tested this product before putting it on the market. The formulation itself isn't the problem, just the application. At first it goes on very smooth and matte, but in just a few seconds a white granular film forms wherever it's been spread. And no matter how much you rub, the granular residue remains. Putting makeup on over this or even just trying to sleep can feel uncomfortable. What could Ortho have been thinking?

The patent for Retin-A, Renova, and Retin-A Micro is just about to run out. That allows other drug companies to produce their own versions of retinoic acid. In the next few years I hope some pharmaceutical company somewhere will formulate a tretinoin product in a gel or liquid base that won't present any risk of clogging pores.

Meanwhile, remember that using any tretinoin product can make the skin more vulnerable to sun damage and sunburn. It is essential to wear an SPF 15 sunscreen that contains avobenzone, titanium dioxide, or zinc oxide as the active ingredient.

Basic directions: *After you have cleaned your face and applied a topical disinfectant, you can spread on a tiny amount of Retin-A, Renova, or Retin-A Micro. If you are going outdoors in the daytime, it is essential to follow this with a sunscreen to protect the face from sun damage. At night you can apply a moisturizer afterward over dry areas or around the eyes.*

Differin

In the world of prescription acne treatments, Retin-A has been in a class by itself for many years. Now it has some stiff competition in the form of Differin, generically known as Adapalene, a new topical acne medication from the folks who make Cetaphil.

Remember, if abnormal skin cells in the layers of skin and in the pores are left to do their own thing, they accumulate inside the pore, creating an environment in which blemishes can flourish. Aside from topical and oral antibiotics that primarily address the issue of killing off the bacteria responsible for producing pimples, Retin-A for years was the only prescription product available that helped exfoliate skin cells (especially inside the pores), literally changing the way they are produced. It works for more than half of the people who can tolerate the treatment, but therein lies the rub: tolerance. Retin-A, Renova, and Retin-A Micro can irritate the skin. Even Dr. James Leyden, an associate of Dr. Albert Kligman, the original patent holder for Retin-A, has said, "Retinoid [Retin-A] therapy ... due to the side effects, has always been a double-edged sword, limiting its use in many patients." (I was one of those patients. Retin-A left my face so red and inflamed I thought it was going to blister, especially in the days when I also used strong astringents and bar soaps.)

Where does Differin fit into this picture? Differin is a retinoid, comparable to Retin-A, but in clinical studies it has proven to be significantly less irritating. According to a study published in the March 1996 *Journal of the American Academy of Dermatology*, Differin was also significantly more effective in reducing blemishes and was better tolerated than tretinoin gel. It seems Differin has a radarlike ability to positively affect the skin-cell lining of the pores, substantially improving exfoliation and helping to prevent blockage. Moreover, Differin comes in a lightweight gel formula that is barely felt on the skin. It contains little more than water and cellulose, a sheer thickening agent.

Should you consider Differin? If you have tried Retin-A and had difficulty dealing with the irritation, or if you just want to see if Differin can work better for you (which it may), and you are not considering Accutane (the only real cure for breakouts and oily skin), Differin is definitely an option. It is priced the same as Retin-A, but like Retin-A it requires a prescription, which means an appointment with a doctor. That adds to the initial cost, but it's the only way to check this stuff out.

Basic directions: *After you have cleansed your face and applied a topical disinfectant, you can spread on a tiny amount of Differin. If you are going outdoors in the daytime, it is essential to follow this with a sunscreen to protect the face from sun damage. At night you can apply a moisturizer afterward over dry areas or around the eyes.*

Azelaic Acid

The introduction of new and reformulated prescription exfoliants in more emollient or nonalcohol bases reflects the demand for medications that meet the needs of older women looking for ways to deal with pre- and postmenopausal acne. Differin, the new tretinoins, and Azelaic Acid all affect the way skin cells are formed and shed in the skin layers and inside the pore lining. The difference is that Azelaic Acid not only exfoliates the skin, it also performs antimicrobial action on the skin.

Technically, Azelaic Acid is a saturated dicarboxylic acid found naturally in wheat, rye, and barley that behaves like a 5% topical benzoyl peroxide gel, a 0.05% tretinoin cream, or a 2% erythromycin cream (a topical prescription antibiotic), meaning it can exfoliate and disinfect the skin at the same time. Unlike the tretinoins, Azelaic Acid is well tolerated and doesn't cause much overt irritation, redness, or swelling, although 5% to 10% of people who have tried it do experience problems. However, unlike the tretinoins, Azelaic Acid is unlikely to cause sun sensitivity. It is most definitely an ally in the battle against breakouts, particularly if skin is naturally sensitive to the sun or irritation is an issue.

Basic directions: *After you have cleaned your face and applied a topical disinfectant, you can spread on a tiny amount of Azelaic Acid. If you are going outdoors in the daytime, it is essential to follow this with a sunscreen to protect the face from sun damage. At night you can apply a moisturizer afterward over dry areas or around the eyes.*

Topical Disinfectants

Some things go hand in hand: bread and butter, love and marriage, Laurel and Hardy. None of these is the same alone. That's also true for exfoliants and topical disinfectants when it comes to reducing or eliminating blemishes. Cleaning the skin without exfoliating and disinfecting is useless. You can get pretty good results using one or the other, but the two together are a formidable defense against blemishes.

For years I have been recommending 3% hydrogen peroxide as the first resort in finding a useful disinfectant to kill the bacteria that lurk in the pores and cause pimples. It is not only inexpensive, it is far less irritating than most other disinfectants, though it is also less effective. Before you try anything else, see how your skin responds to 3% hydrogen peroxide. Dermatologists used to dismiss my recommendation as anecdotal and not effective. A few years later several dermatologists started recommending it themselves. Then I began hearing that hydrogen peroxide was a problem because it released oxygen into the skin and instigated free-radical damage. Recently, putting oxygen into products and using hyperbaric oxygen booths have become popular, and the oxygen issue took another strange turn.

Here are the facts: using 3% hydrogen peroxide as a disinfectant for blemishes does not increase free-radical damage or increase the oxygen content of the skin. The released oxygen molecules are neither penetrating nor lasting; they have no more impact on the skin than does the air around us. Whatever remotely negative impact 3% hydrogen peroxide might have on the skin is outweighed by the positive effects of its ability to disinfect and reduce blemishes. The same is true for benzoyl peroxide (which also releases an extra oxygen molecule) and prescription topical antibiotics.

Benzoyl peroxide is the next best choice after 3% hydrogen peroxide for combating pimples. Benzoyl peroxide solutions range from 2.5% to 10%. For the sake of your skin, start with the less potent concentrations. A 2.5% benzoyl peroxide product is much less irritating than a 5% or 10% concentration, and it can be just as effective. It completely depends on how stubborn the strain of bacteria in your pores happens to be. Benzoyl peroxide not only disinfects, it can penetrate the hair follicle to reach the offending bacteria. Yet, despite benzoyl peroxide's superior disinfecting and penetrating properties, some bacteria just won't give up easily, and in those situations stronger weapons may be necessary.

If your skin doesn't respond to 3% hydrogen peroxide or the various strengths of benzoyl peroxide, the next step is prescription topical antibiotics. Topical antibiotics, like any topical disinfectant, have limitations. They can have difficulty penetrating the follicle, and long-term use can lead to antibiotic-resistant bacteria. The most popular topical antibiotics are erythromycin, tetracycline, and clindamycin. A combination of 2% erythromycin and zinc acetate is available in a product known as Theramycin-Z. Zinc can help with penetration and speed healing. Another option, considered to be quite effective, is a prescription product called Benzamycin, which contains 3% erythromycin and 5% benzoyl peroxide. This combination boosts penetration, because that's what benzoyl peroxide does best, and erythromycin has strong antibiotic action.

For all skin types prone to breakouts, the best over-the-counter topical disinfectants are: Clean & Clear Dr. Prescribed Acne Medicine Extra Strength, and Dr. Prescribed Acne Medication Maximum Strength; Fostex 10% Benzoyl Peroxide Vanishing Gel; Mary Kay Acne Treatment Gel; Oxy 10 Maximum Strength Vanishing Acne Medication, and Sensitive Vanishing Acne Medication; Paula's Choice Blemish/Acne Fighting Solution with 2.5% Benzoyl Peroxide; ProActiv Revitalizing Toner and Repairing Lotion.

Basic directions: *After you have cleaned your face, soak a large cotton ball with the disinfectant and gently stroke it over the areas of the face, neck, back, or chest* *where you tend to break out. If you are using AHAs, BHA, Retin-A, Renova, Differin, or Azelaic Acid, apply those after the disinfectant. During the day, sunscreen goes on next; in the evening, if you need a moisturizer, apply it minimally only over dry patches or dry areas around the eye.*

Oral Antibiotics

If topical disinfectants or prescription topical antibiotics don't provide satisfactory results, an oral antibiotic prescribed by a doctor may be the best option to kill stubborn blemish-causing bacteria. As effective as oral antibiotics can be, they should be a last resort, not a first line of attack. Oral antibiotics used in conjunction with topical treatments that exfoliate and disinfect will control or reduce most acne conditions. However, as effective as this method is, oral antibiotics can produce some unacceptable long-term health problems. Dermatologists tend to give the negative side effects of oral antibiotics short shrift and prescribe them for their acne patients as if they were nothing more than candy.

Oral antibiotics are anything but candy. They kill the good bacteria in the body along with the bad, and as a result they provoke yeast infections, bring on stomach problems, and can also discolor the skin and yellow the teeth permanently. A more serious side effect is that your body will adapt to the antibiotic you are taking, making it ineffective for fighting acne bacteria or any other bacterial infection you might get. This means that, after a relatively short period of time, the antibiotic you are taking for your acne will become ineffective because the bacteria adapts and becomes immune to it. Nevertheless, you and your dermatologist may decide that oral antibiotics are an option, but go for it only after you know all the risks.

The most commonly prescribed antibiotic is tetracycline. Erythromycin is a good alternative, although acne as well as most bacteria seems to develop resistance to erythromycin quicker. Minocycline is widely used for acne that is resistant to tetracycline. A sulfa drug known as Bactrim can be used to fight acne that is unresponsive to other antibiotics. Choosing to use oral antibiotics is a decision that should not be made lightly, but it is an option in the war against blemishes. Which course of action you take should be discussed at length and monitored by both you and your dermatologist.

Birth Control Pills for Acne?

Anyone who has searched for a way to stop breakouts is familiar with the arsenal of acne products, encompassing everything from antibacterial cleansers, astringents, and masks to exfoliating gels, scrubs, and oil-control products. Sadly, independent studies indicate that only 25% of the people who self-treat acne this way are pleased with the results. That leaves 75% dissatisfied and in need of better alternatives. Making an appointment with a dermatologist is often the last resort for those seeking a more flawless visage, though it often should be the first. The success rate for acne sufferers goes up 80% when prescription medications are used and used consistently. Treatments can include Retin-A, Differin, prescription-strength topical antibiotics, and oral antibiotics. Now add to those options Ortho Tri-Cyclen birth control pills.

If you are a woman (sorry, guys) looking for a new way to reduce breakouts, you might want to discuss your skin problems with your gynecologist instead of your dermatologist. The FDA has recently approved a low-dosage birth control pill (trade name, Ortho Tri-Cyclen Tablets; generic name, norgestimate/ethinyl estradiol) to be used in the treatment of acne! Depending on your lifestyle and state of health, you could solve two problems with one prescription.

How does the birth control pill work on acne? Increased oil production can be caused by the body's testosterone production, which can be highest just before menstruation starts. It appears that low-dosage birth control pills can decrease the amount of excess testosterone, thereby decreasing breakouts. For a lot of women this isn't surprising. Many have noticed an improvement in their skin after they started taking birth control pills.

Is taking birth control pills to control acne right for you? There are risks associated with taking birth control pills, and they should be taken into account before you make a final decision. These risks include increased chances of heart attack, strokes, blood clots, and breast cancer, not to mention possible side effects such as vaginal bleeding, fluid retention, melasma (dark brown skin patches), and depression. All that may not be a worthwhile trade-off for clear skin. But if you are already considering or using the pill for birth control, this remedy may be worth looking into.

Accutane

Looking back, my only regret is that I waited so long. I tried. I really tried. I patiently waited for my skin to clear up. Spent untold dollars on dermatologists and followed their instructions. Diligently wiped antibiotic lotions over my face and took oral antibiotics for years. Exfoliated with baking soda, Retin-A, and sulfur masks. Used milk of magnesia masks twice a week, and sometimes wore it under my makeup to soak up oil during the day. For most of that time my skin did improve, but it never really stopped breaking out and I still had to put up with oily, wet-looking skin. Besides, in spite of the improvement I saw from using antibiotics and the other treatments, I didn't want to stay on them forever. Adapting to the antibiotics was a risk I wasn't willing to continue taking. Who knew how much longer I would continue breaking out? It had been going on since I was 11, and by then I was 38.

I had known about Accutane for a long time. I knew it had some pretty serious, even dangerous side effects, and that most dermatologists didn't prescribe it very often, and then only in the most serious of cases. My acne and oily skin were serious to me, but not as bad as the pictures I had seen of the cystic acne cases that responded brilliantly to treatment with Accutane. Then, in 1990, a woman I worked with and two of her friends started taking Accutane, and not only did they live through it, their skin looked flawless. More than flawless—radiant (at least in comparison to what it looked like before).

That was the final straw. I decided to research the topic for my newsletter. What a remarkable decision that turned out to be. A dermatologist I had heard about at my health cooperative, Group Health in Seattle, Washington, told me it was possible, in fact highly probable, that I could have clear skin for the rest of my life if I took Accutane. I told him I had heard controversial things about Accutane and was hesitant to try yet another prescription drug for my acne. And this one sounded even more serious than antibiotics. He responded with a fascinating saga.

Accutane is a natural drug made from the molecules in vitamin A, and is taken orally. It essentially stops the oil production in your sebaceous glands (the oil-producing structures of the skin) and literally shrinks these glands to the size of a baby's. This prevents sebum (oil) from clogging the hair follicle, mixing with dead skin cells, rupturing the follicle wall, and creating pimples or cysts. Normal oil production resumes when treatment is completed and the sebaceous glands slowly begin to grow larger again, but they never (or at least rarely) grow as large as they were before treatment.

In a large percentage of patients who complete a four-month treatment with Accutane, acne is no longer considered to be clinically significant. In other words, for all intents and purposes, *their acne is cured!* Does this mean you'll never break out again? You may once in a while, but an occasional pimple here and there is hardly anyone's definition of acne. Especially anyone who, on a daily basis, had numerous breakouts, lots of blackheads, and oily skin.

The remaining percentage of patients who take Accutane do experience recurrences. For this group, when the breakouts return, typically three to six months after treatment, they are often milder and easier to treat, and can on occasion be cured by a second or third treatment with Accutane. Of course, there is a percentage who receive no benefit from taking Accutane, no matter how many treatments they take.

By the way, dosage and duration depend on the severity of the patient's acne, but treatments generally last 16 weeks. If a second treatment is necessary, an eight-week rest period is required in between. Interestingly, acne continues to improve even after the course of treatment is completed, although doctors do not know exactly why this happens.

So what's the catch with this "miracle" drug and why don't doctors prescribe it to everyone? Accutane is controversial for many reasons, but principally because of its most insidious side effect: **it has been proven to cause severe birth defects in nearly 90% of the babies born to women who were pregnant while taking it.** Before physicians knew about this alarming hazard, when it was first prescribed in France back in the 1970s, before enough research had been conducted to establish its safety, more than 800 babies out of 1,000 births were born seriously deformed. The only way to avoid this risk is to abstain from sex during treatment; if this is not possible, according to the information provided with every prescription, a minimum of two forms of birth control are required. If you are taking a birth control pill, you still need to use a condom or diaphragm. You will need to discuss with your physician how long to continue using the extra birth control precautions after you are done taking Accutane. Generally the effect of Accutane does not last very long once you stop taking it.

If you *aren't* pregnant, are there still risks? Yes, but they are only somewhat more serious than the risks involved in taking antibiotics for acne over a long period of time. Commonly reported, although temporary, side effects of Accutane include dry skin and lips, mild nosebleeds (your nose can get really dry for the first few days), hair loss (I lost a small amount of hair that grew back when I was done with the four months of treatment), aches and pains, itching, rash, fragile skin, increased sensitivity to the sun, headaches (mild to severe—mine were fairly mild), and peeling palms and hands. More serious, although much less common, side effects include headaches, nausea, vomiting, blurred vision, changes in mood, depression, severe stomach pain, diarrhea, decreased night vision, bowel problems, persistent dryness of eyes, calcium deposits in tendons (doctors don't know yet whether this is significant), an increase in cholesterol levels, and yellowing of the skin.

However, as scary as all that sounds, *the majority of patients tolerate Accutane very well.* I experienced some headaches, minor body aches, some hair loss, dry nose, and dry skin. One dermatologist told me that over the past 15 years, he has prescribed Accutane to thousands of patients, and only five have had to stop because of negative side effects.

Understandably, most people, doctors included, are scared off by these side effects, above and beyond the risk to pregnant women. (Doctors are hesitant to prescribe Accutane anyway, largely because they fear a malpractice suit in cases where a patient does accidentally become pregnant.) That's why dermatologists recommend Accutane only to patients with chronic acne (large, recurring cysts or blemishes that can permanently distort the shape and appearance of the skin) or sometimes to people with less severe acne that has not responded successfully to other forms of treatment. Many doctors won't prescribe Accutane at all.

Although the high risk of birth defects and the other side effects should be taken seriously, it seems a shame that Accutane has been kept away from many acne patients. It is the most effective short-term drug for acne available today (all other acne treatments require ongoing, tenacious adherence to the program). The public is largely misinformed about Accutane's potential dangers as well as its potential benefit. Many doctors believe that if it weren't for the proven risk of birth defects, Accutane would be prescribed almost as frequently as antibiotics. Not surprisingly, it is prescribed much more frequently to men.

Given what I have learned, I wish somebody had told me about Accutane 20 years ago! It would have saved me a lot of time, money, and heartache. Although oral and topical antibiotics, exfoliants, gentle cleansing, staying away from products that aggravate breakouts, and using milk of magnesia to absorb excess oil can work for lots of people, for many people the question remains, "When will I outgrow acne and how long will I have to struggle with the pain of breakouts?" Sadly, there is no telling if you're *ever* going to outgrow it. People who don't outgrow it, and lots of women don't, are looking at years of taking topical solutions and oral antibiotics that sometimes work well and sometimes don't.

A new version of Accutane under investigation by the FDA is Soriatane. Soriatane (acitretin), which is now awaiting final approval from the FDA, has a shorter half-life in the body than Accutane. This means it is flushed from the body faster and thus is safer for women with childbearing potential since birth defects are a very serious consideration for all of the oral retinoids. It is primarily used for psoriasis, but it could have applications for acne.

How do you deal with some of the side effects when taking Accutane? It helps to be prepared. If you take Accutane, stay out of the sun! This drug makes the skin photosensitive even if you are wearing sunscreen (and you must wear sunscreen). Any prolonged sun exposure can cause severe redness and fever. **Treat dry areas of the face with a moisturizer such as Cetaphil Moisturizer, Lubriderm Seriously Sensitive Moisturizer, or Eucerin Light. If your nose becomes dry, apply a thin layer of petroleum jelly on the skin inside the nose, and do it frequently. That will make a big difference. Do not use any skin-care products that can cause irritation or dryness. Avoid bar soap, washcloths, AHA and BHA products, scrubs, hot water, and facial masks. If you are using**

Retin-A, Differin, Azelaic Acid, or topical antibiotics I would suggest you stop using them unless your doctor recommends that you continue. Dry eyes can be treated with artificial teardrops; do not use products like Visine that simply constrict blood flow. Headaches and body aches are eased quite nicely with ibuprofen. Be sure to drink plenty of water. If you have any concerns, discuss them at once with your physician.

It is also essential for your doctor to monitor your blood. Cholesterol can shoot up dangerously high for some reason, and that would require stopping the Accutane. It is essential to stay in close contact with your physician during the entire time you are taking Accutane.

Excerpt from Cosmetics Counter Update

Dear Paula,

I enjoyed reading sections of your newsletter and books, but there's something you should know (and report on) about Accutane that you failed to mention. Accutane killed my daughter. You spend several paragraphs painting Accutane as a wonder drug, a panacea for women suffering from acne, but barely two paragraphs discussing Accutane's side effects if a woman becomes pregnant!

My wife's dermatologist prescribed Accutane for her adult acne. He also insisted on birth control, as did Accutane's manufacturers. And even though my wife took a birth control pill religiously during this time, she still became pregnant. As everyone knows, no birth control device is 100% effective. Our daughter was born severely deformed and with several organ abnormalities. She died four days after her birth because of Accutane, yet this drug is still being prescribed.

I'm writing in hopes that in future editions of your fine book you will take the time and effort to tell your readers about the real dangers of this horrible drug. While you mentioned the risk of birth defects, you did not mention the fetal and infant deaths attributed to Accutane. Yes, women of childbearing age are required to use birth control, but, as in our case, that is not always effective. And, as many doctors have told the FDA and Hoffman-LaRoche [the makers of Accutane], any woman of childbearing age should be considered pregnant until proven otherwise.

Name withheld by request

Dear Grieving,

Your letter touched me deeply and I am honored that you chose to share your story with me and my readers. I am fully aware of the statistics and risks to a fetus (baby) if the mother is taking Accutane. Perhaps only women who are pro-choice and willing to undergo an abortion if they become pregnant while taking this drug should be acceptable candidates, but for now that is not the case. Because of the risk of fetal death or deformity, Accutane is prescribed to twice as many men as women, as perhaps it should be, since no birth control device is 100% effective.

However, despite your painful experience, I disagree with your conclusion. I do not feel Accutane is a horrible drug, although, like many drugs and medical procedures, it can have horrible side effects (even the birth control pills your wife took can increase the risk for some cancers). I took Accutane knowing the risks and decided to avoid sexual relations with my husband during that time period. I was not willing to take the chance of becoming pregnant. As I have stated before, Accutane is a serious drug, and it does have deadly side effects to a fetus (baby) if a woman becomes pregnant. Yet, at the same time, it is the only potential cure for acne and the treatment lasts only four months, with no lingering side effects. I believe a dermatologist would be remiss in not letting a woman struggling with acne know Accutane is available, along with stressing all the possible horrendous risks.

With all my heart I pray for your family's emotional healing and am passing your story on to impress upon others the worst side effect of Accutane. It could indeed save lives.

Hormone Blockers for Acne?

Using a testosterone-blocking drug to reduce the hormone levels responsible for activating oil production is an intriguing approach to treating acne and oily skin. The most frequently prescribed hormone blocker is known as Aldactone, the trade name, or spironlactone, its generic name. Obviously it is recommended only for women, because without testosterone men start to develop female characteristics like enlarged breasts and softer skin. But because testosterone can be one of the primary causes of acne, curtailing its presence in the body can have positive results: namely, acne clears up and oil production slows. The statistics are impressive for this somewhat controversial method of treating acne: about 60% or so of those who take it find it effective.

The side effects may not be as traumatic as you might think, at least not for women, according to Dr. James Herndon, past professor of dermatology at the University of Texas in Dallas. He says research does not indicate a link between hormone blockers and cancer rates, although they may minimally reduce your sex drive and your breasts may become sore. However, others in the field disagree, citing studies that demonstrate an increased risk of some cancers with the use of spironlactone.

Using a hormone blocker for acne is not a short-term solution. When you stop taking it, the testosterone returns and so does the acne. Because hormone blockers require repetitive, continuous use, at least for treating acne, I strongly recommend trying Accutane before trying hormone blockers. Although Accutane's side effects can be much more serious than those of the hormone-blocking drugs (those side effects are described in the preceding section on Accutane), use of Accutane is very short term, only four months, and it can be a permanent cure. As Herndon explains, "Some people are just averse to taking Accutane because of the risks involved. It isn't my job to argue with them. My job is to present alternatives, and hormone blockers are a viable alternative."

Well, it is my job to argue and suggest that women and men rethink exactly what the pros and cons are for any acne treatment, whether it is something prescribed by their dermatologist or an over-the-counter remedy. In the case of women who want to try Accutane, it is worthwhile to take a pregnancy test to assure that you are not pregnant before you start using it and then abstain from sex until you are no longer using it.

Special Considerations

In Chapter Five, the section "Skin-Care Plans for All Skin Types" outlines specific skin-care routines based on skin type. The routines below, for people dealing with blemishes and blackheads, are also based on skin type.

Severe oily skin with breakouts

A.M.

1. Water-soluble cleanser
2. Topical disinfectant
3. BHA, AHA (preferably in a gel base or liquid base), Differin, or Retin-A
4. Moisturizer (for dry areas only, specifically around the eyes)
5. Milk of magnesia (usually used as a facial mask only; for extremely oily skin, you can apply an extremely thin layer before putting on your foundation to absorb excess oil during the day)
6. Sunscreen (preferably in an SPF 15 foundation that contains avobenzone, titanium dioxide, or zinc oxide)

P.M.

1. Water-soluble cleanser
2. Topical disinfectant
3. BHA, AHA, Differin, or Retin-A (preferably in a gel base or liquid base)

4. Moisturizer (for dry areas only, specifically around the eyes)
5. Milk of magnesia as a facial mask that is rinsed off (at least three times a week)

Mature oily skin with breakouts

A.M.

1. Water-soluble cleanser
2. Topical disinfectant (if breakouts are present)
3. BHA, AHA (preferably in a gel base or liquid base), Differin, or Retin-A
4. Moisturizer (for dry areas only, including the area around the eyes)
5. Milk of magnesia (apply a thin layer over oily areas only before applying foundation)
6. Sunscreen (preferably in an SPF 15 foundation that contains avobenzone, titanium dioxide, or zinc oxide)

P.M.

1. Water-soluble cleanser
2. BHA, AHA (preferably in a gel base or liquid base), Differin, or Retin-A
3. Moisturizer (for dry areas only, including the area around the eyes)
4. Milk of magnesia as a facial mask that is rinsed off (at least three times a week)

Older dry skin with occasional breakouts

A.M.

1. Water-soluble cleanser
2. Moisturizing toner (over dry areas)
3. Topical disinfectant (over areas that tend to break out)
4. BHA, AHA (preferably in a gel base or liquid base), Differin, or Renova
5. Moisturizer (if needed, over dry patches and around the eyes after the sunscreen)
6. Sunscreen (SPF 15, with avobenzone, titanium dioxide, or zinc oxide, preferably in a foundation or in a light lotion base)

P.M.

1. Water-soluble cleanser
2. Moisturizing toner (over dry areas)
3. BHA, AHA (preferably in a light lotion base), Differin, or Renova

4. Moisturizer (if needed, over dry patches and around the eye area)

Acned oily skin

A.M.

1. Water-soluble cleanser
2. Topical disinfectant
3. BHA, AHA (preferably in a gel base or liquid base), Differin, or Retin-A
4. Milk of magnesia (apply an extremely thin layer before applying foundation)
5. Sunscreen (preferably in an SPF 15 foundation that contains avobenzone, titanium dioxide, or zinc oxide)

P.M.

1. Water-soluble cleanser
2. Topical disinfectant
3. Retin-A or Differin
4. Moisturizer (for dry areas only, including the area around the eyes)
5. Milk of magnesia as a facial mask that is rinsed off (at least three times a week)

Acned dry skin

A.M.

1. Water-soluble cleanser
2. Topical disinfectant
3. Renova
4. Moisturizer (over dry areas only)
5. Sunscreen (preferably in an SPF 15 foundation that contains avobenzone, titanium dioxide, or zinc oxide)

P.M.

1. Water-soluble cleanser
2. Topical disinfectant
3. Renova
4. Moisturizer (for dry areas only, including the area around the eyes)

Cystic acne

A.M.

1. Water-soluble cleanser

2. Topical disinfectant
3. Retin-A or Differin
4. Sunscreen (preferably in an SPF 15 foundation that contains avobenzone, titanium dioxide, or zinc oxide)

P.M.

1. Water-soluble cleanser
2. Topical disinfectant
3. Retin-A or Differin
4. Moisturizer (for dry areas only, including the area around the eyes)
5. Milk of magnesia as a facial mask that is rinsed off (at least three times a week)

CHAPTER SEVEN

Cosmetic Surgery

Cutting and Pasting

(I would like to thank Dr. Paul Weiss, clinical professor of plastic and reconstructive surgery at Albert Einstein College of Medicine; Dr. Ray Geronimus, director of the Laser and Skin Surgery Center of New York and clinical associate professor of dermatology at New York University Medical Center; and Dr. Richard Maloney, from The Aesthetic Surgery Center in Naples, Florida.)

Sometimes money is the root of expensive mistakes. Just because celebrities are doing something doesn't mean you should jump in and do it too. Yes, lots of celebrities have had their looks altered by cosmetic surgery, but often you can tell at a glance who got a bad face-lift, because their faces have been cut and pulled so tight they look constantly surprised or incessantly half-smiling. Michael Jackson is a classic example of facial cosmetic surgery gone amok, but we've all seen others who seem shockingly unattractive. Yes, a large number of famous women have had their chests augmented and enlarged to the point that their breasts enter the room a full minute before they do, or stand out like rocks from the chest, but that doesn't mean you should too.

In short, what you don't know about plastic surgery (namely, the pros and cons and all your options) can hurt you—not just your appearance, but also your health and your pocketbook. I'd like to give an overview of what is available, along with what you need to know about the risks and/or benefits of different procedures.

Before I get to the nitty-gritty, I want to address the most important challenge of all: who should do your surgery, regardless of what you decide to have done. Given the number of doctors with cosmetic or plastic surgery practices (if you live in Southern California, their advertisements are about as prevalent and obnoxious as those for car dealerships), it is very difficult to know where to go and how to get started. Most women use one of four methods for choosing a cosmetic surgeon: reading recommendations in fashion magazines, finding out where celebrities like Barbara Walters or Cher went (everybody loves knowing where the "stars" are going for anything and everything), getting a referral from a friend or a friend of a friend, and, last but not least, checking out the doctors who advertise their services.

Though I wouldn't call these the worst plans of action, they should just be the beginning of the process. You need to know more before you can make an informed final decision. Take the time to gather detailed consumer information and draw up a comprehensive list of questions to ask so you'll know what all your options are, which procedures will meet your needs, and which doctors are performing the safest and most reliable current procedures (the latest method doesn't mean the best when it comes to surgery).

Let me reiterate that being proactive about any surgery is incredibly important, but even more so with cosmetic surgery. After all, this surgery is usually elective and completely up to you; there is nothing life-or-death about these procedures. Furthermore, cosmetic surgery is a very lucrative business—most surgeons get paid up front before you go under the knife or laser. Before you hand over your hard-earned money, your very appearance, and your well-being, you have to feel good about every detail.

Cosmetic Surgery vs. Plastic Surgery

What is the difference between a cosmetic or plastic surgeon and a board-certified plastic surgeon? A lot! Training and credentials in surgery are the issues in contention. Although a doctor may offer cosmetic, plastic, or aesthetic surgery, he or she may not be board-certified to perform that surgery, but might be a gynecologist or pediatrician with no training in cosmetic surgery whatsoever. Board-certified means the doctor has gone through very specific and extensive training in a specialized field and passed a difficult examination by a board of experts in that field. A non-board-certified cosmetic or plastic surgeon may be self-taught and likely lacks formal training in that field. Board-certified plastic surgeons consider this an issue of public safety and I think that's an understatement. They suggest that going to anyone but a board-certified plastic surgeon is a huge mistake, asking, "Would you want your plastic surgery performed by someone who has never had any formal plastic surgery training?" Good question.

According to the American Society of Plastic and Reconstructive Surgeons (a professional association), many physicians who today practice plastic or cosmetic surgery received their formal training in another specialty—often a nonsurgical specialty—or had surgical training for another area of the body. One clear distinction is that a board-certified plastic surgeon will have privileges to perform plastic surgery at an accredited hospital. It is completely fair to ask any doctor you see for cosmetic surgery whether he or she is board-certified and which hospitals he or she is affiliated with. Then check to be sure the hospital is accredited and the doctor's certification is current and recognized by the American Board of Plastic Surgery (ABPS), the only board recognized by the American Board of Medical Specialties (ABMS) to certify physicians for the full range of plastic and reconstructive procedures.

Of course, there are great dermatologists and lousy board-certified plastic surgeons practicing plastic surgery. But the odds of getting someone who is inexperienced are greatly reduced by first finding out if that person is board certified. To be certified by the ABPS, a physician must have at least five to six years of approved surgical training, including a two- to three-year residency in plastic surgery. He or she must also have been in practice for at least two years and pass comprehensive written and oral exams in plastic surgery. Call the ABMS at (800) 776-2378 and ask for the names of board-certified plastic surgeons in your area.

What to Ask

Once you've dealt with the issue of board certification, ask plenty of other questions, and look for answers that make you feel comfortable and make the most sense to you in light of the research you have done. Not all cosmetic surgeons will come up with the same game plan for your face. Each surgeon has techniques he or she prefers, sometimes regardless of whether they represent the best or most current technology. **Some surgeons use the latest technology not because it is better or has proven more effective but due to pressure from their "elite" clients, who expect what's new regardless of the risks.**

One of the most important questions you can ask the surgeons you interview is how often each month they perform the specific procedure or procedures you are considering. It is best (but not essential) to get a doctor who specializes as opposed to a doctor who tries to do it all.

Likewise, it is also imperative to ask how many surgeries the doctor performs in a day. If the doctor schedules more than three procedures a day, most likely another doctor or nurse will do the prep work and/or the finishing work. That may not mean poor results, but it does mean the doctor is not giving you his or her full attention. Make sure the doctor you are consulting will be the only doctor working on your face or body, and that he or she will never leave the operating room during your procedure.

It is also valid to ask if the doctor charges for redos and touchups. Though it isn't something doctors like to admit, going back in for fine-tuning or to correct mistakes is common, and you don't want to be charged to repair what you don't like.

Be insistent about understanding every nuance of the postoperative procedure. Many complications can occur when the patient doesn't realize her part in the healing process. For example, scar tissue can cause problems for a breast implant. One of the ways to minimize that risk is to keep your breasts tightly bound and your arms firmly at your sides, with little to no movement and no lifting for four to seven days.

Negative outcomes are another complex issue. Both patients and physicians have a tendency to ignore the downside of cosmetic surgery. Paying attention to the risks of cosmetic surgery takes the glamour out of the process, so dangers are downplayed almost to the point of being entirely ignored. **Even when a doctor does broach the perils of cosmetic surgery, it is often mentioned in an offhand style or glossed over completely in a vague and patronizing manner.** Do not turn your face over to a surgeon who doesn't discuss—at length—all the risks involved with the cosmetic procedure you are interested in.

For example, if you are interested in a laser peel, you should be told about the risk of scarring. About 1% of the patients who have a laser peel will develop some amount of scarring. There is also a 20% to 30% chance of incurring hyperpigmentation after a laser resurfacing. The discoloration tends not to be permanent, but it could last up to three or four months.

Where to Cut?

The options for changing your body and face are almost limitless, and the results can be stunning. Cutting off leathery, thick, lined, sagging, and discolored skin long abused by the sun can subtract years from a person's appearance. In the past, most people waited until they were well into their late 50s and 60s, with noticeably aged skin, before they jumped into the fray of cosmetic surgery. All that has changed with the advent of relatively noninvasive, low-cost procedures such as laser surgery and endoplasty.

Nowadays, baby boomers in their 40s may want to undergo cosmetic surgery to deal with sagging corners of the mouth, slight pouching or sagging of the chin and jawline, and folds along the forehead. Though hardly aging by some standards, these irksome signs of middle age are easy to modify. **It turns out that a good deal of the skin's tendency to sag, and the deepest furrowed lines on the face (particularly the forehead and the nasal-labial folds from the nose to the mouth), are a result of the face muscles sliding down and in toward the center of the face over time.**

Let's say your jawline is beginning to sag. Using the somewhat simple surgical procedure called endoplasty, the surgeon makes a mere quarter-inch cut underneath the chin and at the edges of the jaw and then, via microsurgery (the surgeon watches what is being done via a television screen), sutures the platysma muscle, which runs from jawline to jawline under the chin, back where it belongs.

Likewise, the deep frown lines and vertical creases in the mid-forehead result from a literal slippage of the forehead muscles downward and inward. The same endoscopic technique used to anchor the platysma muscle can be used for the forehead muscles, and an additional separating of the muscles between the eyebrows can reduce the fold lines there. This operation can be done via three tiny incisions inside the hairline, anchoring the slipped muscles back in place and cutting away a small section of the muscles between the eyes.

While reanchoring the muscles of the jaw and forehead can eliminate or decrease sagging, laser surgery is the treatment of choice for smoothing out fine lines all over the face, principally around the eyes and the mouth. Laser surgery can also slightly decrease sagging, but its main function is to smooth out lines. While laser surgery can take three weeks to heal, endoscopic surgery takes only about 48 hours, although it is often accompanied by a postoperative headache that can last for a few days.

Some cosmetic surgeons suggest that laser surgery, endoscopic surgery, and mini-tucks (doing a section of the face as opposed to an overall face-lift) are the best way to put off the need for a full face-lift or eye tuck. They claim that if you fix problems as they crop up there's less trauma, and because younger people generally have more elasticity in their skin, the results should last longer (however, younger people tend to show more scarring). The notion that minor surgery decreases the need for major surgery down the road is at the least a rationalization and at best a theory, though it certainly increases business.

We are in a new era of accessibility to cosmetic surgery, and baby boomers want it all. I doubt strongly that endoscopic surgery, laser surgery, or mini-tucks will postpone anything. As long as the results are impressive (and they are), people will want to stay young-looking via any procedure that is relatively nonrisky and permanent (although all cosmetic surgery has duration limitations). That's neither bad or good. Just understand that the sales pitch about fending off further surgery by beginning plastic surgery in your 40s is a stretch. **Still, it beats wasting money on creams and lotions that do nothing for the skin. As one plastic surgeon I spoke with noted, "Women have been buying wrinkle creams by the truckload, and yet they still get wrinkles and I'm still in business because none of those cosmetic products work to stop or change wrinkling."**

The Possibilities from A to Z

The cosmetic procedures listed below are performed by physicians all over the world. The first list includes procedures for the neck up; the second list includes procedures for the neck down. Both lists are in alphabetical order. The risks and gains are best contemplated cautiously and from a consumer's point of view, not by how your friend looks who had it done. These procedures are not a guarantee of happiness, just a way to buy the kind of body and face you want (if a designer suit didn't make you happy, don't expect new breasts or a face-lift to provide peace of mind!). **Every plastic surgeon I spoke with suggested that the patients most pleased with the results of their surgery were the ones who had the most realistic expectations. What are unrealistic expectations? Ex-**

pecting to end up looking like a supermodel or believing you will now find the perfect relationship. Plastic surgery is about self-esteem, tied up with societal standards of beauty—nothing more and nothing less.

Important details: Keep in mind that everyone scars differently, and it often has little to do with the skill of the surgeon. You could be left with lines wherever an incision was made. In general, the paler your skin, the more prone you may be to red, weltlike scarring, and the darker your skin, the more prone you may be to thick, dark, keloidal scarring.

There are serious risks with all surgical procedures, and recovering from the more serious operations such as face-lifts, tummy tucks, and breast implants can be a daunting, frightening experience. However, studies indicate that 97% of people who experience some kind of cosmetic surgery are quite pleased with the results, but the 3% who are unhappy can be devastated. Eye tucks can damage the tear ducts or permanently destroy eyelashes, face-lifts can leave painful scars and pockets of dimpled flesh, laser or chemical peels can render skin tone uneven, and breast implants can leak or become encapsulated and painful.

Many doctors love using computer imaging to "close the sale" on the cosmetic procedure they are recommending. A picture of your face or body is taken and scanned into a computer program, allowing the surgeon to then demonstrate how you would look pulled a little here, tucked a little there, and lifted a little all over. As impressive as this is, it is only a computer image and not real life. It is a great tool for getting an idea of what you can expect, but it isn't an exact blueprint. Don't let it be the deciding factor in your final decision.

All cosmetic surgery procedures have limitations as to how long the change will last, depending on skin type, age, the surgeon's technique, and postoperative care (including using sunscreen). Do not expect any cosmetic surgery to be permanent, especially laser peels, fat or collagen injections, chemical peels, and Bo-Tox (discussed later in this chapter).

Note: As indicated below, prices for these procedures vary widely. The region of the country you live in, the popularity of the surgeon, the specific techniques utilized (the more invasive or complex, the more expensive), the combination of techniques, and discounts given for doing more than one procedure can all greatly affect price.

From the Neck Up

Cheekbone (Malar) Augmentation *($2,000 to $5,000)*

The cheekbones may be built up by placing an implant over them. This is usually performed through an incision within the mouth, but it may be done through a lower eyelid or brow incision. Look closely at Michael Jackson to see how this operation can go awry.

Alternatively, the buccal fat pads, which are located above the jawline near the corner of the mouth, just below the cheekbone, can be removed in individuals with an excessively round face. This procedure imparts a more contoured look, sometimes referred to as the "waif look," à la Kate Moss. However, plastic surgeons warn that, in many individuals, removal of the buccal fat pads can lead to a drawn, hollow-cheeked look as aging progresses, because that is what naturally happens to the face.

Chemical Peels *($1,000 to $5,700)*

Fine lines and wrinkles around the mouth, forehead, and cheeks may be improved with a wide range of skin treatments involving a chemical peel, but there are definite drawbacks. In this procedure, a chemical solution is applied to the entire face or to specific areas to peel away the skin's top layers. Often, several shallow to medium-depth peels can achieve results similar to one deep-peel treatment, with less postprocedure risk and a shorter recovery time, though long-term effects of these repeated peels are still unknown. Peel solutions may contain alpha hydroxy acids, tricholoracetic acid (TCA), or phenol as the peeling agent, depending on the depth of peel desired and on other patient selection factors. However, chemical peels take a backseat to the effectiveness and expediency of laser peels (see the "Laser Peels" section).

Peels that use *alpha hydroxy acids (AHAs)* or *glycolic acid* are cosmetic (not medical) procedures and as a result are not regulated by the FDA. There is no long-term evidence as to the effect an AHA peel has on the skin. An AHA peel can improve the texture of skin and encourage cell turnover by removing layers of dead skin cells, but that's about it. AHA peels need to be repeated because the results don't last long, so many plastic surgeons consider them a poor option for long-term benefit, but lots of consumers, doctors, and aestheticians have jumped on this bandwagon for short-term results. This peeling mania can be a problem. These procedures, done repeatedly, say three or four times a year, keep skin irritated for long periods of time, which can possibly result in skin damage. Having a deep AHA peel once a year or once every six months is a consideration because you would avoid chronic irritation.

A lesser-known facial peel option is a *beta hydroxy acid (BHA)* or *salicylic acid peel.* A solution of salicylic acid can work in a similar manner to a glycolic acid peel, but irritation is much reduced. Salicylic acid, as I mentioned in Chapter Two, is a compound closely related to aspirin (acetylsalicylic acid). Salicylic acid retains its aspirin-connected anti-inflammatory properties. A BHA deep peel can be superior for many skin types because the irritation and inflammation are kept at a minimum due to the analgesic action of the BHA compound.

Trichloroacetic acid (TCA) is used for peeling the face, neck, hands, and other exposed areas of the body. It has less bleaching effect than phenol (see next paragraph), and is excellent for "spot" peeling of specific areas. It can be used for medium or light peeling, depending on the concentration and method of application. TCA peels are best for fine lines but are minimally effective on deeper wrinkling.

Phenol is sometimes used for full-face peeling when sun damage or wrinkling is severe. It can also be used to treat limited areas of the face, such as deep wrinkles around the mouth, but it may permanently bleach the skin, leaving a line of demarcation between the treated and untreated areas that must be covered with makeup. Given the positive results that can be achieved with laser surgery and the extreme risks associated with phenol, this method is actively discouraged and rarely used.

Buffered phenol offers yet another option for severely sun-damaged skin. One such formula uses olive oil, among other ingredients, to diminish the strength of the phenol solution. Another, slightly milder formula uses glycerin. A buffered phenol peel may be more comfortable for patients, and the skin heals faster than with a standard phenol peel, but it is still a risky procedure and can depigment the skin.

Chin Augmentation (Mentoplasty) or Reduction *($2,000 to $6,000)*

Chin augmentation can strengthen the appearance of a receding chin by increasing its projection. (Look at pictures of Michael Jackson when he was young, then look at a recent picture; it's hard to ignore his mega-chin implant.) The procedure does not affect the patient's bite or jaw, and can be done using one of two techniques. One approach is to make an incision inside the mouth and move the chin bone, then wire it into position; the other requires insertion of an implant through an incision inside the mouth, between the lower lip and the gum, or through an external incision underneath the chin. Hydroxyapatite granules, a bone substitute made from coral, can be used to enhance facial contours—for instance, to form a more prominent chin or cheekbones. The substance also has reconstructive uses in craniofacial surgery.

On the other hand, while the shape of the chin may not be an issue, excess skin can start pouching along the jawline, creating the appearance of a double chin or a turkey neck. A chin tuck can help to shore up this sagging by cutting away surplus skin and using liposuction to remove the excess fat. The scar is hidden just under the jaw.

Collagen Injections *($325 to $1,400)*

Collagen is an injectable protein, obtained from the deeper layers of cow skin, that can be used to treat facial wrinkles. Patients who wish to be treated with collagen should first be tested for any allergic reaction. The results of collagen injections are not permanent because the collagen is eventually absorbed by the body, and treatments must be repeated periodically to maintain results. However, for a quick lift of deep lines between the eyebrows, wrinkles on the forehead, and smile lines by the mouth, this is a noninvasive, safe procedure. A more elaborate procedure for lifting deep lines involves fat implants (see the "Fat Implants" section).

Cosmetic Tattooing *($750 to $1,500)*

Cosmetic tattooing, or micropigmentation, can be used to create permanent eyeliner, eyebrow color, or lip color. It can also be used for permanent blush or eyeshadow, though this is infrequent. Other uses include re-creating the coloration of the areola around the nipple following breast reconstruction; restoring the color of dark or light skin where natural pigmentation has been lost through such factors as vitiligo (a whitening of the skin from an autoimmune response), cancer, burns, or other scarring; and eliminating some types of birthmarks or previous tattoos. Micropigmentation should be performed only under medical supervision by appropriately trained personnel. This is not a procedure you would want done by anyone other than a plastic surgeon, although it often is, given that anyone can buy a tattoo machine.

However, I do *not* recommend tattooing as a cosmetic way to create permanent eyeliner, eyebrows, or colored lips, and especially not for blush. As seductive as permanent makeup sounds—who wouldn't love to avoid drawing on eyebrows and eyeliner, or constantly reapplying lipstick—remember that fashions change and the face ages. Permanent eyebrows that look nice and even when you're in your 40s can sag as your skin ages, and the same is true for the eyeliner and blush. Additionally, your personal taste for a particular style will undoubtedly change. A pink or red lip color imprinted on your mouth may look good today, but in five or ten years it can look strange and out of date.

Dermabrasion *($950 to $5,100)*

Dermabrasion is a procedure in which a high-speed wheel, similar to a rotary sander using fine-grained sandpaper, is used to abrade the skin. It may be recommended, but rarely, to counter extensive sun damage and heavy skin wrinkling, or to improve the texture of pockmarked skin resulting from severe acne or chicken pox. Following treatment, the skin can appear firmer and smoother, but the risk of permanent pigment changes is fairly high. For this reason, dermabrasion is best only for some types of acne scarring, and then only with extreme warnings about depigmentation problems that have a high rate of occurrence.

Ear Surgery (Otoplasty) *($3,100 to $5,000)*

Otoplasty involves positioning the ears closer to the head by reshaping the cartilage (supporting tissue). This is usually accomplished through incisions placed behind the ears so that subsequent scars will be concealed in a natural skin crease. Otoplasty can be performed on children as young as age five or six.

Earlobe Reduction *($1,500 to $3,000)*

If you've worn heavy earrings for most of your life, your earlobes may be swinging down closer to your shoulders than you ever thought possible. A simple, 30-minute earlobe reduction can be performed in a plastic surgeon's office or at the same time as a face-lift. Aesthetically speaking, or at least to be sure your earlobes don't wobble, the earlobe should not be more than 25% of the total length of the ear. In cases where it exceeds this, an L-shaped wedge is cut away, and the earlobe edges are brought together and sutured.

Eyelid Surgery (Blepharoplasty) *($2,500 to $5,000)*

Eyelid surgery is one of the more popular cosmetic surgeries because it is relatively simple to have done and requires minimal postoperative recovery, and the results can be stunning. This operation involves cutting away the fat that causes bags beneath the eyes and removing wrinkled, drooping layers of skin on the eyelids. Blepharoplasty is often performed along with a face-lift or with other facial rejuvenation procedures, especially forehead lifts. Incisions follow the natural contour lines in both upper and lower lids, and the thin surgical scars are usually barely visible and blend into the eyelids' natural lines and folds, but it depends on how your skin scars.

Transconjunctival blepharoplasty, a variation, is performed by making an incision inside the lower eyelid. It avoids any scarring on the lower lid and may reduce the possibility of the eyelid pulling down, a postoperative complication in some patients. It is a useful technique when fat only, and not skin or muscle, needs to be removed from the eyelid area.

It is important to note that eyelid surgery may not be indicated if a forehead lift can produce a more positive effect without risking the eye area or obvious scarring. This option should absolutely be discussed with your surgeon.

Face-lift (Rhytidectomy) *($5,600 to $15,000)*

A face-lift can dramatically reduce sagging skin on the face, neck, and jaw. As impressive as this cosmetic procedure can be in creating a youthful, taut visage, it can also create an overly pulled, masklike appearance with the face drawn up in a stretched permanent smile. This is one cosmetic procedure for which you want to see the doctor's work on someone else up-close and personal. (Of course, any doctor will show you only his or her best work, so be clear about the kind of look you are trying to achieve.)

During this complicated, elaborate procedure, incisions are made in the hairline both in front of and behind the ears (the exact design of the incisions may differ from patient to patient, and surgeons' personal techniques can vary widely). For younger patients, more-limited incisions may be appropriate. When necessary, fatty deposits beneath the skin are removed and sagging muscles are tightened. The slack in the skin itself is then taken up and the excess cut away. Scars can usually be concealed by hair and makeup.

Most face-lifts also include repositioning the muscles of the cheek that have slipped forward, causing deep lines near the mouth (laugh lines), as well as the muscle along the chin. Be sure to ask your surgeon if he or she is familiar with the techniques to secure sagging muscles.

Face-lifts tighten only the area along the cheek and some of the jaw. Other areas require a forehead lift, chin tuck, or endoscopic repositioning of the muscles. Likewise, fine lines in the mouth and eye area are not affected by a face-lift alone and require additional procedures, such as a forehead lift, a chin tuck, eyelid surgery, or fat implants, that are often done at the same time the face-lift is performed.

Fat Implants *($2,500 to $7,500)*

An alternative to collagen injections, fat implants use fat harvested (extracted) from one part of the body and placed into another to smooth lines in the face or build up other features such as the lips. Fat implants are a very reliable way to change the appearance of skin, but the procedure has definite pros and cons. The risk of rejection, given that the implant (the fat) is your own, is very low. However, fat implants are a more invasive procedure than collagen injections. (During a fat implant, a section of the body is cut to get the fat out; the fat is then processed in order to be utilized, and another incision is made to insert the fat at the new site.) Additionally, a large amount of the injected fat is eventually reabsorbed by the body, and the procedure must be repeated periodically to maintain results. Because of the absorption, many plastic surgeons choose to overcorrect to achieve the desired results. Other negatives with fat implants include the formation of scar tissue and the fact that some of the fat does not get absorbed. Those uncontrollable aspects of the procedure make the final results unpredictable.

Injection of fat to enlarge the breasts is a dangerous procedure and is not recommended because of the possibility of dense scarring that may seriously hinder accurate interpretation of both breast self-exams and mammograms.

Forehead Lift (Brow Lift) *($3,100 to $5,700)*

The forehead lift is designed to correct or improve wrinkling, as well as sagging of the eyebrows, that often occurs as part of the aging process. The procedure may also help to smooth horizontal expression lines in the forehead and vertical frown lines between the eyebrows as well as reduce the sagging appearance of the eyelids. Behind the hairline, incisions are placed above the ear and over the top of the head, although in some cases incisions may be made in front of the hairline. Forehead lifts are often (and usually should be) accompanied by repositioning the muscles of the forehead that are partly responsible for the furrowed lines of the brow.

Laser Procedures *($1,200 to $7,500)*

Laser peels are a new but increasingly popular way to smooth skin at almost any age. In this procedure, the top layer of skin is peeled away like an onion, while the collagen underneath is coagulated (thickened) and re-formed (think of how a steak's texture changes when you cook it). Laser peels are also superior for removing sun-damaged skin, brown spots, and spider veins on the legs and face; eliminating some tightening of the skin (but not sagging); and healing rosacea; and they can be used on all areas of the face and body, from eyelids to legs. New procedures available to physicians show impressive results, but be aware that there is no real information about the long-term effects of these devices, and, depending on your skin condition, the results may last only three to five years. Risks include skin discoloration, scarring, and poor results, and laser treatments can trigger skin sensitivities. One cautionary note: At this point, the entire world of laser surgery is too new to make any conclusive determinations. Although the initial results are impressive, data on the safety and long-term effects of this option are extremely limited. That isn't bad, but there just isn't enough solid statistical information on which to base claims for results and risk assessment.

Lasers come in several varieties, each with its own risks and benefits.

The *pulse dye laser* is used primarily for vascular lesions such as birthmarks, surfaced capillaries or spider veins on the face and legs, and the underlying redness of acne rosacea. The machine is capable of selecting a small target and penetrating only that area, which is why it can hit a tiny capillary so precisely. The pulse dye laser requires no anesthesia, but sometimes a topical anesthetic is used just in case the patient is particularly sensitive or jumpy. (Every time the intense light of a laser penetrates the skin, it can feel like a rubber band snapping against the skin.) Perhaps the most remarkable thing about all this is that the results are instantaneous, meaning the surfaced capillaries, birthmarks, or redness from rosacea are eliminated immediately. One drawback is that the skin can appear darkened and discolored for a period of ten to 14 days; however, there is no wound or crusting. And there is good news for women with acne rosacea: evidence suggests that once the redness is reduced, the breakouts that usually accompany rosacea decrease or go away altogether.

As successful as the pulse dye laser is for these conditions, a new machine seems to do an even better job. This new laser is called a *Photoderm* light device. It works almost identically to the pulse dye laser, but with almost no side effects. While darkened skin is a risk with the pulse laser, the Photoderm light device supposedly limits this risk. Furthermore, reports say the Photoderm leaves you looking as if nothing happened, except that the skin problems you wanted erased are most likely gone. Those who advocate use of this new machine, particularly those selling it, claim that the Photoderm is especially useful for erasing spider veins on the face and legs. However, some plastic surgeons are not convinced by the marketing claims for this machine, and they consider scleratherapy (see "Scleratherapy" in the "Below the Neck" section later in this chapter) a better option for removing surfaced face and leg veins. Based on interviews with a number of physicians, I think that scleratherapy and the Photoderm can both be useful, and for some people the Photoderm may be the best option, particularly for small bursts of surface veins.

When it comes to wrinkles, the *pulse carbon dioxide laser* is the machine of choice. It works well for vertical lines around the mouth, crow's-feet near the eyes, and lines on the cheeks. It can tighten the skin, and it may even increase the production of collagen and elastin. How it does that doesn't sound very appealing, but remember that the results are impressive and the risks are small. The pulse carbon dioxide laser removes the top layer of the dermis, just above the papillary dermis layer. Heat generated from the laser is approximately 60 to 80 degrees Centigrade. At that temperature the collagen and protein in the skin coagulate and then very quickly re-form. For unknown reasons, possibly in direct response to the heat trauma, the skin generates new collagen and elastin.

What makes the pulse carbon dioxide laser unique is the width of the laser beam as it hits the skin. Standard lasers used in laser-peel procedures emit a very thin beam of light, but the pulse carbon dioxide laser emits light in varying widths. That means the surgeon has to make fewer passes over the face to connect each section of skin being treated. Ultimately, that can translate to a smoother result. Ask if your surgeon is using this type of machine. However, the carbon dioxide laser does not work for extreme sagging, such as a turkey neck, serious jowling, or deeply furrowed wrinkles. It also does not affect the forehead or the frown lines between the eyes that are the result of repeated muscle contractions.

In addition to the skill of the physician performing the laser peel, postoperative techniques are important in the success of the procedure. One complication of laser surgery is home care. The side effects of a laser peel can be daunting. The skin oozes, crusts, and needs to be cleaned and dressed for about two weeks before you look even vaguely normal. Because the top layer of skin has been stripped away, the raw exposed skin needs to be cleaned and treated very carefully. This handling by the patient can easily be done incorrectly, causing infection, delayed healing, and irritation.

Although it may sound weird, some physicians require patients who have undergone a laser peel to wear a clear silicone bandage (much like Saran Wrap) over the entire treated area for five to seven days. The silicone bandage prevents any interference from the patient except for gentle cleaning around the mouth, eyes, and nose, which are understandably left unbandaged. But there are problems with this type of wrapping. It can be uncomfortable for the patient, oozing can occur at the edges of the bandage, and it just plain looks strange. (On the other hand, peeled skin looks strange no matter what you do to it.)

Postscript: Laser technology sounds so medical and, well, high-tech that the consumer is easily enticed into thinking it will perform miracles, regardless of the application. Thermolase Corporation thinks so too, and has applied for and received approval from the FDA for its *Soft Light* patented hair-removal machine, but that is a use patent only; the company cannot make any claims about permanent hair removal because the machine has no proof it can do that.

Soft Light is a laser device that is supposed to remove unwanted hair. It can be used by a nonmedical technician, which means anyone from a receptionist to an aesthetician or nurse; however, in most states the presence of a physician is required, not necessarily in the same room or building, but at least somewhere, though sometimes in name only. For a fee of $1,000 and up you receive a series of treatments but, alas, no guarantees. Thermolase plans to open spas all over the country, and the company has been making headway in cities like New York, Houston, Los Angeles, and Chicago.

According to the FDA, the Soft Light machine was approved because "it was substantially equivalent to other dermatological lasers that remove tattoos and spider veins, which have been around for quite a while." What is the patent all about? It covers the process of using this already well-accepted laser device with a heat-conducting topical ointment that sends the laser beam down the hair shaft to zap the follicle. The cream, which contains microrefined carbon, is applied over the unwanted hair and absorbed into the hair shaft. Once the laser is trained on the hair, it super-heats the carbon and supposedly kills the follicle. At least, this is the theory. There is no proof yet that this process works.

Thermolase Corporation submitted three-month clinical studies to the FDA. None of these studies substantiated or proved that the Soft Light machine provides permanent hair removal, nor did they demonstrate that the process is painless. As a result, the company can make no claims about long-term effectiveness, lasting removal, or pain-free treatment. Thermolase is very sensitive to these claim limitations, but plans to submit more data to the FDA that it hopes will demonstrate permanent hair removal. If you think this sounds expensive, you're right. Your $1,000 buys a one-time leg and bikini treatment; it's $5,200 for a series of four to six treatments. For this kind of money, *permanent* removal should be more than just a hope, but that's yet to be seen.

By the way, the Soft Light laser is also being used on the face as an alternative to high-concentration AHA peels, accompanied by a not-so-surprisingly-high price tag. Does this laser facial make a difference in the skin? Yes. Peeling the skin always makes a difference, but the results are strictly superficial, more due to swelling than to cell turnover. This laser facial is not the same as laser surgery; it is strictly peeling away a very superficial layer of skin with laser light instead of chemicals. What are the long-term results? Who knows? Not only is this technique brand-new, but the consumer is the guinea pig.

For all forms of laser peeling, there is no long-term research on what happens to the skin in the long run, whether it's done with a pulse dye laser or the more superficial Soft Light laser. Data indicate that a large number of women experience wonderful wrinkle-smoothing results, while some see no change and others have problems with skin discoloration afterward and require extensive skin-lightening treatments. What happens ten or 20 years down the road? What if the woman gets repeated laser treatments? No one knows. Lasers haven't been around long enough for anyone to know.

Lip Augmentation, Lift, or Reduction *($1,000 to $5,500)*

One of the most effective methods of augmenting the lips is to surgically advance the lip forward via incisions placed inside the mouth. While thin lips may not seem like a cosmetic issue, for some women looking for perfection, fuller lips are considered more attractive. Fat implants (see the "Fat Implants" section) or collagen injections (see the "Collagen Injections" section) may then be positioned under the lining of the lip to add additional plumpness. Neither collagen nor fat is permanent, however, and the procedure must be repeated periodically to maintain results. Fat injections are considered risky and are best undertaken only by doctors aware of the risks involved.

A lip lift is a technique that surgically lifts the corners of an aging mouth to eliminate the pronounced droop and unhappy facial expression that often develop with advanced age. Cutting away small diamonds of skin just above the corners of the mouth raises the border of the lips into a slight smile.

If thin lips have a fashionable downside, it isn't hard to believe that overly full lips can also be viewed as unattractive. In lip reduction, a small section along the top lining of the lip is surgically removed to narrow the lips to the desired proportion. The small scars on the outside of the lips are often barely noticeable, but it all depends on how you scar.

Nose Reshaping (Rhinoplasty) *($4,000 to $9,500)*

Rhinoplasty is usually performed to alter the size and shape of the bridge and tip of the nose. Reshaping is generally done through incisions inside the nose, but sometimes an incision across the central portion of the nose between the nostrils is also made. Narrowing the base of the nose or reducing the size of the nostrils involves removing small wedges of skin at the base of the nostrils. The nose is reduced, or sometimes built up, by adjusting its supporting structures, which involves either removing or adding bone and cartilage. The skin and soft tissues are then redraped over this newly created structure.

An open rhinoplasty technique can sometimes benefit patients who need more complex correction or who are undergoing a secondary rhinoplasty procedure. A small incision is made outside the nose across the columella (the tissue that divides the two nostrils). This enables the plastic surgeon to turn the outer tissue of the nose back, providing a view of the structures inside. Additional incisions, like those used in the traditional closed approach, are made inside the nose as well. The scar from the incision on the outside of the nose eventually becomes barely visible.

From the Neck Down

Arm Lift (Brachioplasty) *($3,000 to $6,000)*

All the weight-lifting in the world won't build up enough muscle to pick up the excess skin that can hang and flap under the arm, particularly if you have extra weight in that area. Excess fat in the upper arms can sometimes be reduced through liposuction alone, but loose, drooping skin may need to be excised. To that end an arm lift is an impressive way to shore up that area, making the skin smooth and taut again. Incisions are hard to hide for this operation, which can run lengthwise from the armpit to just above the elbow.

Breast Implants or Augmentation (Augmentation Mammoplasty) *($4,500 to $8,500)*

Breast augmentation is typically performed to enlarge small breasts, underdeveloped breasts, or breasts that have decreased in size after a woman has had children. It is accomplished by surgically inserting an implant behind each breast. The implant is soft and pliable, and is something like a plastic bag filled with water. An incision is made either under the breast, around the areola (the pink skin surrounding the nipple), or in the armpit. A pocket is created for the implant either behind the breast tissue or behind the muscle between the breast and the chest wall. Not surprisingly, a recent psychological study of women who have undergone breast augmentation concluded that 83% were satisfied with the overall result of surgery (10% were neutral, 7% dissatisfied), and 94% reported increased self-confidence.

Textured-surface breast implants are made with the same silicone elastomer used for the shell of other types of breast implants, but a special manufacturing process creates a textured surface. Some studies have suggested that the textured surface may help to reduce the incidence of capsular contracture—tightening of the naturally forming scar tissue around the implant—which can make the breast feel firmer than normal. (Capsular contracture is discussed in more detail later.)

The controversy surrounding implants over the past several years has to do with serious health risks associated with silicone gel–filled implants leaking into the body. Although the final word on breast implants is still not in, large-scale epidemiological studies conducted independently by leading research institutions have provided some reassuring data. A large-scale epidemiological study conducted by the Mayo Clinic and published in the June 16, 1994, issue of the *New England Journal of Medicine* found no connection between silicone breast implants and connective tissue diseases such as rheumatoid arthritis and lupus. Similar findings have been reported by researchers at the University of Michigan and by a major Australian study. Large-scale studies of implants and cancer have shown a reduced incidence of breast cancer in women with silicone breast implants, but it isn't clear why that was the case.

Despite the controversy, the FDA has made it illegal to use breast implants with silicone gel. Saline-filled breast implants are the only type widely available in the United States for cosmetic augmentation, due to restrictions imposed by the FDA in 1992. However, silicone gel–filled implants are still available in many foreign countries.

The FDA recently approved clinical trials of a breast implant filled with a soybean oil derivative, which developers say may allow better detection of breast masses through mammography than either silicone gel or saline fillers. Currently, there is no scientific evidence that women with either silicone gel or saline breast implants are diagnosed with breast cancer any later than other women, or that their prognosis for recovery is any worse than for other women.

Be sure the physician you see is familiar with the differences between saline, soybean oil, silicone gel, and textured surface implants. Also, your physician should be aware of the need for strict postoperative treatment and should explain it to you at length. For example, it is essential that there be no movement of the hands or arms above the waist for at least four days after surgery. Also, the breasts must be bound for between several days to three weeks after surgery. All this assures healing and minimizes the chances of the implant being encapsulated.

Occasionally the implant is rejected by the body, or scar tissue builds up and pushes against the implant. This can create a capsule around the implant, causing rock-hard, painful breast tissue. Capsular contracture is the most common problem associated with breast implants. It is not a health concern, but moderate to severe contracture can make mammography more difficult and possibly damage the implant. (Mammoscopy, done with an endoscope, can determine whether breast implants are intact or ruptured.) Following strict postoperative instructions from an attentive physician may prevent capsular contracture.

Enlarging the breasts by fat injection is an experimental procedure that produces temporary benefits and poses serious long-term risks to patients, possibly making future detection of breast cancer difficult or impossible. Plastic surgeons strongly discourage any woman from undergoing this procedure.

Although the idea of having large, full, Pamela Anderson–type breasts can be tempting, be sure your physician is sensitive to your body type and will veto your preconceived notion of what a desirable body looks like if it is not appropriate for your size and shape. It is best to have breasts that look like they are a part of you and not two huge blimps pointing straight out and up from your chest.

Breast Lift (Mastopexy) *($3,000 to $5,000)*

Frequently, a woman elects this surgery after losing a considerable amount of weight, or after losing volume and tone in her breasts after having children. The plastic surgeon relocates the nipple and areola (the pink skin surrounding the nipple) to a higher position, repositions the breast tissue to a higher level, removes excess skin from the lower portion of the breast, and then reshapes the remaining breast skin. Scars occur around the areola, extending vertically down the breast and horizontally along the crease underneath the breast. Variations on this technique, in some cases, may result in less noticeable scarring.

Breast Reduction (Reduction Mammoplasty) *($5,000 to $14,000)*

Perhaps no other form of elective cosmetic surgery is more life changing than a breast reduction procedure. A woman with massive breasts struggles with the extra bulk, which is extremely uncomfortable and awkward and curtails physical activity. Additionally, because of the substantial extra mass, detection of breast cancer is compromised and the skin tissue under the breast area can be incessantly lacerated and infected by rubbing, irritation, and perspiration. With the development of successful reduction mammoplasty procedures, there is no reason for any woman to struggle with this kind of physical distortion.

Unlike most other types of cosmetic surgery, breast reduction is normally classified as a reconstructive procedure, since oversized breasts greatly interfere with normal daily activity and physical activity, and pose health issues such as infection and difficulty in breast cancer screening. Depending on your insurance company's policy regarding breast reduction, the entire procedure may be paid for in full by your health insurance provider. Generally, the determination is made according to how much tissue by weight is removed. A certain gram weight is needed to prove to the insurance company that the procedure is corrective and not just aesthetic. However, regardless of the insurance company's position, there is an important aesthetic component to the operation, since the plastic surgeon can improve the shape of the breasts and the nipple area, and a woman's physical profile is enhanced.

Breast reduction involves removing excess breast tissue and skin, repositioning the nipple and areola, and reshaping the remaining breast tissue. Some of the risks are fairly serious, including noticeable scarring, loss of sensation, and the inability to breast-feed. But for women with heavy, pendulous breasts, a breast reduction can be a godsend. Women who wear double or triple D or E bras often experience chronic back and shoulder problems, and because the skin under the breast is never exposed to air, it can become raw and prone to skin infections.

Buttock Lift *($4,500 to $7,000)*

Excess fat and loose skin in the buttock area can be reduced by performing a buttock lift in combination with liposuction (see the "Liposuction" section). Incisions required for skin removal can often be hidden in the fold beneath the buttocks. Though the results are impressive, the scarring can be quite noticeable, meaning you'll look great in pants but in the buff your backside might look like a road map.

Calf Augmentation *($3,000 to $5,000)*

Can you believe people do this? Increased fullness of the calf can be achieved using hard silicone implants, which are inserted from behind the knee and moved into position underneath the calf muscle.

Cellulite Treatments

I thought I would throw this in for the sake of making a point. Cellulite is a cosmetic term referring to the dimpled-looking skin that often appears on the buttocks, thighs, and hips. This is not a result of excess fat; rather, it occurs when connective tissue in the thigh allows fat deposits to poke through. (That is why cellulite creams don't work; the appearance of dimpling is a result not of fat but of the skin's structure.) At this time there is no treatment that will eradicate this problem because there is no way to change the thigh's structure. Liposuction can get rid of excess fat and improve the contour of the leg, but even the thinnest women can have cellulite because it is caused not by the presence of fat but by the nature of the skin's structure.

Laser Surgery

See "Laser Procedures" in the section "From the Neck Up" earlier in this chapter, and the "Scleratherapy" section.

Liposuction *($4,900 to $8,000)*

Liposuction allows the plastic surgeon to remove localized collections of fatty tissue from the legs, buttocks, abdomen, back, arms, face, and neck using a vacuum device that literally cuts up and then sucks up fat tissue. Depending on the area treated, the procedure leaves only minute scars, often as short as one-half inch in length or less. The use of refined equipment allows removal from delicate areas such as calves and ankles. Liposuction removes fat, but it cannot eliminate dimpling (cellulite) or correct skin laxity, which is a result of the skin's structure and not due to the presence of the fat itself. If a patient's skin has lost much of its elasticity, the plastic surgeon may also recommend a skin-tightening procedure such as a thigh lift, buttock lift, or arm lift, all of which leave more extensive scars. Liposuction is considered a low-risk procedure with impressive results. If there is any downside to this procedure it is on the part of surgeons who do not screen their patients. Liposuction does not take the place of a diet. If someone is obese, gains and loses weight frequently, or has an eating disorder, he or she is not a good candidate for liposuction.

There is much talk nowadays about ultrasonic liposuction. This form of liposuction uses high-pulse sound waves to liquefy excess fat, which is then removed. The procedure is considered controversial because, although it's been available in Europe for quite some time, it has lost a great deal of its initial popularity. The equipment for ultrasonic liposuction is cumbersome and time-consuming to use, plus one notable study demonstrated there was no difference in outcome between regular liposuction and ultrasonic liposuction.

Scleratherapy *($250 to $1,000)*

While lots of women worry about cellulite, I worry about the road map of veins running all over my thigh. It's not that I don't have cellulite, but it just doesn't bother me as much as these surfaced veins. They are not swollen or raised, but they are not a pretty sight. The most typical treatment for large red and blue varicose veins is scleratherapy. Laser surgery doesn't work well, if at all, on larger veins.

In scleratherapy a saline solution is injected into the thighs to collapse the walls of the veins, destroying the source of the problem. Actually, no one uses normal saline anymore. One alternative is polidocanol (aethoxysclerol), which was originally developed as a local anesthetic. Polidocanol turned out to be undesirable as an anesthetic because it shut down veins wherever it was injected, but it was perfect for scleratherapy. It is virtually painless. It is also one of the few drugs you can inject into the skin that doesn't leak into the other veins, so it affects only the vein you are going after. That means there is little to no risk associated with this treatment. Your doctor will want to choose the best option for your condition, but make sure he or she is familiar and skilled with all available options. For more serious, larger varicose veins, a more potent choice is sotradecol. It is somewhat similar to polidocanol, but sotradecol can cause sores (ulcers) if it leaks.

It is best to determine the underlying cause of a problem before treating it, but that isn't always possible. A surfaced vein is distended and visible because it is connected to a high-pressure system that has gone wrong. These surfaced veins are similar to the experience of driving along and all of a sudden finding heavy traffic backed up several miles from the actual problem. When veins work normally, they collect blood from tissues and pump it around the body in an even flow, without hitches, stops, or sudden starts. When things go wrong, the blood can actually go in the wrong direction. This occurs because the valves in the vein no longer function properly or because blood volume in the vein increases (often because of trauma); usually both conditions occur together and are interrelated. This misdirected blood flow can build up pressure, creating tortuous swelling and protrusions. A vein that becomes permanently dilated is called a varicose vein. Theoretically any vein can develop varicosity, but certain veins, such as those in the legs, are more likely to. This can be due to an injury; or pregnancy hormones, which make the valves in the veins soft and floppy, causing damage; or being overweight; or just bad veins. And the problem can spread from even just one bad vein, affecting a multitude of veins.

The first course of action is scleratherapy. If you don't find that effective, surgery is the next step, although 25% to 30% of the time the problem can recur. If the problem originated with an injury, the veins should stay clear as long as there are no further injuries. If the problem was caused by excessive hormones or excess weight, no further treatment should be required once things go back to normal. But if the problem is genetic, more surfaced veins will develop over time.

Varicose veins that become raised and swollen should not be ignored. This is more than just a cosmetic problem. Venous thromboses (blood clots), which are tender and painful, may develop and break off and become obstructions elsewhere, particularly in the pulmonary arterioles, causing heart failure.

Thigh Lift *($5,000 to $7,500)*

Losing a lot of weight or suffering a lot of sun damage can cause the thigh area to sag, making cellulite look worse and excess weight more noticeable. Liposuction alone won't lift up skin that hangs down, causing pouching and folds. A thigh lift can be performed, along with liposuction, to tighten sagging muscles and remove excess skin in the thigh area. Because a thigh lift leaves noticeable scars in the inner or outer thigh area, it is not a frequently performed procedure.

Tummy Tuck (Abdominoplasty) *($5,000 to $10,000)*

Sometimes, after multiple pregnancies or major weight loss, a person's abdominal muscles weaken and skin in the area becomes flaccid and hangs below the pubic bone. For many women this is not a pretty sight. Abdominoplasty can tighten the abdominal muscles and, in some instances, banish stretch marks because they are cut away, never to be seen again. In both men and women, the procedure removes excess skin and fat. Generally, an incision is made across the pubic area just above the bikini line and around the navel. The skin is lifted up and away from the sides of the body and just under the breasts, then pulled down and reshaped firmly along the body. Liposuction may be used to remove excess fat along the back area just in front of where the skin is lifted away from the body. Often the stomach muscles, which may have separated and pulled apart, are stitched back together, re-creating the natural girdle you had when you were younger. The excess skin is then cut away, and what remains is stitched back together at the original incision above the pubic bone.

Caution!

Bo-Tox. Bo-Tox is an abbreviation for botulism toxin—that's right, botulism, the acute disease that paralyzes the muscles of anyone who ingests the toxin. A relatively new cosmetic procedure uses Bo-Tox to paralyze the muscles of the forehead, which prevents frowning and thereby eliminates wrinkles. Twenty-four to 48 hours after ultra-minute doses of Bo-Tox are injected into the muscles of the forehead, most of those muscles can no longer be used. That makes squinting or raising the front half of the eyebrows impossible. The result? A smooth forehead with no squint lines. (Remember, most of the deep horizontal and vertical lines on the forehead are a result of frowning, not sun damage.) Bo-Tox treatments last about six months and are not considered dangerous. Ophthalmologists have used Bo-Tox for several years to treat eye tics and they report no ill side effects, yet many plastic surgeons I have interviewed are opting not to use it. Why? Because Bo-Tox can migrate to forehead muscles you don't want affected, like the muscles that support the eyelids. That can result in having drooping or closed eyelids for several months. Also, because the injections have to be repeated to maintain results, the risk of affecting other muscles increases.

Laser-assisted aesthetic surgery. At present, there is no evidence that using lasers for aesthetic procedures such as eyelid surgery and face-lifts, instead of using conventional scalpel surgery, has any effect on the final surgical outcome. The debate on the benefits of laser surgery for these procedures centers around blood loss, bruising, swelling, pain, and length of recovery. Further study is needed to document any measurable decreases due to the variations between different types of laser instruments, physician technique, and varying skin types of the patients who have the procedure.

Liquid silicone injections. Clinical investigation of liquid silicone injections for the correction of facial deformities took place from 1978 to 1988 under an FDA-approved and -monitored protocol. The injections were used by some physicians for the treatment of facial wrinkles, creases, and scars. However, alternative treatments for these problems are available, and the FDA currently considers liquid silicone injections to be in violation of federal law. Plastic surgeons have reported seeing patients with severe complications from having their breasts injected with liquid silicone in the 1950s. Note: The silicone gel in some breast implants is not associated with the complications caused by free injection of liquid silicone into the breast.

CHAPTER EIGHT

Makeup Application Step by Step

My Makeup Philosophy

I believe that beauty is more than skin deep. I believe with all my heart that physical beauty has little meaning compared with the importance of an individual's contribution to the world we live in. A capacity for compassion, kindness, creativity, and an abiding respect toward our fellow beings, the environment, and all living creatures is infinitely more meaningful than how we look. While this is my fervent belief, I also know that appearance has enormous consequences in life. Whether you can or should judge a book by its cover, for the most part, we all do. I don't know if Mel Gibson, Matthew McConaughey, Cindy Crawford, and Elle Macpherson are good people, but they are simply stunning to look at. Looking beautiful has power in our society and often determines the way people relate to each other. Ignoring the significance of that impact may be virtuous, but it is utterly unrealistic.

There are plenty of studies demonstrating that people assume an attractive individual is more successful, more intelligent, and happier than a less attractive one. Attractive people are more likely to get the jobs, pay raises, and career advancement they want, and are given authority faster than people who are considered less attractive.[1] I know that when I am nicely dressed and have my makeup on, people who don't know me treat me better than when I am dressed down. My older sister, who is a doctor of psychology, occasionally reminds me that in many cases the first sign of mental health problems is a deteriorating appearance. Conversely, one indication that a person is doing better emotionally is increased attention to how he or she looks.

Being attractive translates into power and a sense of well-being and self-esteem for both men and women. There are many ways in our culture to feel and look beautiful. Even if your features are less than perfect, your looks will be

---

[1] An article in the Marketplace section of the August 12, 1997, *Wall Street Journal* described a study in which researchers discovered that companies with executives who were highly rated for beauty and good looks had higher revenues than companies with fewer "beautiful" executives. They used 1,282 photos of people who worked for 289 Dutch advertising agencies (the study was conducted by Dutch and American economists) and had a panel rate the photos for beauty. The researchers had already done studies showing that good-looking people earn higher wages, and they wanted to see if these people were actually worth what they were being paid. According to the study, they were. The researchers think beautiful people may attract more clients to a firm and they also may improve the productivity and well-being of the people around them by giving them something attractive to look at!

enhanced by regular aerobic (exercise that raises your heart rate) and anaerobic exercise (weight-bearing exercise that tones or builds muscle); a healthy lifestyle (meaning no smoking; eating fruits, vegetables, and generally low-fat foods; maintaining an appropriate weight; and staying out of the sun); well-groomed hair; a classic, neat wardrobe; good posture and poise; and, for women, well-applied makeup. The latter is the subject of this chapter.

Applying makeup is about looking well groomed and feeling more beautiful. Wearing makeup can be exciting and fun. It can also express a great deal of personal power and élan. In the following pages I explain how to apply makeup with panache and sophistication so you can, if you choose, add to or improve this concept of beauty in your life. I personally feel less is best when it comes to makeup, but I know women's choices and tastes range from no makeup at all to the whole nine yards. Whatever your choice, if you do want to wear makeup, applying it deftly can make the difference between looking attractive and looking out of date, out of place, or just plain silly.

Throughout this chapter, I try to guide you through the maze of options and help you create a beautiful makeup look for yourself that feels comfortable and fits like a glove. **Although fashion statements can be taken to extremes—from following the whims of everything the fashion magazines portray or your favorite celebrity decides to get into, to holding on to looks that are long out-of-date—ignoring fashion is a mistake. Finding a balance between fashion, comfort, and personal style is the most logical and beautiful choice.**

Excerpt from Cosmetics Counter Update

Dear Paula,

Being female in our society is hard enough, but it is made worse by the media. It is almost impossible not to let the media and their idea of beauty drive you crazy. Because of their constant and often conflicting messages about what is beautiful and fashionable, it is difficult to decide whether you can be beautiful. I, like other girls my age [17], sometimes become a slave to what I read or see. Why don't they just leave women alone? Men don't have to go through this.

Recently, I was flipping through a magazine and it was explaining how men prefer women with long hair to women with short hair. Does that mean we should all have long hair? Women with low self-esteem who have short hair are bound to feel terrible about how they look and may very well decide they are no longer beautiful or desirable. And what makes this magazine think women have hair only to attract a man?

Looking at and reading a magazine can be fun, but it isn't easy to stop yourself from feeling inferior, because you can't live up to their retouched standards of beauty. Women, including myself, should come to realize that our differences are what make us unique and special. The world wouldn't be as interesting if we all walked around looking like Cindy Crawford or Kate Moss.

Tara

Dear Tara,

Your point is well taken. It isn't easy being bombarded with so many messages about what is beautiful. The media's idea of an attractive woman is more often than not one whose breasts spill out from her neckline and who wears a skirt so tight she can barely walk and shoes so impractical they are like Chinese foot-binding. Women are extremely vulnerable to the notion of being beautiful and glamorous, and even more anxious about being sexually attractive. Many are driven to spend a good deal of their lives preoccupied with grooming and with what the fashion pundits decide is good taste. Yet following the direction of most fashion designers results in making women little more than sex objects. If you don't believe me, just turn on MTV or flip through a fashion magazine; the repetitive, incessant image of women we see is strictly sexual and, as far as MTV is concerned, close to pornographic. Where are the positive images of family woman, businesswoman, volunteer, athlete, politician, or decision maker?

Finding a balance between personal style and what is fashionable takes a great deal of self-awareness and style savvy. It isn't easy. Just keep working on what is best for you, stay aware of what it means to be a powerful, influential, assertive, successful, joyful woman (only you know what that means for you), and you will find yourself making wise decisions when it comes to how you want to look and how you want to be seen.

Dressing Your Face

In many ways, makeup application is infinitely less complicated than skin care. Caring for your skin involves complex technical, medical, and physiological issues to sort through, while makeup is a more subjective and introspective art form. Makeup has little to do with facts and everything to do with skill and fashion. Discovering your personal preferences and honing your application technique are the essence of makeup application. **For the most part, makeup application is about experimentation and self-determination, because there are essentially no dos or don'ts, no have-tos, and no absolute rights or wrongs.** By way of illustration, you may decide that blue eyeshadow, dark brown lipstick, white foundation, and false eyelashes create the fashion statement you want to make, while I unequivocally recommend you avoid doing any of that. Yet wearing that makeup combination won't hurt you in the least. It may prevent you from being taken seriously or from getting the job you want, but that depends on whether you want to be taken seriously or what your career choices are.

When fashion is the topic, there are enough opinions and viewpoints to fill thousands and thousands of pages in hundreds of women's magazine every single month, 12 months a year. With such sweeping options screaming at us from the pages of *Vogue, Glamour, Marie Claire,* et al., choosing a direction may seem impossible. One model may wear a minimal sweep of tan blush on her cheeks, a hint of lipstick, taupe eyeshadow used on both the lid and crease, and a thin coating of mascara. Another model may have on an elaborate blend of contour shading; blush on top of that; an array of eyeshadow colors; dramatic, thick liner across the upper lashes and another thick sweep of liner along the lower lashes; and lots of mascara. The variations are endless. To make things even more confusing, each month there are new announcements about what is fashionable and what isn't. One month red lipstick is hot, the next month it's mauve, and the next brown, and then you read that blue eyeshadow is coming back and you have to avoid wearing anything more than a hint of blush.

Where do you fit in? Of course, that's completely up to you. **I want to show you how to build a basic and classic makeup application, one that most, if not all, makeup artists use repeatedly in one form or another.** Once you get these basics down—how to choose and apply concealer, foundation, powder, contour (if you want), blush, eyeshadow (one is plenty, but you can choose more), eyeliner (optional), eyebrow color (if needed or desired), mascara, lip liner (optional), and lipstick—wearing as little or as much color or as many of these products as you feel comfortable with is completely up to you. That's not to say I won't be throwing in my opinions of what I think works and looks best. If you use lip liner that smears, eyeshadows that streak and flake, mascara that clumps, blush that goes on choppy, eyeliner that smudges, or concealer that creases into the lines around your eyes and mouth, you and your makeup will not look beautiful in the least—and the goal is to look and feel more beautiful.

The pictures in this chapter show me doing my own full makeup application, and depict a progression of colors—neutral tones across the cheeks and eyes going from light to dark—that can fit most any face. Makeup professionals the world over use this pattern time after time, and you can see it on the covers of most fashion magazines and on news anchors, TV personalities, and celebrities. It can be adjusted in a wide variety of colors and intensities to achieve the look you want. This type of makeup application has been around for more than 25 years, established by makeup artist extraordinaire Way Bandy back in the early '70s and utilized today by most professional makeup artists.

Does Makeup Change with Age?

Should you be doing something different now that you are 50 instead of 20 or 30? That completely depends on what you were doing at 20 or 30. If you've been wearing a classic makeup application with neutral, nonshiny eyeshadows; soft shades of taupe, brown, or dark brown eyeliner; a sheer foundation that matches your skin exactly; a sheer powder that doesn't change the color of your foundation; a neutral shade of lipstick or a lipstick color that complements your blush; a softly blended blush color that coordinates with your lipstick; and a softly blended contour, there is absolutely nothing you need to change. This style of makeup is stunning at any age.

However, if in your youth you wore shiny, pastel eyeshadows; shiny, obvious blush; heavy foundation (in hopes of covering up blemishes or other imperfections); overly lined lips with greasy lip gloss or lipstick applied inside that line; and eyeliner in swoops of color around the eye; or if you try to reproduce whatever fad or style is the current rage, from a retro Marilyn Monroe look with wings of thick black eyeliner to the failed Evita image with overly tweezed brows, no blush, and overexaggerated lips, then yes, you need to change and go to a classic, well-blended finish, where no one aspect of your makeup is more prominent than any other.

Full, bold, blood-red lips, with minimal eye makeup and pale to almost nonexistent blush, or thickly lined eyes with flecks of gold eyeshadow, no blush, and brown lipstick, can look great on an 18-year-old model but strange on a mature woman going to the office or grocery shopping. Trying to look 20 is always a mistake for an older woman. You can end up looking like Bette Davis in *What Ever Happened to Baby Jane?,* which is probably not the fashion statement you're trying to make.

Being over 50 doesn't mean you have to overdo or undo your makeup. At any age, you need to find a style that makes you look and feel beautiful, and that means finding colors that enhance your appearance and blending techniques that make it all look natural and smooth instead of contrived or painted on.

Is Blue Eyeshadow Coming Back?

Every fall, winter, spring, and summer, fashion editors tell you what's hot and what's not. I want to remind everyone: you don't have to change what you are doing with every headline or forecast. Fashion pronouncements rarely have anything to do with improving your appearance or advancing your career, but everything to do with increasing cosmetics sales and finding something new for a journalist to say on a very old subject. Individual cosmetics lines, celebrity makeup artists, and elite fashion designers all want you to wear makeup (or clothes) according to their rules and regulations. We often obey their mandates, worrying that if we don't acquiesce, we'll look out of date. Regardless of how uncomfortable, bizarre, inappropriate, childlike, or outlandish the fashion statement, we often dutifully follow or worry that we should. Blue eyeshadow might come back, but who does that help? Dark brown lipstick may be in style, but does it make you look more attractive or just trendy? Shiny, iridescent eyeshadow may be all the rage, but wearing party makeup to the office won't help you gain stature in most jobs.

The truth is, if we don't like what we see on the fashion pages and don't buy it, the fashion designers lose their control over our lives, the control of giving us colors or products that take away our professional, successful, and beautiful image. Actually, the designers are no longer quite as much in control as they used to be. As it turns out, the majority of us won't invest heavily in trends anymore and instead stick mostly to classic looks.

All this reminds me of the baby-doll dresses that bombed at the department stores a few years back because most women wouldn't buy them regardless of how fashionable they were at the time. (Teens and young adults bought them in droves, but they absolutely did not belong in the "women's" department.) The beauty industry can keep manufacturing false eyelashes, orange foundations, shiny blue and green eyeshadows, dark brown or black lipsticks, and greasy lipsticks, telling us these are the hottest new looks, but if we don't buy them, the manufacturers will have to concentrate on what women really need to be beautiful and successful in the world.

As you look at fashion magazines and study the various makeup applications, styles, and images portrayed, decide which ones will help you with your career or any other aspect of your life that is important to you. The world is complicated enough; who needs to waste time wondering what to wear every season? It is far more powerful and beautiful to stick with classic looks that facilitate and enhance your ability to handle job interviews, get ahead in your career, raise a family, and concentrate on financial matters than to chase every new trend that comes along. The fashion headlines may look beautiful, but if they don't fit with your lifestyle and goals, let them be beautiful for someone else who has time and money to waste.

Excerpt from Cosmetics Counter Update

Dear Paula,

I've just read the latest issue of your newsletter and noticed that, once again, you're having a go at blue eyeshadow. When I first saw your book *Blue Eyeshadow Should Be Illegal*, I thought the title was simply a catchy pull, but after years of reading your books and newsletters, I have realized you are absolutely serious.

Paula, there are millions, nay, squillions of women of makeup-wearing age, with skin, hair, and eyes of every conceivable color, tone, and hue. How can you say with such certainty that none of them, not even one single woman, looks good in blue eyeshadow?

Your objection seems to be on two fronts: (1) it is out of date, and (2) it makes a woman look painted and not suitable for business.

That it is out of fashion (but apparently coming back) is of little concern to anyone but the dedicated fashion watcher. All colors come and go; brown eyeshadows were the thing in the '80s but are dull and drab in the '90s.

That it makes women look like painted dolls may or may not be true; it depends entirely on whether blue suits the woman in question and whether she has applied it well. Of course, it can look dreadful, but so can any wrong color, so why pick on blue? Why not violet or green?

You also seem to have the same hang-up about shine. Again, I have to say that some folks look quite good in matte makeup and some look better with a more lustrous finish. A totally matte makeup can look dull on some people, particularly on mature skin.

Sandra

Dear Sandra,

Much like any critic, I spend a great deal of time researching and analyzing the issues and try always to state clearly the criteria on which I base my comments. I try not to be capricious or glib, but sincere and earnest. In terms of blue eyeshadow, yes, there are "squillions" of women and they can wear whatever they like, but I can nevertheless say "Don't wear it" with the same certainty that I suggest not wearing spiked orange hair or black lipstick. At least not if your goal is to be taken seriously in a career or any kind of job save in a punk rock band. Blue eyeshadow or any other obvious color on the face is a fashion mistake. The most successful and respected women in a wide variety of careers are not wearing colorful makeup applications. Bold splashes of color are used for shock value, not for sophistication or finesse.

Lord knows the cosmetics industry loves supplying women with ill-conceived products—peach foundations, greasy eye pencils, mascara that smears, and greasy, gooey lipsticks—but that's what an open market is all about.

Brown eyeshadows dated? Not in any fashion magazine I've read over the past 15 years. Quite the contrary: if there is one aspect of fashion that has hung on the longest, it is the classic or understated makeup look—neutral eyeshadows, soft neutral blush and muted lipstick, and natural-looking foundation. In my books, I state at length what else should be illegal besides blue eyeshadow, and that includes pink, violet, green, and shiny eyeshadows (they make skin look wrinkly), bright pastels, and on and on.

By the way, I've worked with dozens of makeup artists, but I have met none over the past five years who even owned any pastel or shiny eyeshadows, much less used them.

I agree that a slight sheen helps older skin look moist and smooth, but why produce it artificially with shiny powders when using a foundation that leaves the skin looking dewy can do the same? Sometimes just leaving powder out of the makeup routine can leave the entire face looking very moist, and then shiny eyeshadows and blush are unnecessary.

Where to Begin

Three of the most difficult aspects of makeup are choosing the right colors, discerning the differences between products, and learning the correct application techniques. Though these issues need to be addressed, they are only part of the picture. Wondering where to put your blush or how to blend your foundation before you know what type of foundation or what color of blush you should be wearing is putting the cart before the horse. Before you choose specific makeup colors, discriminate between products, or deal with application, it is important to have a clear idea of the makeup look and style you want to create. Just as you would choose clothes to wear that are appropriate for where you are going—you wouldn't put on a jogging suit to go to a formal dinner or wear a long gown for running—the same guidelines are true for makeup.

Color, style, and fashion are all essential elements in clothing, and they are also essential to putting together a great makeup look. Too often women shop for or apply makeup with only one of those things in mind. Shopping for a lipstick or eyeshadow color without taking into account the other items in your makeup wardrobe is a mistake. Decide what kind of makeup wardrobe you want to create and then go about choosing compatible colors, products, and application techniques to fit that concept.

The way you see yourself, the way you want to be seen, what you do for a living, what you do in your leisure time, what colors are in your wardrobe, what style of clothing you are comfortable in, and how much time you are willing to spend creating a particular look all affect the way you choose and wear makeup. Those elements should set the course for choosing the right colors and products. So let's think a bit about the image you want to create.

Choosing Makeup According to Your Image

The first part of this makeup self-analysis is to take a close look at yourself. How do you want to be seen? What do you do for a living? What occupies most of your time during the day? The external image you want to project in your business life and personal life is what wearing makeup is all about. Too often we dress our face without thinking about how it affects our image. One vivid example of this can be seen in the movie *Working Girl,* which stars Melanie Griffith and Harrison Ford. Griffith's appearance changes dramatically as her character decides to become more "professional" in order to enhance her career aspirations. In addition to changing her wardrobe, she changes the way she wears her makeup. In order to look more polished and put-together, she softens her makeup look. Griffith goes from wearing strong pastel-colored eyeshadows to taupes and browns. She stops wearing heavy black eyeliner on the lid and lower lashes in favor of a more subtle shade of dark brown. Her lipstick changes from cranberry red to a neutral coral-tan, and her boldly applied blush is replaced by a soft neutral tone. The striking difference in her looks is a beautiful example of how makeup can affect the image you project.

Rather than just randomly selecting a lipstick, stop and consider not only whether it's the right color for the outfits you wear, but also whether it is too soft, too sheer, too noticeable, too sexy, not sexy enough, or just right to support the image you want to project. **Problems with how you apply makeup can be solved via technique, but understanding how you want others to see you comes from a sense of purpose and an understanding of what you want out of life.**

Before You Start

Because makeup goes on poorly over unclean skin, the first step in applying beautiful makeup is to start with a clean face. Wash your face with a water-soluble cleanser and follow it with an irritant-free toner (completely optional) or topical disinfectant (depending on your skin type), an exfoliant, and sunscreen (unless your foundation contains sunscreen). Then you can start applying your makeup. Women with dry skin should also wear moisturizer under their foundation (preferably a moisturizer with a good SPF if the foundation doesn't contain an SPF). Women with normal to oily skin should avoid wearing moisturizer under their foundation. Moisturizer of any kind only adds to an active oil flow, and will make skin look greasy that much sooner. (It is, however, completely acceptable to wear a minimal amount of moisturizer over dry areas such as the under-eye area or cheeks.)

The only reason to use a moisturizer is to smooth and lubricate dry skin or dry areas. In spite of what you hear from cosmetics salespeople, moisturizer does not and cannot protect the face from a foundation, nor is that necessary. It's a good sales gimmick, but not the truth. There is nothing "bad" inside a foundation that your face needs to be protected from. Moisturizers are absorbed into the skin, and once they are, to all intents and purposes they're gone, and they can't prevent anything else you put on the face from going where it wants. Whatever protection you think you're applying when you put on a moisturizer is wiped away as you apply your foundation.

I know this idea of wearing a moisturizer only when you have dry skin borders on heresy, but in the long run it makes the most sense for your skin, especially if you are wearing a water-based or emollient foundation. What you might not know is that most water-based foundations, and definitely emollient foundations, contain exactly the same ingredients as your moisturizer, so it isn't necessary to double up products. If you wear at the same time a moisturizer that contains an SPF 15 and a water-based foundation without an SPF, your face can become too slippery and the rest of your makeup will tend to slide right off by lunchtime. If you feel a moisturizer helps your foundation go on more smoothly, the problem could lie in the way you apply your foundation, the type of foundation you're using, or your skin-care routine, which may be drying out your skin and leaving a rough feeling rather than a smooth one.

A good way to judge whether your skin needs moisturizer during the day is to notice how long your skin feels dry after you wash your face. Some amount of dryness immediately after you wash your face is typical. However, if this feeling lasts longer than 15 or 20 minutes, you should wear a lightweight moisturizer under your foundation. If your skin tends to feel extremely dry after you wash your face, wear a more emollient moisturizer under your foundation. If your skin tends to become drier as the day goes by, that too is a good reason to wear a moisturizer.

Important note: Either your daytime moisturizers or your foundation must be rated SPF 15 (SPF 8 and over will do, but most dermatologists and oncologists encourage SPF 15) and contain either titanium dioxide, avobenzone, or zinc oxide. There is no reason to wear two products, a sunscreen and a moisturizer, when so many products combine both beautifully.

Less Is Best!

Never use more than you have to, either in the intensity of the colors you choose or in the number of products you wear. Many steps in applying makeup can be consolidated or eliminated without affecting your overall makeup look in any way.

Frequently a salesperson at the cosmetics counter insists that you need an absurd number of products in order to be properly and attractively made up. My job is to make things less complicated, because more complicated doesn't mean you will look any better. If anything, a more complicated makeup routine can mean more mistakes, causing you to look overdone as well as wasting your valuable time.

Speaking of doing too much, so-called submoisturizers, eyelid foundations, blemish cover-ups, and color correctors—to name a few—are, with few exceptions, completely unnecessary. They complicate the process of applying makeup by requiring additional blending and allowing too many colors and products to interact on the skin at the same time, leaving a thick, gunky mess and contrasting colors on the face. Your SPF 15 foundation (or foundation with an SPF 15 sunscreen/moisturizer underneath) can quite nicely accomplish all the functions those extra products are supposedly designed to handle without any of the fuss and expense.

Submoisturizers are an interesting breed of moisturizer on the cosmetics scene. You find them mostly in the higher-priced cosmetics lines. Perhaps women who can afford to waste money are more easily convinced to waste it. These products are sold rather persuasively as being needed "to prepare and help the skin absorb the moisturizer." These submoisturizers all contain standard moisturizing ingredients, usually the same ingredients found in most irritant-free toners or lightweight moisturizers. They do not prepare the skin in any way and they do not help the skin to absorb moisturizer any better, they only oversaturate the skin. If the moisturizer you are using doesn't take care of your dry skin, you need to change moisturizers instead of applying additional products.

Eyelid foundations are sold to the consumer to help eyeshadows stay in place longer. The eye area is indeed a tricky place to get color to last, but there are ways to make it stay without special eyelid foundations. Besides, most eyelid foundations are very similar to regular foundations. Placing face foundation on your eyelid and putting loose powder over it works just as well. Also, if your eyeshadows smear or slip into the eyelid crease, the problem will be greatly reduced if you do not place a moisturizer or greasy foundations on your eyelid.

Blemish cover-ups are sold to consumers solely on the basis of something I call acne anxiety. The promise conveyed by the word "cover-up" is that this product really can hide a blemish, but nothing could be further from reality. Most cover-ups are heavier than your foundation, and over a blemish they look thick and obvious. And if the blemish cover-up doesn't match your foundation exactly (most don't), it will look like a different layer of color (usually a shade of peach) placed over the blemish, bringing more attention to the very problem you are trying to hide. Even if the cover-up is the same color as your foundation, you will probably place too much extra makeup over the lesion. Your foundation all by itself is more than sufficient to cover the redness without bringing more attention to the area. I totally understand the desire to want these facial sore spots to disappear. Unfortunately, there is only so much you can do to cover up a blemish before you start making matters more obvious by layering on too much makeup.

It is especially problematic to apply concealer only over blemishes and nowhere else, without any foundation. Natural color and texture of your skin does not resemble foundation or concealer. Spot application looks spotty. That doesn't hide anything, but can look very strange in daylight.

Some concealers and cover-ups are dubbed "medicated" and meant to cover blemishes, but they are in no way any better for blemishes. They don't disinfect or exfoliate, and they don't cover any better than normal concealers.

Color correctors are those bottles of pink, lavender, or yellow liquid meant to be worn under your foundation to alter skin color. These little gems are hard to find anymore, but some cosmetics lines are steadfast in making you believe you need them. The notion is that if your skin is pink or ruddy, you need to tone it down with a yellow-tinted color corrector. If your skin is olive or sallow, you would use the pink or lavender color corrector. It's an interesting concept, but a waste of time.

The ingredient lists for most color correctors are very similar to those for moisturizers, which means they are easily absorbed into the skin. Once they are absorbed, you are left with a slight tint of pink, lavender, or yellow on the face. Supposedly this means you have now changed your skin tone for the better. In fact, once the liquid has been absorbed, the result is often so minor as to have little to no real effect on skin tone at all. For the sake of argument, though, let's say there is a noticeable effect. The tint of the color corrector on your skin would mix with your foundation and you could end up with a very strange shade of foundation. A good foundation in a neutral, yellow-tone base should be able to correct and even out all skin tones without adding another layer of makeup on your face.

The Classic Face

Basic, classic makeup encompasses all of the following elements: concealer/highlighter, foundation, powder, contour (optional), blush, eyeshadow, eyeliner (optional), eyebrow color (if needed), lip liner (optional), and lipstick. For each of these steps, you want to find a corresponding product type that is best for your skin type and the coverage or look you want. Each step also requires an application and blending tool so you can achieve a smooth, flawless appearance. **Along the way, you can eliminate steps that seem excessive or too complicated, and decide how much makeup you want to wear and what colors are suitable to your needs.** Do you want an evening look, a business look, a trendy fashion statement, or a casual, sporty appearance? With those decisions in place, accompanied by a deft technique, your makeup can go on relatively quickly and easily.

The first two steps in applying a complete makeup are to reduce the darkness under the eyes and apply a foundation to even out the skin (it's sort of like putting on panties and a bra). Once that is done, the eyeshadows and blushes can blend on smoothly over an even palette instead of over varying skin textures and colors. Whether you start your application with the concealer or the foundation depends more on personal preference than anything else, although the color of the concealer is another factor. For the sake of organization, I'll start with the concealer.

Concealer (Highlighter)

Generally, a concealer is thought of as a product that covers blemishes, while a highlighter is a product that covers dark circles under the eyes or highlights certain areas of the face, and is a lighter texture than a concealer. Despite the names, highlighters and concealers vary in consistency and usage from product line to product line, but are truly interchangeable depending on the effect you desire. Regardless of the name, concealers or highlighters with thicker consistencies are best for covering problem areas such as dark circles under the eye or extreme redness on cheeks or noses. Concealers or highlighters with a lighter or thinner consistency are better for minimal coverage and creating highlighted areas of the face you want accented. Throughout the rest of this book I refer to all products that provide extra coverage (over and above what foundation can do) or make certain areas of the face lighter as concealers.

The primary purpose of concealers is to offset the natural shadows that occur under the eyes and, in more elaborate makeup applications, to highlight certain areas of the face such as the center of the nose, forehead, top of the cheekbones, or center of the chin. Principally, the under-eye area needs concealer most because the eye is set back in a socket, which lies in a shadow created by the surrounding bone structure. In addition, the skin around the eye tends to be thinner than the skin on the rest of the face, so pigment discolorations and surface veins easily show through, making the under-eye area look dark and dull. The first thing you need, then, is a light flesh-tone highlighter that is a shade or two lighter than your foundation (see the picture on page 269).

However, if you don't have dark circles under the eye area, you don't need a concealer. If your foundation is opaque enough to even out the skin tone under the eyes, you don't need an extra product for that area.

The logic behind using a lighter flesh-tone color is the same basic rule you learned in Art 101: when you need to make paint a lighter color, you add a lighter color than you started with. Any other color, or the same color, or a darker color would defeat the purpose. Blue, yellow, or regular shades such as your foundation color will not make the under-eye area lighter. Standard shades can cover discolorations, which is fine, but applying a lighter shade is the only way to correct the darkness caused by shadows. Also, a slightly lighter under-eye area can make the face look brighter and translucent. **(However, foundation may be all you need to even out minimal discolorations under the eye, cheeks, or nose, or for minor facial discolorations.)**

When you shop for an effective concealer, it is critical that the concealer be the same basic, natural skin tone as your foundation, only one or two shades lighter. That way you will be assured of having the foundation and concealer blend together under the eye. If you choose a concealer that is a very different color than your foundation, you will simply end up with a third color where they overlap and intersect.

The only time you wouldn't use a lighter concealer is when the area under the eye is naturally lighter or the same color as the rest of the face. In that case, it is fine to apply your foundation there with no concealer. In fact, it may sometimes be necessary to apply a concealer that is slightly darker than your foundation to avoid having a whitish goggle effect around the eye.

I prefer applying concealer first and then the foundation. If you are using the new ultra-matte foundations, getting this step blended on first prevents streaking and staining. (It's hard to blend anything over ultra-matte foundations.) You can apply your foundation in a small arc around the inside corner of the eye or, for a more involved makeup application, you can apply it in a sweep under the entire eye and out on the upper cheekbone. Blend this out evenly, being sure not to spread it onto areas where you don't want it. The foundation is then applied lightly over this area and blended out over the face.

There are times when I choose to wear as little makeup as possible, and in those situations I use only a minimal amount of concealer that is closer to my true skin tone than the concealer I normally use, or I use a lighter shade of foundation than I normally do and apply it only in the under-eye area. The trick in this case is to blend extremely well so that there is no discernible edge between the concealer and the part of the face where there is no makeup.

In the past it was almost impossible to find concealers in a good selection of colors that also didn't crease into the lines around the eyes. Now the tide has turned and many cosmetics lines have lovely shades and textures to choose from. When shopping for a concealer, the primary things to look for are (1) a neutral skin tone that is one or two shades lighter than your foundation, but not so light that it looks obvious when blended under the eye area, (2) a smooth texture to assure smooth blending, and (3) staying power so it doesn't crease into the lines around the eyes.

Types of Concealer

Concealers come in four different forms: stick concealers, creamy liquid concealers, cream concealers, and the new ultra-matte or stay-put creamy liquid concealers, which blend on smoothly and creamily and dry quickly into an unmovable layer.

Stick concealers: Stick concealers come in tubes like lipsticks.

Application: Stick concealers are applied to the under-eye area much the way a lipstick is applied to the mouth. They can be applied over or under your foundation, depending on how much coverage you want—under the foundation provides less coverage and over the foundation provides more. Dab the stick over the area in dots and then blend. Avoid wiping it on like a matte streak of color. That tends to build up too much makeup and it also pulls the eye area, causing sagging. If the skin under the eye area is dry or wrinkled, it does help to first apply a lightweight moisturizer and then apply the concealer. Be careful the moisturizer isn't too greasy or put on too heavily, or it will assure slippage of the concealer into facial lines.

Pros: Depending on their consistency, stick concealers can provide more complete coverage and control for very dark circles under the eye. They tend to go on thickly and don't spread easily, which means you can better control the application.

Cons: The texture of many stick concealers is rather dry and thick, which makes them difficult to blend without overpulling the skin under the eye. They also go on too heavily, which can create an obviously made-up look. Some stick concealers are also quite greasy, which can look less obvious, but can also slip too easily into the lines around the eyes.

Creamy liquid concealers: Creamy liquid concealers generally come in small squeeze-tube containers or long, thin tubes with wand applicators.

Application: Use your finger or the wand applicator to transfer the liquid concealer in small dots or a light coat of color under the eye area. Blend gently along the under-eye with either your finger or the sponge applicator, concentrating the amount of concealer over the darkest areas. If the skin under the eye area is dry or wrinkled, it does help to first apply a lightweight moisturizer and then apply the concealer. Be careful the moisturizer isn't too greasy or put on too heavily, or it will assure slippage of the concealer into facial lines.

Pros: Depending on their consistency, creamy liquid concealers provide very light, even coverage and have the least tendency to crease into the eye area.

Cons: Depending on their consistency, creamy liquid concealers can have too much movement and be hard to control. It is important when applying an under-eye concealer to keep the color just where you want it. If the concealer is too greasy or loose, it can spread too easily, highlighting parts of the face you don't want highlighted. Some liquid concealers go on too thinly, offering very little coverage, but if you don't want a lot, these are the way to go.

Cream concealers: Cream concealers usually come in small pots and typically have a smooth and creamy texture. Occasionally these may also have a dry, thick texture.

Application: Depending on their consistency, cream concealers can go on easily with your fingertips or a sponge, placing the color in dots under the eye area. Blend the concealer out under the eye area, concentrating the application over the darkest areas. If the cream concealer has a dry, thick texture, it can be very difficult to blend and can look heavy and obvious on the skin. If the skin under the eye area is dry or wrinkled, it does help to first apply a lightweight moisturizer and then apply the concealer. If the cream concealer is very emollient, use minimal moisturizer under the eye area and dab off the excess. Most moisturizers can make these types of concealers slip even more easily into facial lines.

Pros: Cream concealers can have a very pleasing, creamy, and moist consistency, but they can also be rather thick and heavy. Depending on the consistency, they can go on well and provide even coverage. They are especially good for someone with very dry skin who wants more coverage.

Cons: If the cream concealer is too thick or greasy, it will crease into the lines on your face. If it is dry and thick, it can be difficult to blend and can easily crease into facial lines.

Ultra-matte or stay-put creamy liquid concealers: The new ultra-matte concealers generally come in thin tubes with wand applicators.

Application: Use your finger or the wand applicator to transfer the liquid concealer in small dots or a light coat of color in the under-eye area. You must blend these on very quickly and accurately because they dry within seconds. Once these ultra-matte concealers are dried in place, they don't budge, so you could end up with streaks or patches of color. There is no way to adjust blending after they have dried into place. Once stay-put concealers dry, they do what they say they do! If the skin under the eye area is dry or wrinkled, it does help to first apply a lightweight moisturizer and then apply the concealer.

Pros: Depending on their consistency, ultra-matte concealers provide very light, even coverage and, if blended on correctly, they absolutely will not crease into the lines around the eyes. They are great if you tend to lose makeup during the day or have problems with makeup slipping.

Cons: Because ultra-matte concealers stay so well and are so matte, they can make lines under the eyes look worse. It doesn't help to apply moisturizer underneath because that can only make the concealer streak and look stained. It is important when applying under-eye concealers to keep the color just where you want it and to blend quickly.

Techniques for Blending Concealer

Regardless of the type of concealer you use, the application remains basically the same. Dab the color on with either your fingertips, the wand applicator, or the tube concealer itself in a half-inch crescent from the corner of the eye out to approximately one-third of the way under the eye. Apply the concealer only where the eye area is dark. If the eye area is dark all the way out under the eye, then that's where the concealer should go. You can apply concealer to the eyelid too if that area is also dark and could use some lightening.

If you want a more elaborate makeup application, you can apply the concealer along the flat bridge of the nose, along the laugh lines, out along the entire under-eye area and on the top of the cheekbone, and in the center of the forehead and chin for accent and enhancement (see the picture on page 269). These options tend to be complicated and time-consuming, even for women adept at applying their makeup, and you can get the same results by applying the rest of your makeup correctly. I used none of those techniques with my makeup as it appears on the cover of this book, and all those areas appear nicely highlighted because of the way I applied the rest of my makeup. However, in the pictures that follow, I used the more formal technique to show some of that application placement. If you do choose to highlight these areas, place your highlighter in dots over or under your foundation in these areas and blend well, controlling the color so it does not spread all over your face.

Whether you apply the concealer first and then the foundation or the foundation first and then the concealer over that, carefully blend the concealer out and under the eye in a dabbing motion, with either your finger or sponge (I prefer using a sponge always), making sure you cannot see the edge where the concealer stops and the foundation starts. The trick is to keep the concealer blended only over the area where it is needed.

Concealer Mistakes to Avoid

1. **If you have noticeable lines around the eyes, do not wear a concealer that goes on too thickly or too drily; it can cake under the eye and exaggerate wrinkles.**
2. **Consider my recommendations in *Don't Go to the Cosmetics Counter Without Me* for specific concealers that don't crease into the lines around eyes. If you buy a concealer that's not in my book, be sure to test it first by wearing it for a while under the eyes to be sure that it doesn't crease and that it works with the foundation or your skin tone.**

3. **If the concealer is obvious, you've chosen the wrong shade.**
4. **Do not wear a peach, orange, rose, or ash shade of concealer.**
5. **If the skin is dry, apply a lightweight moisturizer under the eye to prevent the concealer from caking or making the wrinkles look more noticeable. A moisturizer that is too heavy or emollient can make almost any concealer slip into the lines around the eyes.**
6. **Do not forget to blend the foundation and concealer together so there are no edges where one stops and the other starts.**

Foundation

Personally, I've never been fond of the whole process of smearing foundation all over my face or even part of my face. I totally understand when women complain about feeling "made up" when they wear a foundation. So why do I recommend using foundation at all? Because of the flawless, even base a foundation can provide. If the skin has a uniform color, texture, and appearance, the blush and eyeshadow colors you apply will look smooth instead of choppy. **However, to the extent possible, the face should never look like it has a layer of foundation on it.**

If you are already blessed with a totally even, perfect complexion, you will nevertheless want to consider wearing a foundation because of how it helps eyeshadows and blushes go on more evenly. If you try to blend blushes and eyeshadows without foundation, they will most likely go on choppily or wear unevenly during the day. Foundation keeps those powdered colors in place. Skin itself has no real adhesive properties (think about what would adhere to it if it did). Foundation therefore gives the rest of the makeup something to hold on to evenly. Blushes and eyeshadows have some ability to cling, but not much.

Finding the Perfect Foundation Color

I cannot stress this point enough: your skin and foundation should match exactly. If you are pale, that's OK—accept the fact that you are pale and buy a light foundation that matches exactly. **Whether you have red hair and fair skin or black hair and dark ebony skin, the foundation must match your underlying skin color exactly. Do not buy a foundation that will make your face look even a shade or two darker or lighter.** Even with a difference that slight, you run the risk of a more obvious makeup application than you really want, particularly in daylight. Find a foundation that matches your skin perfectly and goes on sheerly and smoothly.

When I tell you to match the foundation with your underlying skin color, you may be asking yourself, "Exactly what is meant by skin color?"

Traditionally, skin color has been defined by underlying skin tones described as olive, when the skin appears ashen or green in color; sallow, when the skin has a yellow or golden shade; and ruddy, when the skin has overtones of pink or red. These categories hold true for all women, including women of color; your underlying skin color will always relate to one of those skin tones. You may have been told that you are a particular "season" and your wardrobe and foundation color should be a specific undertone, either cool (blue tones) or warm (yellow tones). Unfortunately, all this information surrounding skin tone can be misleading when it comes to choosing a foundation color.

If you are told your face has cool undertones, meaning blue undertones, should you wear a blue-toned foundation? Of course not. If your skin color is ashen, choosing an ashen foundation will make you look more green. If your face is strongly pink or red, applying a pink foundation all over will make you look like you're wearing a pink mask. None of those would look natural and flawless the way foundation should look, and none of them would come close to matching your skin's underlying, basic color.

When purchasing a foundation, it is important to identify your overall, exact skin color and find a foundation that matches it, regardless of the underlying tone. **For the most part, regardless of your race, nationality, or age, your foundation should be some shade of neutral beige, tan, dark brown, chocolate brown, or ebony with an undertone of yellow but without any orange, pink, green, or blue. There are no orange, pink, green, or blue people, and buying foundations in those colors is absurd.** Why a yellow undertone? Because skin color almost always has a yellow undertone: that's just what the natural color of melanin (the pigment in the skin) tends to be. There are a few exceptions to this rule. Native North American or South American women, a tiny percentage of African-American women, and some Polynesian women do indeed have a red cast to their skin, and in those instances this information about neutral foundations should be ignored. Because their skin has a slightly reddish cast, they need to look for foundations that have a slightly reddish cast to them, but that's only a hint of brownish red, and not orange or peach.

A few makeup lines are aimed at the Asian woman. These boast a "unique collection of yellow-toned foundations" appropriate for all skin types, but most specifically the Asian woman. I concur that most skin types, including Asian women, are better served by yellow/neutral-based foundations and powders. However, plenty of lines have awesome yellow/neutral-based foundation colors. The same is true for African-American women. There are many lines claiming to meet the needs of darker skin colors, but more often than not, these lines have poor color selections or poor foundation types. It is best to find a foundation color and type that works for your skin type rather than limiting yourself to a special line claiming to serve a specific skin color.

Question: If all the fashion magazines and makeup experts talk about foundations being sheer and matching the skin exactly, why do so many women of all ages wear heavy-looking, obvious foundations? It may be confusion about skin tone and foundation color; it may be failure to check the foundation in daylight; and, in some cases, it may have something to do with the fact that many women hate their skin and think a layer of foundation looks better than what exists naturally. Rather than arguing about the emotional ramifications of disliking your skin, let me just say that covering your face with an obvious layer of foundation only makes matters worse. **It is essential to an attractive makeup application of any kind to start with a good, sheer foundation; otherwise you will look as if the makeup is wearing you.** Even if you feel that you are in need of a foundation that provides good coverage, *obvious* coverage is a monumental mistake and can negatively affect the entire makeup application.

An Exception to the Rule

Although you are attempting to exactly match the skin color of your face when you choose a foundation, in some cases it is more important to match the foundation to the color of your neck. If your face is darker than your neck and your foundation matches the face, it will look like a mask because of the difference in color. The opposite is also true. If your face is lighter than your neck and you put on a foundation that matches the face, it will still look like a mask because of the difference in color. In this situation, match the foundation more to the neck color or to a color in between the color of the neck and the face.

For some women who have serious facial discolorations or scars, and need a heavy foundation application that provides opaque, full, concealing coverage, a heavy or thick foundation is the only way to achieve this effect. Foundations making claims about superior coverage that also looks natural are not telling the truth. You can't cover your face with foundation and camouflage imperfections without seeing what is providing the coverage. It doesn't mean you shouldn't consider a heavier foundation; just be aware that you are exchanging one problem for another. It's the lesser of two dilemmas to choose between, and you are the best judge of what works best for you.

The Final Decision

Once you have selected a foundation color, there is only one way to be absolutely sure it is right for you: apply the color all over your face and check it outside in the daylight. Check it from all angles and decide if it matches your skin exactly. If you applied it carefully but there are lines of demarcation at the jaw area; if it looks too thick or too greasy; if it gives the face an orange, pink, rose, or ashen tint; or if it looks heavy and opaque instead of sheer and light, go back to the testers. In fact, you may need to test several types before you find the right foundation.

One popular technique for narrowing down your choices is to test several different colors that look like good possibilities by placing them in stripes in a row over the cheek area. The best choice is the one that blends almost perfectly with your skin color. The wrong choices will stand out, with obvious edges that don't disappear into your skin. This procedure is a reliable method for eliminating choices, but I've also seen it go wrong more times than I can count because it doesn't go far enough. Use it only as an elimination process; it does not replace the need to check out the color on the face in the daylight.

Keep trying on foundations until you find the best one. **Once you've made a selection you feel good about, apply it all over your face, wait at least two hours, and check it again in the daylight. How a foundation wears during the day—does it change color or become too greasy or dry as the day passes?—can be evaluated only after you've worn it for a while.** Once you've assessed all these details in the daylight, you can safely make a final determination as to whether this is the right color or type of foundation for you. Please take the time to follow this procedure. It is the only way to make sure you've found the right foundation. This advice will lead you in the right direction. If you rely only on the salesperson and the lighting at the cosmetics counters, it will be pure luck if you end up with the right color. And if you get the foundation wrong, regardless of how perfectly you choose and apply everything else in your makeup wardrobe, it will all look wrong.

Custom-Blended Foundations

If a foundation is blended for you and you only, will that get you the best shade? This style of selling makeup is very enticing. The customer-service interaction is impressive. Your foundation is supposedly mixed and matched for your exact skin color and needs. The premise is that there are only so many ready-made shades and you might be better off having one custom-blended. Unfortunately, it sounds like a better idea than it is. The major problem with custom-blended cosmetics is that the success of the match depends on the expertise of the salesperson—and there are huge variations in skill.

As nice as custom-blended foundations sound, the formulations are not necessarily superior to or even as good as standard products. The foundation may be too greasy or too dry and it might turn to rose or peach as you wear it. With so many off-the-shelf foundation products available, in many excellent colors, custom blending turns out to be more an expensive gimmick than anything else.

When should you try a custom-blended product, particularly foundation? When you have tested many standard foundations and are still frustrated with the color of your foundation.

Types of Foundation

Now that you know how to find the right foundation color, figuring out the type of foundation best suited to your skin type is the next hurdle. Cosmetics counters carry a mind-boggling assortment of foundations these days, including oil-free and matte foundations, ultra-matte or stay-put foundations, water-based foundations, oil-based foundations, pressed powder–based foundations, cream-to-powder foundations, so-called self-adjusting foundations, and foundations that have shine. Given this range of options, narrowing down your choices can be tricky.

Oil-free and matte foundations: These almost always contain oils (even though the names don't sound as though they would) or ingredients that act like oils. These oils and oil-like ingredients are not necessarily bad for any skin type, but their presence demonstrates that the term "oil-free" is another cosmetics industry contrivance that won't necessarily help you find the best product for your skin type. Regardless of the formulations, what most of these foundations have in common is that they blend on in a matte finish, with no shine or dewy appearance whatsoever; at least, that's what the good oil-free or matte foundations should do. Oil-free, matte foundations come in two types: one looks like a bottle of colored water that contains mostly talc, alcohol, and coloring agents; the other looks like a traditional liquid foundation.

Application: See the "Blending Foundation" section later in this chapter.

Pros: These foundations are the best choice for women who want balanced coverage with no shine at all, and who like a smooth, matte look. They last much longer on oily skin than most other foundation types (except for the ultra-matte foundations), which for some women is a very desirable, if not essential, effect.

Cons: The disadvantage of using oil-free, matte foundations is that some of them can go on rather heavily and masklike, leaving the skin feeling quite dry and taut. In order to get this makeup on evenly, you must blend quickly or it will dry in place before you know it, and then it can be difficult to blend further. You have to get it on right the first time, because once it's on, it doesn't move easily. This foundation can be hard to work over when applying eyeshadow and blush. Oil-free, matte foundations have less movement than more emollient foundations, which means eyeshadow and blush have a tendency to stick to them, which can make blending and correcting mistakes a bit irksome.

I never recommend alcohol-based foundations because of their poor coverage and the irritation alcohol can cause the skin.

Women of color should be careful when choosing an oil-free or matte foundation. Even if it is the right color, these foundations can tend to look gray and ashen after being applied to darker skin tones. Skin that shows no shine or reflection in general tends to look dull gray with this kind of foundation, and that effect is even more pronounced for women of color.

Ultra-matte or stay-put foundations: These are an amazing new breed of foundations that truly stay put. Most have a very liquidy consistency and are blended on like any other foundation. The only trick is to blend these on as quickly as possible because once they dry into place, they cannot be budged or smoothed. If you end up with a streak or smear, it will be almost impossible to blend away. These foundations have the most amazing staying power. Try them if you have exceptionally oily skin, live in a humid climate, or prefer an ultra-matte finish; you'll be impressed.

Application: See the "Blending Foundation" section later in this chapter.

Pros: These foundations are a superior option if you have seriously oily skin, have trouble with makeup slipping or disappearing as the day goes by, live in a humid climate, exercise but still like having your makeup stay put, or like a completely matte finish. Ultra-matte, stay-put foundations will outlast any other foundation, with no slippage or movement. If you have oily skin, these are an absolute must to try.

Cons: The disadvantage of using ultra-matte foundations is much the same as for the oil-free and matte foundations, so refer to those warnings and increase them twofold.

Water-based and standard liquid foundations: Water-based does not mean oil-free, even if the label says so; it generally means the first ingredient is water and the second or third ingredient is some kind of oil or emollient slip agent. These foundations look like a somewhat thick liquid and pour slowly but easily out of the bottle. They are perfect for women with normal to dry skin.

Application: See the "Blending Foundation" section later in this chapter.

Pros: Most water-based foundations are best for those with normal to dry skin. They are perfect for wearing without a moisturizer for these skin types, or they can be worn with a basic moisturizer or a moisturizer that contains sunscreen. The oil or emollient part of these foundations gives them good movement, which makes blending a pleasure and allows blushes and eyeshadows to blend on effortlessly and evenly over the face. Mistakes are easily buffed away with the sponge.

Cons: If you have oily or combination skin, this is not the foundation type for you. The little bit of oil or emollients in a water-based foundation show shine almost immediately if you have oily skin. Those who do not have oily skin but have a paranoia about any shine on the face will not like the effects of a water-based foundation either; the small amount of oil or emollients in this cosmetic may make you nervous. For the most part, I personally don't feel there are any disadvantages to using water-based foundations and I recommend them wholeheartedly. Water-based foundations are also a great option for women of color. The slight amount of oil these contain help create a nice glow on the skin, preventing darker skin tones from appearing dull or ashen.

If you are concerned with the small amount of shine that water-based foundations leave behind on the skin, try adding a light dusting of loose powder. After you've blended the foundation in place, you can apply the powder all over the face to reduce the shine.

Oil-based foundations: Oil-based foundations have oil as their first ingredient and water usually as their second or third ingredient. Oil-based foundations feel greasy and thick, look greasy and thick, and go on greasy, but can blend out quite sheerly and softly. You can blend an oil-based foundation to a very thin, subtle layer of makeup.

Application: See the "Blending Foundation" section later in this chapter.

Pros: Oil-based foundations can be very good for women with extremely dry skin or wrinkled skin. The emollient ingredients help the skin look very dewy and moist, which can minimize wrinkles.

Cons: Oil-based foundations tend to be very greasy, thick, and heavy, and can look that way on the skin unless you are very adept at blending. They also have a tendency to turn orange on the skin because the extra oil affects the pigments in the foundation. This can be true for women of color: oil-based foundations can look orange after they are worn for a while. The typical recommendation for using oil-based foundations is to add water to your sponge so that it goes on thinner, more like a water-based foundation. But that can be tricky to gauge and can cause the makeup to streak. Why not just use a water-based foundation in the first place and skip the negatives of the oil-based foundation? That would be my recommendation. Additionally, if you wear face powder over this type of foundation, the oil grabs the talc and the face can appear coated and heavily made up even if you blend it on thinly. The same is true for blushes and eyeshadows—they will go on more heavily because of the increased oil on the skin, and they will also become darker once applied.

Pressed powder–based foundations: These foundations are relatively new on the cosmetic scene in the past several years. They come in a compact and look and go on like a thicker pressed powder, which is really all they are, but with a bit more tenacity and coverage. Almost all of them have a superior creamy, silky feel, but when applied to the skin, they blend on as easily and lightly as any pressed powder.

Application: You can apply these foundations with either a sponge or a brush all over the face, including the eyelids. This is the easiest way to get a smooth, light, and fast application. You might have to worry about a smooth application if you have dry skin, but these powder-based foundations go on evenly for other skin types, providing extremely sheer, light coverage. For more specifics about blending techniques, see the "Blending Foundation" section later in this chapter.

Pros: Powder-based foundations are great for women with normal to oily skin. They blend on easily and quickly, last all day, generally don't change color, and feel exceptionally light on the skin. They are best for those who want a minimal feel and appearance from their foundation.

Cons: Women who have dry skin should not wear powder-based foundation. This is also not a good option if you have any amount of flaky skin, regardless of your skin type. The powder content makes this type of foundation too drying for someone with dry skin, and the way it goes on can make the skin look more dry and flaky. Also, women with oily skin might want to be cautious because powder-based foundations can take on a thickened, pooled appearance as oil resurfaces on the face during the day.

Cream-to-powder foundations: These foundations are an interesting cross between a pressed powder and a creamy liquid foundation. They come in a compact and have a very creamy, almost greasy appearance. When you blend them on, the creamy part disappears and you are left with a slightly matte, powdery finish. Cream-to-powder foundations provide much better coverage than pressed powder-based foundations.

Application: Cream-to-powder foundations are best applied with a sponge. Some women have success using a brush, but I think this is a difficult, messy technique. See the "Blending Foundation" section later in this chapter.

Pros: Cream-to-powder foundations blend on quickly and easily and provide a semi-matte, soft, medium coverage. They work great for someone with normal to slightly dry or slightly combination skin. The consistency doesn't require powdering after you apply it.

Cons: Cream-to-powder foundations can blend on slightly thickly, providing a made-up look rather than a sheer, natural appearance. They don't work well for someone with oily skin because the cream components can be too creamy, and they don't work well for dry skin because the powder part can be too powdery. Essentially, they are best for normal skin types.

Self-adjusting foundations: These foundations supposedly can absorb oil, stop oil production, and also prevent moisture loss. I've yet to see one perform as promised, though it would be great if someone ever came up with one that could.

Foundations with shine: A definite trend in the world of makeup is having your entire face shine, either with a makeup primer that shines, a foundation that has shine, or a powder that shines. This seems an ironic turn of events, given the manic desire until recently to eliminate any shine on the face. Shimmering shine (as opposed to naturally produced shine) seems to be "in" and I have to admit that it does look great in pictures. In real life, it tends to look sparkly, and if you have normal to oily skin, it looks like the very oil you were trying to do away with. Try this one and check it out in daylight before you splurge. It works better for an evening look than a professional, classic daytime look.

Blending Foundation

When it comes to blending foundation over your face, keep one mantra in your head: blend, blend, and blend again, and then, just to be sure, blend one more time. All the other details are, well, just details, and not anywhere near as important as buffing off the excess foundation and smoothing out the edges to be sure you have the thinnest possible layer of foundation over the skin (see the picture on page 269).

Keep in mind that the goal of wearing foundation is to create the illusion of smoother-looking skin, not a mask of foundation. Of course, the best place to check your blending technique is in broad daylight. Unfortunately, most of us apply foundation in bathroom light, with only minimal exposure to sunlight. Once you get into daylight, even on a cloudy day, the areas you missed, particularly next to the ears, mouth, jawline, sides of the nose, and temples, often look streaked, have a line of demarcation (even when the color matches perfectly), or appear blotchy or smudged. This is not the effect you are trying to achieve. Smoother-looking skin takes diligence and daylight; even expensive, bright, interior lighting does not really duplicate the painful but necessary clarity of daylight.

Do not use cotton balls or cotton pads to apply foundation; they deposit tiny fibers all over your face. Also, when you try to blend with a cotton ball, you end up wiping more foundation off than on because of how well cotton absorbs. I also never recommend blending foundation with fingers. Instead, use a sponge. **Painting a wall with your fingers would leave streaks and lines, and the same is true for applying foundation to your skin. Using the flat, smooth surface of a sponge is the best way to get a smooth application.** The best tool is a flat, square, or round one-quarter-inch-thick sponge that doesn't have holes and is not made out of foam rubber. The shape and density of this kind of sponge provide the smoothest application possible.

Be good about cleaning or changing your sponges frequently, particularly if you tend to break out or have rosacea, psoriasis, seborrhea, or eczema. While sponges are great blending tools, they love holding on to bacteria, fungi, and yeast that can make those conditions worse.

The sponges frequently found for sale or in use at most cosmetics counters are the thick wedge-shaped foam rubber sponges. These sponges are compact, but they drag over the skin, which makes blending difficult; and because they're so thick, most of the foundation is absorbed into the sponge, where you can't get to it, which can waste a lot of product. Wedge sponges are used for traditional theatrical makeup. They are great for applying grease stick or pancake foundations, which require more "pull" across the face in order to apply them evenly, but that is the last thing you need when wearing a water-based, lightweight foundation.

To achieve an even application with your nice, thin, flat, square or round sponge, shake some of the foundation from the bottle onto the sponge, then transfer the foundation to the face and over the eyes by dabbing the sponge over the skin. You can also use your fingers to transfer the foundation in dots from the bottle to the face and then use the sponge to blend the dots. Start by placing the foundation generously over the central area of the face, including the eyes but avoiding the sides of the face near the hairline, jaw, and chin. The foundation can go on in large patches or small dots all over the nose, eyelids, cheeks, and forehead, but only in this central area. Avoid placing the foundation all over the face unless you want a very full makeup application. If you concentrate the foundation over the center part of the face, as you blend down and out from the center there will be less foundation at the jaw and hairline.

Once the foundation is on your face, begin using your sponge to blend evenly. **Holding the sponge between your fingers and thumb, spread the foundation down and out over the entire face with a stroking, buffing motion, going in the direction of the hair growth.** (Going against the direction of the hair growth on your face coats the hair with too much foundation.) The idea is to blend the foundation color from the center of the face, where you initially placed it, to the perimeter of the face, leaving no line of demarcation at the jaw. Use the edge of the sponge without foundation (or turn the sponge over to the clean side) to dab or buff away any of the excess that tends to collect under the eye or around the nose. You can also use the sponge to wipe away any of the excess that gathers at the jaw or hairline. When blending the foundation, do not try to force it into the skin. There is a fine line between blending something on and wiping something off. Instead, blend a thin layer over the face, smoothing it with your sponge as you go. At this point your sponge should not be full of foundation; if it is, you've used too much.

If you did not apply a concealer before the foundation, you can now apply it and blend that into place. Apply the concealer, which is a shade or two lighter than the foundation, over the under-eye area and other areas you want to highlight, then dab it into place with your finger or sponge.

Watch out for the jaw and neck. This is very important. **Never, ever put makeup of any kind on the neck; you do not want your makeup to end up on your collar.** Always double-check your blending. Places on the face that you are likely to miss with foundation include the corners of the nose, the tip of the nose, the corners of the eyes (especially over the concealer), and the edge along the lower eyelashes. Also, some places are likely to end up wearing foundation that shouldn't, including the ears, the jawline, and the hairline, especially blonde hairlines. Be careful to remove this foundation if you've gone past your mark. Both situations can make your makeup appear sloppy.

Your sponge is an exceptional blending tool that you should keep near you at all times. When the edges of your blush or eyeshadow need softening, you can blend out the hard edges with the side of the sponge that was used to spread the foundation over the face. Using the side of the sponge that has foundation on it as opposed to the dry edge allows the sponge to glide over the blush or eyeshadow without streaking or rubbing it off.

Applying a Mini-Application of Foundation

If you dislike the feel of foundation as much as I do or if you want to wear the least amount of foundation possible, yet you want the benefits that wearing a foundation provides, mainly helping blush and eyeshadows go on more evenly, there is an alternative. The thing most women don't like about foundation is how it feels all over the face. One way to solve that problem is to not wear foundation all over the face, because basically it isn't necessary (unless your foundation contains your sunscreen, which does require applying it evenly all over the face). Remember, unless it is the source of your sunscreen protection, foundation is primarily needed to give the blush and eyeshadows something to adhere to. If the foundation color matches the face exactly—and after you finish this section, it will—you can apply a mini-application of foundation over the areas where you will place the blush and eyeshadows. This way you won't feel heavily made up and the blush and eyeshadows will still go on evenly.

For a mini-application, place the foundation only over a mask-shaped area between the eyes and mouth, including the nose and cheeks. Coverage is not needed on the chin, forehead, or jaw area. Be sure to blend the edges carefully with your sponge. Apply the concealer the same way you would for a full makeup application.

Blending Over Those Fine Little Wrinkles

Whoever came up with the term "fine wrinkles" should be shot. There's nothing "fine" about them!!! Nevertheless, if you've started to notice that foundation or concealer is sinking into some of those little wrinkles on your face, especially the laugh lines, lines under the eyes, or near the crow's-feet (no mercy either for the person who came up with the term "crow's-feet" to describe the lines extending from the back corner of the eyes), you have to be even more meticulous about how you blend your foundation into place. In this regard, less is best. Blend, blend, and blend again, being sure to remove the excess in those areas with the clean side of the sponge. Continue blending intermittently while you apply your lipstick, blush, and/or eyeshadow to ensure that you have removed the excess.

Minimize your use of moisturizers over the areas where you have lines, and use a foundation or concealer that's neither greasy nor too emollient. Anything with movement and slip gives the foundation a free ride into the lines.

About those concealers and foundations that claim to deflect, reflect, or somehow improve the appearance of wrinkles: they don't. And the cosmetics lines that sell foundation primers, which are usually just moisturizers with extra film-forming agents (hairstyling-type ingredients), don't work all that well either, plus it is just too many layers for any one face. Talk about suffocation and pore-clogging ingredients. **The truth is, a face without foundation always looks less wrinkled. I'm not sure why this has to be so, but it is. You can test this for yourself.** Go to the cosmetics counter, find the most expensive foundation with the most elaborate claims about making the skin look less wrinkled, apply a sample to one side of your face, and leave the other side naked with just a dab of moisturizer over dry areas. Then check out your face in the daylight. You will be amazed how much more noticeable the lines on the foundation side of the face are. Of course, the foundation side will look smoother and will have a more even tone, the redness and blotchiness will be gone, and the pores will have virtually disappeared. But the wrinkles will be more noticeable than on the side without foundation. The agony and ecstasy of foundation.

Blending the New "Stay-Put" Foundations

I have to admit, I'm in love with the new "stay-put" foundations, all of them (well, almost all of them). **Estee Lauder Double Matte, Almay Amazing Lasting, Maybelline Great Wear,** and **Lancome Teint Idole** are just great, and they do stay put! But their strong point is also their drawback. Once these foundations are blended into place, they dry quickly and don't budge. That means if you accidentally leave a streak, smudge, or buildup of foundation, there it will stay, no matter how hard you try to blend it away.

The trick to blending these foundations is twofold: you have to be quick and you have to be meticulous. One morning, in less than perfect light, I blended on my Almay Amazing Lasting Foundation; two hours later I noticed a strange smudge of makeup alongside my nose. No matter what I did to blend and smooth it into place, I only made matters worse and I never corrected the problem. Now I apply this foundation in bright daylight and blend systematically, starting with the left side of my face and working across to the right.

You also have to be very careful about using a moisturizer under stay-put foundations. If you use too much, if it's too greasy, or if you don't allow it to be adequately absorbed, it can make the foundation gunk up or streak. It may take a bit of experimenting to get it right, but if you have oily skin or live in a humid or hot climate, these foundations are worth the effort.

Blending Ultra-Matte, Stay-Put Foundations with Stay-Put Concealer

If you are using one of the new stay-put concealers, the same blending concerns for the stay-put foundations apply, except more so. The stay-put concealers tend to dry in place even faster than the foundations do, so you have to be really quick, and there's no second chance.

If you are also using a stay-put foundation, blending concealer into place can be problematic. Once the foundation is blended on, it doesn't necessarily like having other things blended over it, particularly liquid-type products like a concealer. I personally use **Almay Time Off Concealer,** which is much less dry than the **Almay Amazing Lasting Concealer** or the **Maybelline Great Wear Concealer.** (These last two are both excellent, but they make the lines under my eyes look more prominent than I care for.) Applying the Time Off Concealer after the Almay Amazing Lasting Foundation caused streaking and was not a pretty sight. The problem was eliminated when I applied the concealer first and then the foundation over that.

A general problem with concealer is getting it applied smoothly in the under-eye area and without making it look too white. It is important to always blend the edge of the concealer away from the eye until it disappears. Also, try to concentrate the concealer along the inside corner of the eye and down, as opposed to out. The less concealer you put at the back corner of the eye (unless that area is dark), the less likely you are to look like an albino raccoon.

If you don't have to use a concealer with an ultra-matte foundation, often the foundation provides enough opaque coverage to cover just about anything; that would be the best option.

FOUNDATION MISTAKES TO AVOID

1. **Do not buy a foundation before trying it on and checking it in the daylight.**
2. **Do not wear foundation unless it matches your skin color.**
3. **Do not wear a foundation that is lighter than your skin, or you will end up looking chalky or pale.**
4. **Do not wear pink, coral, orange, or ash-colored foundation.**
5. **Do not wear oil-based foundations unless you have very, very dry skin. Oil-based foundations can look greasy and appear more orange and pink than other types of foundations.**
6. **Do not wear oil-free or ultra-matte foundations unless you have very oily skin. Oil-free and ultra-matte foundations can look quite thick and matte and make lines on the face more evident.**
7. **Cream-to-powder foundations work best for normal skin. The cream part can be too greasy for oily skin and the powder can be too dry for dry skin.**
8. **Use foundations that have shine for a special evening look.**
9. **Do not apply a thick layer of foundation; thin and sheer are the operative words when it comes to applying foundation.**
10. **Do not use your fingers to blend your foundation over the face.**

Brushes

Before we go on to powders, eyeshadows, and blushes, it is crucial to discuss the most important blending tools you can use, besides the sponge for blending on foundation: brushes. Brushes are simply the best way to apply powders of any kind. You would be hard put to find a makeup artist anywhere who disagrees. After years of struggling with tiny, prepackaged sponge eyeshadow applicators and doll-sized blush brushes, we now have a profusion of brushes to choose from. From M.A.C., Trish McEvoy, Prescriptives, Bobbi Brown, Maybelline, and Nordstrom S.A.N.E. to Joan Simmons, Aveda, The Body Shop, and BeneFit, good brushes are available in an impressive array of sizes, shapes, and sensual textures that facilitate makeup application in ways that feel artistic and effortless. But, as usual, a high price does not always mean superior performance. And having more brushes does not mean you will be able to apply your makeup better.

Choosing a personal set of brushes is determined strictly by how you apply your makeup. If your makeup application is elaborate and nuanced, involving several eyeshadows, contour, and highlighting, you need a variety of brushes. If your makeup application is uncomplicated and basic, you need fewer brushes. It's that simple. (The reason makeup artists carry an arsenal of brushes is because they see a vast assortment of eye and face sizes. All you need is a group of brushes that match the areas of your face and the kinds and colors of makeup you apply.) All of the brushes I recommend are depicted in the pictures on pages 314 and 315.

I do not recommend buying a packaged set of brushes. More often than not, you end up getting brushes that you will never use or that are incorrectly shaped for your face. Instead, select individual brushes based on the shape of your face and the way you wear your makeup. A full makeup application can require three basic eyeshadow brushes, an eyeliner brush (for liner and brows), blush brush, contour brush, large powder brush, lash brush (an old clean mascara wand will do), brow brush (a toothbrush will do nicely), and a lip brush.

The general rule to follow is: **the size of the brush should match the size of the area you are working on.** Too small and it will take longer to apply your makeup and it can end up looking striped. Too large and you can end up with a messy application. If you are lining the eye, a tiny thin brush with few hairs that doesn't scratch or feel stiff is best. If you are filling in the brow, a small angled brush with a slight amount of stiffness to control the color is best. (It should be small and stiff enough to fit through the spaces in the hair and follow the edge of the brow with pencil-like control.) For the eyelid, choose a brush size that fits the curve of your lid, and the same reasoning applies for the crease area. Both are determined by the size of your eye and not by some cosmetics company's standard sizes. To highlight along the brow, a soft, small wedge brush (less stiff than the brow brush), fitting just that area, is best. Try not to use the same brush for both lighter and darker shades of eyeshadow.

How many and which brushes do you need? Here is a good basic group to consider. I recommend **two or three eyeshadow brushes,** including one for the lighter eyeshadow colors and one for the crease. If you want to save time and money, you can use the edge (side) of the eyeshadow brush you use for the lid to place a light color under the brow. If you want the perfect tool, a small, soft **wedge brush** for that area is best. If you are shading the back corner of the eye with a dark eyeshadow, you may want to select a **smaller eyeshadow brush** than the one you use for the lid or crease. Again, the size is determined by the shape of your eye. That means testing the brush before buying to see if you can work with it.

If you aren't using a pencil, a **tiny, thin eyeliner brush** is best for building either a thick or thin line along the upper and lower lashes. While some makeup artists use thicker brushes that are more square or wedge-shaped for this purpose, I think they are harder to control (they can make a thick line, but it's hard to get them to create a thin line, while a tiny, thin brush can do either). A **wedge-shaped brow brush** can be used just for the brow to apply eyeshadow powder or to smooth out the line of an eyebrow pencil. Personally I use a tiny eyeliner brush to fill in the brows to keep the shading soft by creating hair-thin strokes. An old **toothbrush** is still the best tool for combing through the brows. For combing through the lashes, I strongly recommend a good, densely packed **used mascara wand** that you wash clean, like the ones in L'Oreal Voluminous or Accentuous mascaras, Maybelline Illegal Lengths, and Lancome Defincils. The bristles of most lash brushes sold separately are too far apart to be helpful for easy unclumping and separating.

Both the **blush brush** and **powder brush** should have a soft, firm texture and not splay when placed on the skin or into the color (no brush should be so loose as to splay when used either on the face or in the product). They should also feel soft and silky, yet hold their shape. If a brush is too wobbly, it will be hard to control the color. I often recommend getting two good blush brushes in the same size and using one for powder and one for blush (you don't want to dust color over the face). Many powder brushes, though they may feel incredibly soft and luxurious, are too large, cumbersome, and hard to control. It's nearly impossible to maneuver some of these behemoth brushes under the eye, along the corner of the nose, or along the cheek without hitting other areas of the face that may not need powder, and using too much powder is extremely likely.

If you are looking for a **contour brush** to shade along the temple, jaw, or cheekbone, a smaller blush brush is a great choice. Brushes specially designed for this area come in a variety of sizes, but the flat edge of these specially designed brushes, though impressive in appearance, can create just that, a hard edge, which takes more blending to soften than necessary. Simply use a small, half-inch-wide version of your blush brush; the idea is that this contour/blush brush should fit the hollow of the cheekbone.

I'm not one who diligently applies lipstick with a **lipstick brush.** I just don't have the time. Generally, I save this precision for special occasions or when I want to use up every last drop in the tube. Look for a brush with bristles that are strong and slightly stiff. Tug hard on the brush and make sure it doesn't move in the least. Look for a brush the size of your lips. Too small and it can take forever; too big and you'll be applying lipstick to your face. You know those retractable metal brushes you see almost everywhere and in every price range? They are all the same, and they are excellent! Retracting the bristles neatly back into place beats trying to keep the little plastic protective cap on a wood-handled brush (they never stay on and lipstick ends up getting all over your purse and makeup bag!).

You may notice that some brush collections sport a white, thin, slightly stiff brush sold as a **concealer or highlighter brush.** If you use a concealer or highlighter for smile lines, under the eyes, on the corners of the nose, in the center of the chin, a dab in the middle of your lips over lipstick, or to spot-cover a blemish, this brush is a consideration. Many makeup artists use this type of brush to do things that most people (including me) do with their finger or their foundation sponge. Supposedly it allows better blending with less drag. It definitely prevents drag and it does tend to help you use less product. One thing it does not help in the least is keeping the concealer or highlighter from creasing into lines.

As you check out the different lines of brushes, the first thing you will hear about is the so-called quality of the bristles, and the salespeople will use this to justify the cost. Although the issue of animal testing is increasingly important to most cosmetics consumers, and therefore most cosmetics companies, that goes out the door when the subject is cosmetic brushes. Depending on the line, you will hear pretentious claims about squirrel, sable, pony, goat, and several other animals that did not give up their coats voluntarily. Now, I am not one to eschew leather shoes, nor am I a 100% vegetarian, but hasn't anyone else noticed the inconsistency in this arena?

While natural bristles are definitely softer (and more expensive) than synthetic, it does not take sable to make the perfect brush, and a mixed-hair brush of both natural and synthetic fibers can make for a stronger, pliable brush that doesn't lose its shape. Natural hairs tend to get softer over time, which means a firm, well-controlled brush can eventually become floppy and too soft. Salespeople who encourage you to buy the expensive brushes will claim that synthetic hairs get coarser and stiffer, and fall out after a year or two of usage, but I have not found that to be the case.

Ignore the claims about hair quality and trust your own **touch and feel tests.** Brush the bristles along the nape of your neck and ask yourself, "Is it smooth? Do the bristles hold their shape? Does it feel too loose, too stiff, or too soft? Does the brush feel densely packed, meaning lots of hairs, or flimsy?" Once you decide which feel you prefer, you can determine which brushes you want to work with.

Now that you have a sense of the feel part of the test, use the touch test to ascertain how the brush will hold up. Simply tug at the bristles, away from the handle, to see if there is any give. Do any hairs fall out? If you feel any release whatsoever, this is not a well-constructed brush. Some brushes are poorly anchored and bound into the base of the brush. For example, Maybelline's incredibly inexpensive brushes beautifully pass the feel test (they are wonderfully soft and firm) but fail the touch test (the bristles tend to pull out). In the short term they are a superior bargain, but they won't hold up over the long haul.

Several cosmetics lines still sell the bamboo-handled brushes with white bristles. These are often the sparsest of brushes and not constructed very well. They are a great example of the type of quality to avoid, because, although they are attractive, they are a waste of money.

When it comes to the **shape of the brush,** avoid blunt brushes and brushes with the bristles lined up flat. For most brushes—eyeliner, lip, eyeshadow, blush, and powder—look for ends that are more dome-shaped. Not only do these have a softer feel, but they allow for a softer, less hard-edged application, which is almost always the goal. The only exception is the wedge brush for the brows or under the eyebrow.

When I'm doing my own makeup for media appearances or doing someone else's makeup, I personally favor brushes with long, elegantly tapered wood handles. None of those stout, metal, modern-art-looking tools for me. But once I try to squeeze these long-stemmed beauties into the small makeup bag I keep in my purse, I realize what a joke they can be. For women who want to invest in only one set of brushes, short handles are not only more convenient, they are essential.

When it comes to **caring for your brushes,** some people claim you must wash them frequently. If you are a makeup artist working on lots of people, I suspect you should be washing your brushes somewhere between every day and once a week. But for those of us who are working on ourselves only and not changing colors on a daily basis, once a month is just fine (and I won't tell anyone if you don't do it that often). Especially for natural-hair brushes, frequent washing breaks down the hair shaft and breaks down the hair. Also, washing too often can loosen the glue in the handle that holds the bristles together and keeps them in place. When you clean the brushes, concentrate your effort on the bristles, not the handle.

It is best to use a regular shampoo instead of a special brush-cleaning solution (which is just shampoo anyway). The shampoo shouldn't contain any conditioning agents, which can build up on the brush just like they do on the hair. L'Oreal Colorvive Gentle Shampoo is an excellent option. A conditioner is not necessary when caring for your brushes. Brush hair is extremely healthy. It isn't damaged from dyeing, perming, styling, brushing, and the other things people do to their own hair, which then requires the use of conditioners. When washing your brushes, carefully follow these steps:

- Gently but thoroughly wash the brush in tepid water.

- Meticulously rinse the brush.
- Carefully press out the excess water and dab the brush dry.
- Arrange the bristles back into their original shape.
- Let the brush air-dry on a towel without the help of a blow dryer, which can damage bristles.

Brush Techniques

For the most part, brushes are foolproof tools for applying makeup, but it is definitely possible to use brushes incorrectly. I've seen enough women use their brushes in a rubbing or wiping motion on the face to know how often it can happen. Many women beat at their faces with a wild brushing motion as they attempt to apply their blush and eyeshadows. There truly is an easier way. When you wipe, beat, or rub the brush against the face, it may be removing what you just put on, not to mention wiping off the foundation underneath. Instead, brush in short, light, purposeful motions that glide over the skin.

If there is a distinct line where the brushstroke was placed or if you feel an urge to use your finger to blend what you've just applied, most likely you are not using the brush properly or your brush is too stiff for a soft application. (You may also have applied your foundation too thickly or used a foundation that is too greasy, which means you need to read the "Foundation" section again, or the blush color you've chosen is too strongly pigmented for your skin color.) You should not be blending anything with your fingers—only with your brush or the flat, square, thin sponge you use to apply your foundation. Remember, use your sponge for applying foundation and softening edges of your blush, contour, and eyeshadows.

Something else that is critical to using brushes effectively—even though it may seem insignificant at first—is the way you pick up the powder on your brush before you apply it. **Never smash or rub your brush into the powder. Rather, place your brush into the powder gently, without moving the bristles.** You don't want to see the brush hair bend or splay. Always stroke through the powder evenly and always knock the excess powder off the brush before you apply it to the face. This prevents you from applying too much color to the first place your brush touches.

Brush Mistakes to Avoid

1. **Do not use hard or stiff brushes.**
2. **Do not use a brush that is too big or too small for the area of the face you are working on.**

Step-by-Step Makeup Application

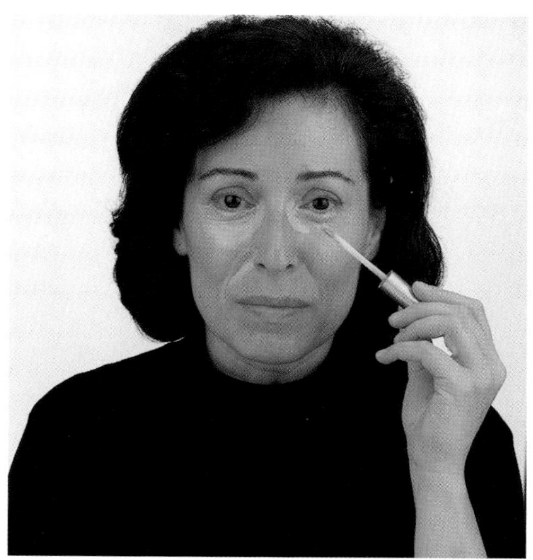

1. Place concealer along the inside corner of the eyes and over dark areas under the eyes.

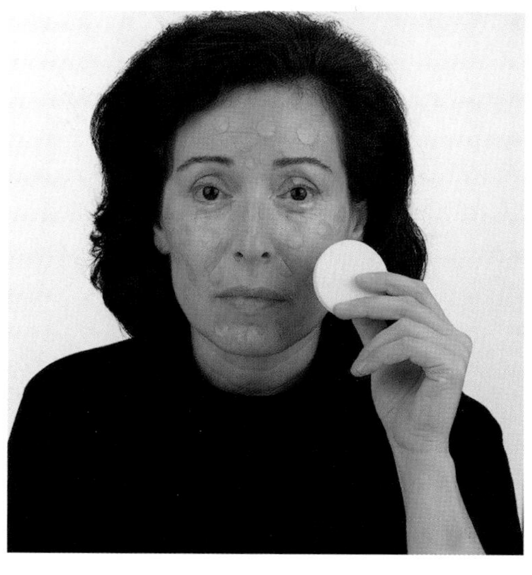

2. Dot foundation over the central part of the face, including the eyelids. Blend the foundation down and out with a smooth sponge.

Step-by-Step **Makeup Application**

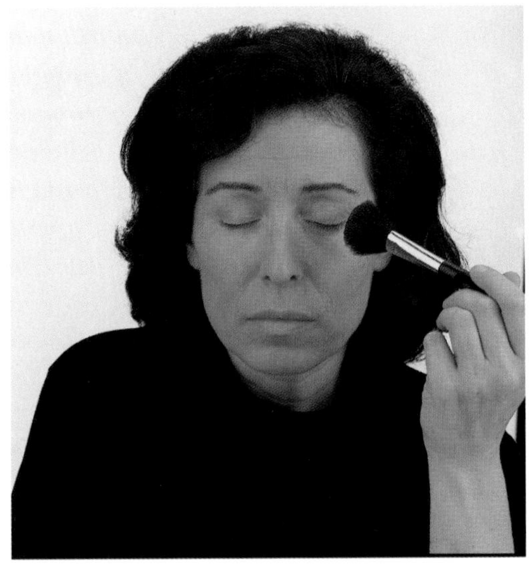

3. Dust a light layer of powder over the face, including the eyelids. (Depending on your skin type and the type of foundation you use, powdering is an optional step.)

Step-by-Step **Makeup Application**

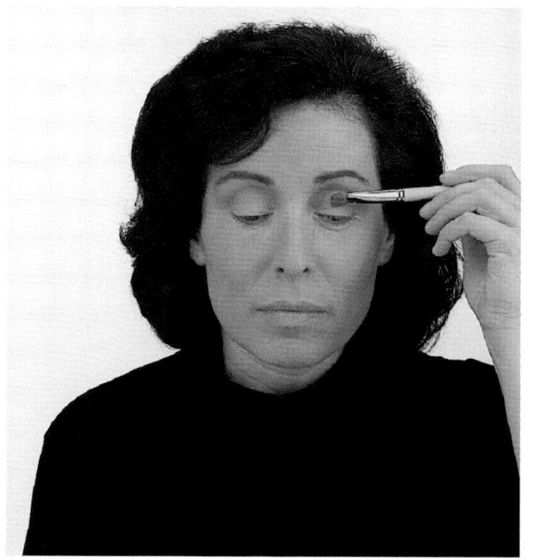

4. Apply lid color.

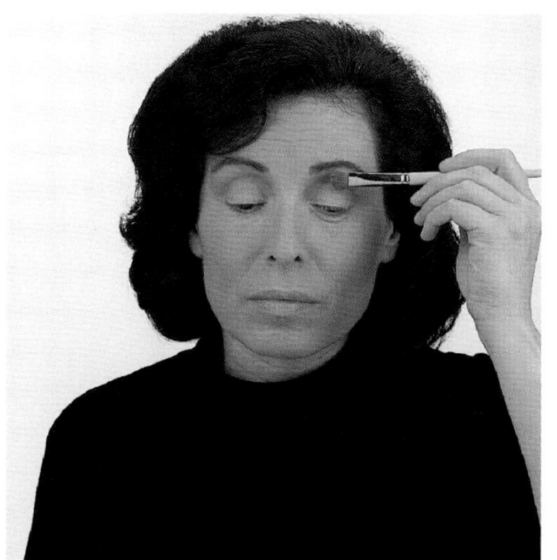

5. Apply under-brow color, over the entire area between the crease and the brow.

Step-by-Step Makeup Application

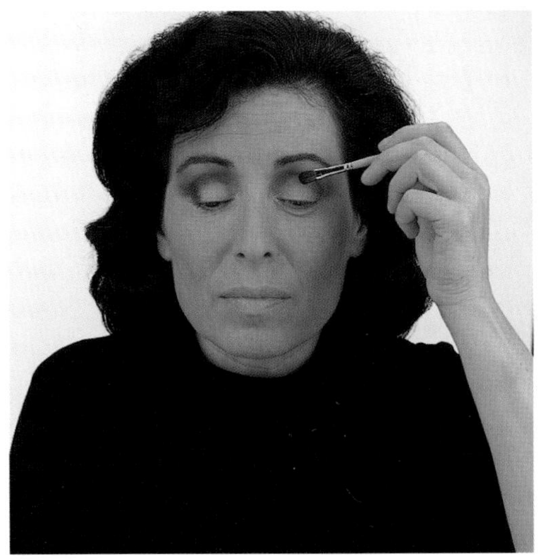

6. Apply crease color and/or shade the back corner of the eyelid with a darker color.

Step-by-Step **Makeup Application**

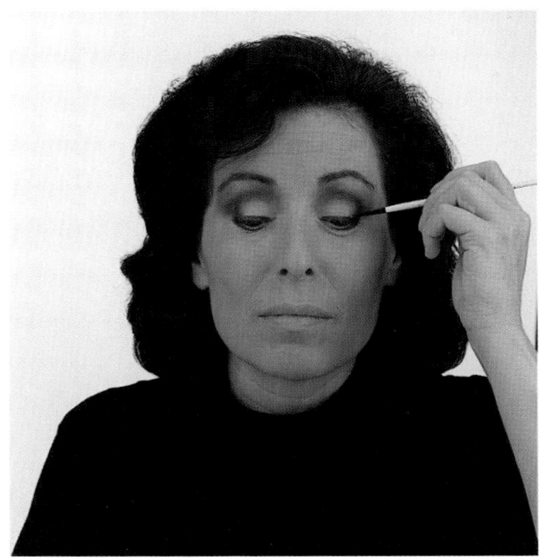

7. Using a dark shade of eyeshadow, wet or dry (or eye pencil if you prefer), draw a line as close to the lashes as you can get. Generally, match the width of the line to the size of your eyelids. If you have small eyelids, apply a thin line; if you have large eyelids, you can apply a wider line.

Step-by-Step Makeup Application

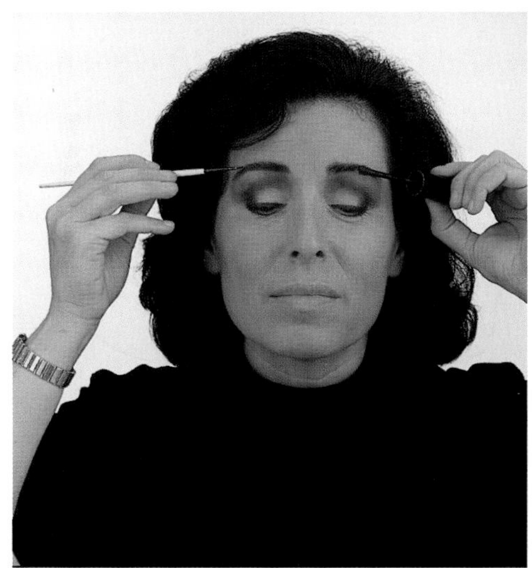

8. Fill in the eyebrows using brow gel, eyeshadow, brow powder, or an eye pencil.

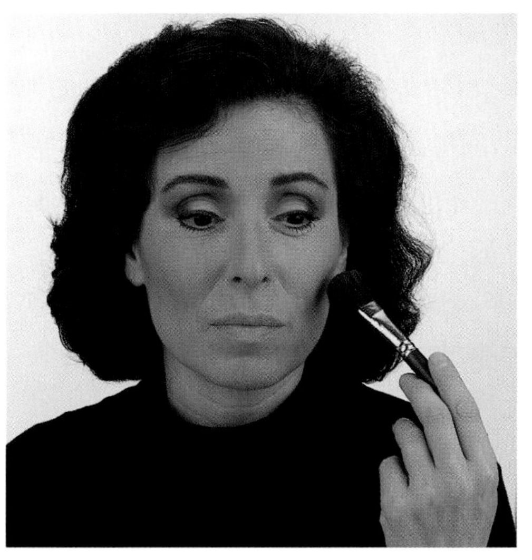

9. Apply contour under the cheekbones, along the temples, and under the jawline. (Contouring is a completely optional step and is most appropriate for an evening look, if done at all.)

Step-by-Step **Makeup Application**

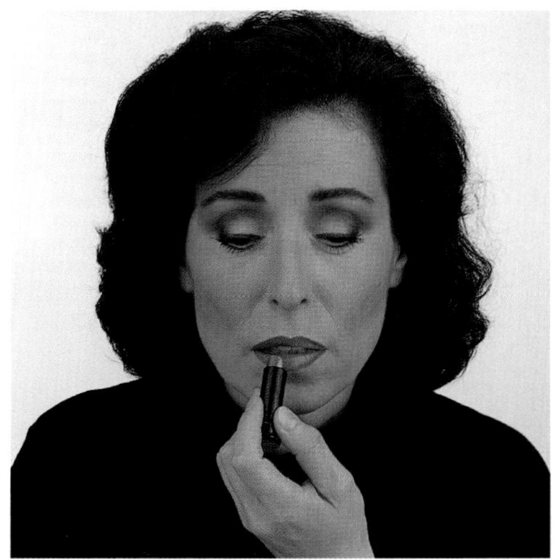

10. Apply lip liner following the actual outline of your lips and then fill in the lips with a matching or slightly lighter lip color.

Step-by-Step **Makeup Application**

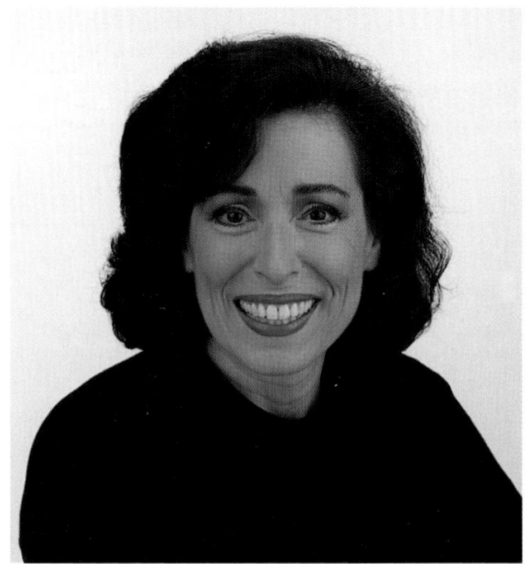

11. Apply the mascara last. All done. (Remember, you don't have to use all of these steps.) Be sure to check for mascara smears and eyeshadow drippies. Also double-check your foundation and soften any edges that look too obvious.

3. **Do not use brushes that are too soft or whose bristles are too sparse.**
4. **Do not forget to knock the excess powder off the brush before you apply the color to your face.**
5. **Do not wipe or rub the brush across the face; instead, gently brush on the color with short strokes.**
6. **Do not forget to use your sponge to blend out hard edges and soften your color application.**

Powder

Classic makeup application requires powdering after you've applied your foundation, but powdering doesn't work for all types of foundation. Powdering after applying foundation works best with the water-based and oil-based foundations, and with some matte foundations that aren't all that matte. It is either unnecessary or problematic to apply powder over most oil-free or matte foundations, all of the ultra-matte foundations, and all of the pressed powder–based and cream-to-powder foundations.

If you are using a water-based or oil-based foundation, you may indeed want to apply powder to absorb any excess moisturizer or emollients that may make the face look too moist or too dewy. However, the less powder you build up on your face, the less made-up you will appear. Also, I am convinced that overpowdering makes the face look dull and dry, especially if you have dry skin or darker skin tones. Some amount of natural, dewy shine to the face is very attractive. **I think it is a 1950s notion that the face should not shine at all and that a woman must constantly wipe powder over her face to reduce the shine (and then apply shiny eyeshadows, blush, lipstick, or powder so the skin shines, but artificially).** After a foundation is applied, the slight shine that is left behind (except with oil-free, matte, ultra-matte, and pressed-powder foundations) gives the face a radiant glow. Powder is great for touch-ups as the day goes by to dust down excessive shine (see the picture on page 270). Just avoid overpowdering.

Types of Powder

Loose powder and pressed powder: Are exactly what the names suggest. Loose powder tends to provide a more sheer, light application and can be best for someone with normal to oily skin. Pressed powder is merely loose powder with added waxes to keep the powder in a solid form. While pressed powder is heavier than loose powder, it is more convenient and less messy. Even if the pressed powder is labeled as oil-free, the ingredients that keep the pressed powder in its pressed form can add an extra layer of makeup to the skin. Both loose and pressed powders are perfectly fine options and it is a matter of personal preference which you use. What is essential, though, is to choose a powder that is the same color as your foundation. If your powder is lighter than your foundation, you can end up looking pasty and pale; if your powder is darker, you will look like you're wearing a mask.

Someone with oily skin would do better with loose powder or pressed powder that contains no oils. Check the ingredient list to be sure no oils are listed (and remember that some oils do not include the word "oil" in their name).

Application: Apply the powder with a large, full, round brush. Avoid using a sponge or powder puff, which can put too much powder onto the face. Pick up some of the powder on the full end of the brush, knock off the excess, and brush it on using the same motion and direction as you did the foundation. Keep everything going in the same direction to help retain a smooth appearance.

If you are touching up your makeup later in the day, before powdering use your sponge, a facial tissue, or special oil-absorbing paper (perm roller papers that you buy in a drugstore work great for this) to dab away excess oil from the face. Then apply the powder.

Some makeup artists do use a powder puff to press the powder into the skin for a very flat, matte finish. As professional a touch as this may be, it is best only for photographs. A powder puff places too much powder on the skin and can look thick and heavy in real life.

Pros: If you want to reduce shine or moisture on the face, powdering is the fastest, easiest way to get the job done.

Cons: There are really no negatives to wearing powder, except overdoing it, using the wrong color, and building up too much powder on the skin. There are also some powders that have sparkles or shine added to them. I have even seen some matte or oil-free powders that contain shine. If powdering is meant to reduce the shine produced from your oil glands or from your foundation or moisturizer, it is a huge mistake to apply a shiny powder. Clearly that would defeat the entire purpose. If you do want to use powder to add shine, see the next entry, "Powder that shines." That concern aside, powdering is a basic step to help keep makeup looking fresh during the day for most all skin types.

Powder that shines: If you want to make the skin look luminescent and shiny, one of the best ways to do that is with powder that has shine. Apply this after your foundation and regular powder, and dust it only over the areas you want to glow, such as the cheeks, chin, center of the forehead, shoulders, neck, and décolletage.

Powdering Mistakes to Avoid

1. **Never buy powder without testing it over your foundation before you buy it. Even if the powder is translucent, it always has some amount of color to it, and that color and the extra texture over the skin can greatly affect the appearance of your foundation. Powder should match the color of your skin (and foundation) and not change the color of either.**
2. **Never powder with a color that is lighter or darker than your foundation; powder should match your foundation color exactly.**
3. **Never powder with a white, orange, pink, or coral shade of powder; it will make you look either pale or overly made-up.**
4. **Don't forget to dab off excess oil from the face before you apply your powder, to help prevent buildup.**
5. **Do not apply more than the sheerest layer necessary to take away excess shine; the face can handle only so much powder before it starts looking thick and heavy.**
6. **Do not powder more than necessary during the day. Powder only once or twice a day to prevent buildup.**

Eyeshadow

I've been watching and evaluating other makeup artists and their eyeshadow techniques for years. Though there are myriad alternatives, eyeshadow design is usually built on an application sequence that allows you to create a flow of colors in either one, two, three, or four steps. The four steps are applied in a succession of colors that can be anything you want them to be, but if the goal is a classic makeup application, the colors proceed from light to gradually darker. The basic technique is to apply the lightest shade either just on the eyelid or all over the entire eye area (including the crease and up under the eyebrow) and then place each progressively darker shade in a more specific section of the eye area, such as the crease and/or the back corner of the eye (see the pictures on pages 271 and 272).

Types of Eyeshadow

In addition to powders, eyeshadows are available in tubes, pencils, and creams. Though these can be fun and easy to use, they are hard to blend and control. Makeup artists rarely if ever, use them, and I don't recommend them. I admit they're fun; I just wish they worked better to create a more sophisticated blend of colors.

Using Brushes to Apply Eyeshadow

Eyeshadow is applied exclusively with brushes. It is best to use brushes that are designed specifically for eyeshadow. Never use sponge-tip applicators; they drag across the eye and tend to blend colors in streaks. Once you get used to good brushes, you will never go back to sponge-tip applicators again.

When applying eyeshadow, use the flat side of the brush against the eye. Gently wipe the brush across the eyeshadow, knock the excess off the brush, and apply it with long stroking motions across the eyelid or crease, or under the eyebrow area. This motion of laying strips of color that overlap and blend together over the eye is the way to achieve an even, well-blended design, as opposed to beating the brush back and forth across the eye.

Remember that the size of the brush should match the size of the eye area you are working on. If you have a large eyelid area, use a brush that is wide and full. If your eyelid is small, use a smaller brush that's the same width as the lid. The same is true for the crease area (if a specific color is being placed just there) and the under-eyebrow area. Using brushes that match the job is essential to getting makeup on effectively and efficiently. Do not purchase or use brushes that have hard, coarse bristles, or you will end up with hard edges where the eyeshadow couldn't be blended, not to mention irritated skin.

Designing the Eye Makeup

Makeup books and cosmetics salespeople describe and demonstrate all kinds of eye makeup designs—say, a dab of yellow in the center of the lid, teal across the crease, taupe above the teal, pink above the taupe, and gray in the back corner of the lid. Not only do I think those designs are too complicated, I've never, at least not that I can recall, seen a model on the cover of any fashion magazine wearing a multicolor pastel eye design. In fact, even the cosmetics lines that sell these pastel color sets, including Lancome, Estee Lauder, Elizabeth Arden, Max Factor, and Borghese, rarely apply them on the models in their ads. The same is true for vivid eyeshadow colors such as jade green, purple, or cranberry.

The most beautiful makeup applications, the ones you see and admire the most on models and actresses, are neutral, not colorful. Look at any fashion magazine. You're not going to see pastel or vivid eyeshadows on many faces, unless it's a purposely eccentric or bizarre montage. Too many competing pastel or vividly colored shadows make the eye design distracting. Pastel colors are hard to blend together, so they stand out. Besides, the purpose of eyeshadows is to shape and shade the eye, not to color it. **The only way to shape the eye is by shading it with neutral tones such as taupe, brown, gray, ash, beige, tan, ma-**

hogany, redwood, sable, charcoal, and black. Eyeshadows are called "shadows" for a reason: they build shape and interest via shading, not via color.

The list of appropriately neutral colors and tones available is actually quite extensive. Color on the eyelid is best kept as subtle as possible, or you will end up creating an eye makeup design that is more noticeable than your eye. **Color on the face is provided by the lips and cheeks. More color standing out around the eyes can be overkill.**

Be cautious about thinking you must choose a design based on the need to correct a perceived facial problem, such as your eyes being too close together, too far apart, too round, or not round enough. There are no standard facial dimensions that define how attractive you or your eyes are.

The best way to choose which design to wear is to decide what image you want to project. The more shading you use, the more dramatic and formal the eye makeup design; the less shading, the more subtle and casual the design. Other considerations for choosing one eye makeup design over another include your skill at applying makeup, your personal preference, and the amount of time you want (or have) to spend. For example, if you are new or unaccustomed to wearing makeup, keep your entire makeup look simple until you become adept at the different application techniques. Also, if you have only a few minutes in the morning to get your makeup on, it is best to keep your routine simple. Trying to apply full makeup very quickly can result in mistakes or a sloppy application.

Applying an Eye Makeup Design

Options for building an eye design are almost too numerous to list. The basic concept is to shade the eye to accent its shape or change its shape by using a progression of light to dark colors across the eye, blending one over the other so that you can't see where one stops and another starts. Here I explain, step by step, how you can use one eyeshadow or several different eyeshadows to create a well-blended, beautiful eye makeup design. Even for the most formal eye makeup design, four different colors should be plenty. Whether you use one, two, three, or four different eyeshadows, they become a full design when worn with eyeliner, temple contour (see the "Contouring" section later in this chapter), and mascara.

One-color eye makeup design: This design blends one soft, subtle color all over the eye area, from the lashes to just under the eyebrow, with no patches of skin showing through. You should not wear only a splash of color over the eyelid and ignore the rest of the eye area.

Application: When applying this single color, first place it from the lashes to the crease, being sure that you do not extend the color into the inside corner of the eye (off the lid area) or out beyond the lid onto the temple. Also be certain there are no patches of skin showing through on the lid next to the eyelashes. The entire lid at this point is one solid color.

Next, place the color from the crease up to the brow, following the entire length of the eyebrow from the nose out to the temple area. Avoid leaving a hard edge at the back corner of the eye where the eyeshadow stops. Because the eyeshadow for this one-color eye makeup design is so soft and subtle, blending and application are quite easy. The best colors for this design include light tan, neutral taupe, beige, pale mauve brown, pale gray, golden brown, camel, and light auburn. Whatever the color, it should definitely not be obvious.

Two-color eye makeup design: You can approach this design by applying the lighter color to the eyelid and the deeper color from the crease up to the brow, or you can apply the deeper color to the lid and the lighter color from the crease to the brow. Generally speaking, the under-eyebrow color should be a shade or two darker than the lid color. You do not want it to be a distinctly different color, just a different shade. The lid can be taupe, beige, tan, camel, gray, light auburn, golden brown, or any light neutral shade, and the under-eyebrow color would be a deeper shade of the same color. Women with darker skin tones can wear muted rose, mauve, or peach as long as it doesn't make their eyes look irritated or isn't too obvious. Bright, shiny, or whitish shadows can look dated and make the brow bone look more prominent and heavy.

Which color and what shades go where? **The general rule is that the larger or more prominent the eyelid area is compared with the under-brow area, the darker or deeper the eyelid color can be; the smaller the eyelid area is compared with the under-brow area, the brighter or lighter the eyelid color can be.** The notion is that if the eyelid area is already prominent or large, it isn't necessary to make it appear any bigger by applying a light color to it. If the eyelid area is small, it is appropriate to make it more prominent by wearing a lighter color.

Application: Whichever way you choose to apply this design, the lid and under-brow shades should meet at the crease but not overlap. As an option for the two-color eye makeup design, you can apply the light shade to the lid, and the darker shade from the crease up to the brow. Then, using a small wedge brush, you can use the light color again as a highlight just along the lower edge of the eyebrow. This can bring dramatic but subtle attention to the shape of the brow and the eye without requiring another eyeshadow color.

Three-color eye makeup design: Start by applying either of the two-color eye makeup designs mentioned above. Once you have done that, the third shade, an even deeper color than the two previous colors, is added to the back corner of the lid or in the crease or over both the crease and the back corner of the lid.

In this design, the lid and under-brow colors are softer and less intense than the color at the back corner of the lid or in the crease. Regardless of where you place this third, darker color, it can be a beautiful deep shade of brown, charcoal, mahogany, sable, red-brown, slate, chocolate brown, camel, or black.

Application: If you apply the third eyeshadow in the crease, the trick is to not get the crease color on the lid, but rather to blend it slightly up into the under-eyebrow area and out onto the temple. Be sure, when sweeping the crease color across the eye, not to follow the movement of the eye down. Notice in the picture on page 272 that I blend the crease color out and up into the full back corner of the eye, and up onto the back of the brow bone.

When you apply the crease color, be sure to watch the angle of your brush as you blend the color from the crease out and up toward the under-brow area. If you place your color straight up at a 90-degree angle, you will look like you have drawn on wings. The softer the angle and the fuller the sweep, the softer the appearance, so be certain you blend out and slightly up from the lid area toward the under-brow area.

If you apply the third color at the back corner of the eye, the color hugs a small section of the lid, blending out and up into the crease and temple area. I explain this step in more detail for the four-color eye makeup design.

Four-color eye makeup design: In this design, you again start with the one- or two-color eye makeup design, then add a darker color to the crease and an even darker color such as black to the back corner of the eye. Shading the back corner of the eyelid involves the art of placement and blending. Because this area almost always requires a dark color, blending is essential to make it look soft, with no hard edges.

Why bother with a crease color and more shading at the back corner of the eye? The best part of this full eye makeup design is that it shades, defines, and creates movement by adding a shadow in a curved flowing motion that follows the natural shape of the eye. The difficult part of this design is blending this crease color across the entire length of the eye without making it look obvious, choppy, or smeared. The goal is to tuck the color just in the crease at the fold nearest the nose and have it hug the crease until you get to the back corner of the eye, where you start the movement of the eyeshadow up and out onto the brow bone. Again, this sweep of color should not look like a stripe across the eye.

Application: **Be sure to knock the excess eyeshadow off your brush, and apply the color with very small strokes over the back corner of the lid only.** The problem is keeping the color on the back of the lid only. If you don't know how to handle the brush, the back wedge can take up more than half of the eyelid (looking more like a mistake than carefully blended shading) or look like a stripe across the temple.

When you apply the crease color, be sure to watch the angle of your brush as you blend the color from the crease out and up toward the under-brow area. If you place your color straight up at a 90-degree angle, you will look like you have drawn on wings. The softer the angle and the fuller the sweep, the softer the appearance, so be certain you blend out and slightly up from the lid area toward the under-brow area.

The center or fold of the crease area is always the darkest, so start your brush there and blend out in each direction. Concentrate your efforts on how much of the crease area you want to shade. You can start all the way at the front part of the eye area under the front third of the brow, then follow the crease through the center, blending slightly up toward the brow. As you approach the back corner of the eye, begin your movement up and out toward the temple, aiming toward the eyebrow.

Eye Design Mistakes to Avoid

1. **Do not overcolor the eyes: too many bright colors can be distracting, not attractive.**
2. **Do not create hard edges: you should not be able to see where one color stops and another starts.**
3. **Do not wear bright pink or iridescent pink eyeshadows; they make eyes look irritated and tired. Muted pink is an option, but be very, very careful. If it makes the eye look irritated or "red," it isn't the color for you.**
4. **Do not wear shiny eyeshadows of any kind if you are concerned about making the skin looking more wrinkled.**
5. **Do not apply lipstick or blush over the eye area; it might sound like a time-saver, but if you have a lighter skin tone, it can make you look like you've been up all night crying.**
6. **Do not match your eyeshadow to your clothing or your eye color. If you have blue eyes, blue eyeshadow would make the blue of your eyes look duller. And complementing your clothing is at best dated; besides, what do you do if you're wearing red or black?**

Eyeliner

Let's take a short trip down eyeliner memory lane. Between 1960 and 1974, we progressed from wearing heavy liquid liner that swept over the eyelid and ended in wings at the back of the eye, to wearing Twiggy lashes, which were pointy lines drawn vertically from the lower lashes, with false lashes worn on the lid. Then, somewhere around 1976, smudge pencils became the fashion.

The smudge sticks were great; they were fast and convenient and, sad to say, did just what their name said they would do; they smudged all over the place. Smeared eye makeup was a definite problem.

In the early 1980s, fashionable eye makeup design meant one with liner placed on the inside rim of the eye. Placing the pencil here was supposed to make the white of the eye appear whiter. Nothing could be further from the truth. Constant application of a foreign substance resulted in irritation that left the eyes bloodshot and tearing. Liner on the inside rim lasted only about one hour anyway, and then the color clumped up at the inside corner of the eyes and smeared under the eyes. During the mid-'80s, eyeliner became a more specific, though soft, line around the outside of the eyes, and the pencils were thinner and more reliable. Unfortunately, thin eye pencils, even if they don't smudge as much as fatter pencils do, can still smear and wear off.

Do you need to wear eyeliner? As with any makeup step, eyeliner is completely optional. From an artistic perspective, if you are wearing eyeshadow, I almost always recommend wearing eyeliner, unless your eyelids and eyelashes are obscured by your brows. Eyeliner is a basic part of an eye makeup design because it shapes and defines the eyes and makes the eyelashes look thicker. If you are wearing only mascara and not eyeshadow, or if you want an extremely soft look, eyeliner is not necessary. If you do decide to wear eyeliner when you are wearing mascara and no eyeshadow, be sure to line the eyes with only a very soft, well-blended eyeshadow color.

Types of Eyeliner

Today you can choose from among several styles of liner, but be aware of which should be avoided and which have the best staying power. What kind of eyeliner should you use? Because of all the problems I just mentioned regarding pencils, I rarely recommend them for eyelining, even though they are assuredly easier to apply. Not only do even the best pencils smear, but they are also hard to sharpen, making it difficult to keep a good point intact and making it harder for you to control the thickness of the line.

None of that is true for a brush and an appropriate eyeshadow powder. I strongly recommend using a dark-toned eyeshadow color (almost any eyeshadow color can work) and a tiny brush. A tiny, thin eyeliner brush allows absolute control over the thickness of the line around the eye. Another benefit of using powder and a brush is that you can use the powder as an eyeshadow by just changing the brush size.

Should you apply 1960s-style liquid eyeliner? Unless you are in your 20s and going out for the evening, overexaggerated eyeliner with wings beyond the corner of the eyes is not a good idea. Depending on the effect you are trying to create, you can use a more definite eyeliner look most any time of day. But for a more classic look, it is best to keep eyeliner soft by using powder or by using a pencil and then applying powder over it.

Which eyeliner color should you use? For a classic eyeliner application, choose dark brown, slate gray, or black eyeshadow for the upper lid and a softer shade of those—chocolate brown, soft gray, or soft black—along the lower lashes. Eyeliner is meant to give depth to the lashes and make them appear thicker. If the liner is a bright color or a true pastel, attention will be focused past the lashes to the colored line as opposed to the more subtle flow of color from dark lashes to dark liner. Test it on yourself. Line one eye with a vibrant color, the other eye with brown or black, and see which one looks like it has thicker lashes. Then, if all my attempts to convince you have failed, and you still prefer to use bright pastel liners, go for it.

Application: Choose a dark shade of eyeshadow. Always line the eyes last—after all the other eyeshadows have been applied. Use a tiny, thin, slightly stiff brush. Whether you use your powder wet or dry (either is fine, but dry is softer and wet is more dramatic), stroke the brush through the color, keeping the bristles together. Do not dab or rub the brush into the color. Move the brush across the eyeshadow in the direction of the bristles, making sure the form of the brush is not destroyed. Knock the excess color from the brush, then apply the color to the eyelid next to the lashes and under the eye near the lower lashes (see the picture on page 273).

Make the line along the eyelid a solid, even line, starting thin at the front third of the lid and becoming slightly thicker at the back third of the lid. You can line all the way across the eyelid if you like, from the inside corner to the outer edge, or you can stop the line where the lashes stop and start. Along the lower lashes, line only the outer two-thirds of the eye. **Be sure the lower liner is a less intense color than the upper liner. Also make sure that the two lines meet at the back corner of the eye.** Never line all the way across the lower eyelashes. Always leave some space on the inside corner of the eye where the lashes end near the tear ducts. Wrapping a complete circle of eyeliner around the eye tends to create an eyeglasses look and can make the eyeliner a stronger statement than the eye itself.

Some makeup artists recommend that women over 40 should not line the inner corner of the eye either on top or on the bottom. I think that is a fine suggestion.

How thickly can you line the eye? As a general rule, for a classic look, the thickness and intensity of the eyeliner is determined by the size of the lid: the larger the eyelid area, the thicker and softer the eyeliner should be. The smaller the eyelid area, the thinner and more intense the liner should be. If your lid doesn't show at all, forget lining altogether.

You may have seen or heard a dozen other ideas as to how to apply eyeliner. Halfway across the lid, or one-third, or one-fourth, and three-fourths of the way under the lower eyelashes, or one-third, or one-fourth, and on and on. You are more than welcome to experiment with all these placements, but I encourage you to try the classic way first and see how you like it. Because the major reason to wear eyeliner is to shape the eye and make the eyelashes look thicker and deeper, I feel it is important to line where the lashes are and not just arbitrary sections of the lid. You can always line with a very soft color if you are concerned about overdefining the eyes, but I am not convinced that these "adjusted" lengths of placement look very natural.

If you do choose to wear pencil eyeliner, as many women do, remember the following rules.

- Self-sharpening pencils are by far the product of choice. Sharpening regular eye pencils is difficult, and keeping the point without chewing up the pencil can be tricky.
- It is easier to apply pencil along the lower lashes than on the upper lid, because the eyeshadows on the lid are harder for the pencil to stick to. You may want to consider using a greasy pencil for the lid and a firmer, less greasy pencil for the lower lashes. (If a pencil flattens when you press it, it will blend on more easily—and also tend to smear more easily.)
- You can warm the pencil between your fingers to apply a softer line of color; however, this is not a surefire way to get a smooth application.
- To get a more precise line, if you have the time, leave the pencil in the freezer for a minute or two.
- Apply eyeshadow over pencil to get the best of both worlds.

Checking for Mistakes

After the eyeshadow and eyeliner are completed, check for drippies under the eye and on the cheek. Drippies are those little powder flakes that fly off the brush and land on the cheek. Knocking off the excess from the brush every time helps prevent drippies, but there will always be flakes that end up where they don't belong. The best way to go after drippies is to use your sponge and simply wipe them away. If you do this, your next step is to touch up your foundation if that has gotten smeared.

If you do choose to wear pencil eyeliner, check for smears under the eye as the day goes by. This is annoying, but letting it go without blending away the smears can make any well-applied eye makeup design look like a mess.

Eyeliner Mistakes to Avoid

1. **Do not use greasy pencils to line the lower lashes; they smear and smudge.**
2. **Do not use brightly colored pencils or eyeshadows to line the eye; they are distracting and automatically look like too much makeup. All you'll see is the color and not your eye.**
3. **Do not extend the eyeliner beyond the corner of the eye (no wings).**
4. **Do not make the eyeliner the most obvious part of the eye makeup design.**
5. **Do not line the rim of the eye; it is out-of-date, messy, and unhealthy for the cornea.**
6. **If you do use pencil to line the eye, apply a small amount of eyeshadow over your eyeliner pencil to help set it and keep it from smearing.**
7. **Do not apply thick eyeliner to small or close-set eyes.**
8. **Do not use eyeshadow as an eyeliner without the proper brush.**
9. **Do not line the eye with a circle of dark or bright color. Both are too obvious and create an eyeglasses-style circle around the eye.**
10. **Do not overblend, spilling your eyeliner onto the skin under the lower lashes; that makes dark circles look worse.**

Mascara

Mascara is an amazing invention and is considered basic to any kind of makeup application. Many makeup artists, including myself, say that if you're not wearing any other makeup but still want to wear something, wear mascara. On the other hand, many of us—and I'm guilty of this too—get carried away and wear way too much mascara.

Women overdo mascara in part because the cosmetics industry tells us loudly and clearly that long lashes are to be coveted, but even unadvised we covet someone else's long, beautiful lashes. When we apply mascara, visions of longer, thicker lashes immediately come into view and then we get carried away and decide to apply more. Unfortunately, applying too much mascara increases the chances that the mascara will flake, chip, or smear, and that the lashes will appear hard and spiked. Also, the eyelashes can take only so much weight, and excess weight can break them. Gunked-up lashes with tons of mascara do not resemble long, thick lashes—they resemble gunked-up lashes.

The desire for longer, more noticeable lashes brings up the ever-popular device that curls the lashes by squeezing them into a bent-upward shape. The problem with curling lashes is that it can bend the lashes into a severe angle, which looks unnatural, and while it may make lashes more noticeable (in an odd sort of way), it ends up breaking and pulling them out. Doesn't that defeat the purpose of making your lashes look longer? If you're still gung-ho on doing this, curl lashes only before you apply mascara, never after, or you will absolutely end up with broken, strangely bent lashes. The best lash curlers are the ones with a sponge-tip section where the eyelashes are squeezed for protection. Squeeze gently with even pressure. Hold for a few seconds and release slowly.

Types of Mascara

Mascara comes in two basic types: waterproof and water-soluble. Mascaras should not smudge, flake, or clump. It is not your fault if they do. Price does not tell you anything about a mascara's application. Drugstore mascaras can be as good as anyone else's, and sometimes even better. **Regardless of where you buy your mascara, you might find that upon opening it, it already seems dried up. Buying an already dried-up mascara is a recurring problem in the cosmetics world. Take it back immediately and get a refund or another tube.**

Can you extend the longevity of your mascara? If you want to, there are a few possibilities. First, do not overpump the wand into the tube in an attempt to build up mascara on the brush. All that really accomplishes is pumping air into the tube, which makes the mascara dry up faster. Another solution is to avoid mascaras with a wide-bristled brush. In order to accommodate the wider brush, the tube opening needs to be larger, and this allows more air to get inside, again causing the mascara to dry out faster. Don't be fooled by the promise that wider bristles will make lashes longer. If anything, big brushes are clumsy to use, and they make it harder to get the lashes at the corners without making mistakes.

Many experts say you shouldn't add water to your mascara tube and that is probably a good recommendation. However, personally I do on occasion stretch the life of my mascara by adding a mere drop of distilled water to the tube. I've increased the life of my mascara for at least a month or more by doing this. (This of course applies only to water-soluble mascara.)

Water-soluble mascaras: The problem with some water-soluble mascaras is that they don't come off all that easily with water, even though they should. You want to avoid using an eye makeup remover and wiping at the eye, which causes sagging. Luckily, there are great water-soluble mascaras that build long, thick lashes without clumping or flaking and that come off easily with a water-soluble cleanser. I recommend many excellent mascaras in a variety of price ranges in my book *Don't Go to the Cosmetics Counter Without Me.*

Waterproof mascaras: These cause problems because in order to remove them you must pull and wipe at the eyes, which sags the skin and can pull out lashes. I understand the desire to go swimming while wearing your makeup or to cry at weddings and not have mascara streaming down your cheeks, especially if you're the bride. Waterproof mascara is fine for occasional use, but wearing it every day can cause more headaches in the long run. Another drawback is that although most waterproof mascaras hold up well under water, they can still break down and smear due to oil from your skin or emollients from your moisturizer or foundation. Do not make the mistake of thinking that waterproof means smearproof.

Applying Mascara

Apply mascara to the lower lashes by holding the wand perpendicular to the eye and parallel to the lashes, which prevents you from getting mascara on the cheek. It also makes it easier to reach the lashes at both ends of the eye. Combine this technique with the traditional upper-lash application method of rotating the mascara wand by round-brushing from the base of the lashes up to get all the lashes around the entire eye. **Keep an old, cleaned-up mascara wand in your makeup bag to be used for removing mascara clumps (it can happen with the best mascaras) and separating lashes.**

Have you ever had mascara end up on the eyelid or under the eye while you're applying it? Wait until it dries completely and then chip it away with a cotton swab or your sponge. Most of it will just flake off, with very little repair work needed. Always check for mascara smudges; they can look very sloppy and distracting.

Mascara Mistakes to Avoid

1. **Do not wear colored mascara such as blue, purple, or green if you're trying for a professional daytime look.**
2. **Do not wear mascara that smears; there are lots that don't, so don't put up with smearing.**
3. **Do not use waterproof mascaras on a daily basis; they are too difficult to remove.**
4. **Do not forget to apply mascara evenly to lower lashes.**
5. **Do not overapply mascara; your lashes will look clumpy or like thick-barred windows.**

Eyebrow Shaping and Shading

No aspect of makeup has gone through such dramatic fashion changes as eyebrow styles. Eyebrows are as representative of each fashion decade as clothes are. We've gone from overtweezed, pencil-thin, tortured brows to overdrawn, thickly penciled brows to a full, bushy natural look, and now we've settled on very soft, full, but definitely shaped brows. The idea is for the eyebrows to be natural in appearance but not bushy or thick, with a defined but not pointed arch.

Shaping the Eyebrows

Full, softly shaped eyebrows are easier to keep up, but there is a balance between overtweezing and no tweezing. We are talking about natural, not Neanderthal. There is a middle ground between Groucho Marx and Greta Garbo when it comes to the appearance of your brows.

Discovering the best shape for your eyebrows without sacrificing a natural appearance is what you want to accomplish. The eye is framed by the arch, length, and thickness of the eyebrow. Just as the shape of a mustache can change the appearance of a man's face, the shape of the eyebrows can affect the appearance of the eyes. For example, if you tweeze too much off the front part of the eyebrows, the eyes will appear smaller. If you tweeze too much from under the eyebrows, increasing the distance between the eye and the eyebrow, you can look permanently surprised.

Deciding which hairs to leave and which ones to remove makes the difference between attractively shaped brows and misshapen ones. And go slowly; for some reason eyebrow hair does not always grow back after it is tweezed. You can use an eyebrow pencil and a diagram to help you line up the following parameters for shaping your eyebrow.

The beginning of the brow should be in alignment with the center of the nostril, the arch should fall at the back third of the eye, and, although the eyebrow should be as long as possible, it still shouldn't extend into the temple area (see the diagram on page 316). **The basic rule is that the front part of the brow should never drop below the back part of the brow.** Allowing this to happen, either with the way you tweeze your eyebrows or the way you draw them on, makes you look like you're frowning and overemphasizes the downward movement of the back part of the eye.

The best tweezer is the one from Revlon with a tip that is slightly rounded to a soft point. Tweezers that are too pointy can stab the skin; too flat across the top, and they can grab skin along with the hair. There are lots of other tweezers around in all kinds of shapes or with handles that snap together, but these all pose problems when it comes to reliability and ease of use.

Steps to Shaping a Perfect Brow

1. **Before you start tweezing, use a lip or brow pencil to heavily draw on the shape you want; you can adjust it as you decide on the look you want.**

2. **Once that shape is drawn on, tweeze any hairs that fall outside the line of the brow.**
3. **Next, brush the brows straight up with an old toothbrush. Any hairs that are too long and floppy should be trimmed with a small scissors.**

Types of Eyebrow Products

What color eyebrow shadow or gel should you use? Generally, you should match the exact color of the brows rather than your hair color or a color you think would look better than what already exists. You don't want to see a difference between the eyebrow hairs and the shadow or gel used to fill them in. However, if you have pale eyebrows and want to darken the brow color, use a soft shade of brown that is as close to your brows' natural color as possible. If you have red hair and brown eyebrows, using a red pencil or red-brown powder will look unnatural; stick with brown. If you have blonde eyebrows, you could use a slightly darker blonde or taupe color on your brows to make them visible.

What if you don't have any hair at all where the eyebrows are supposed to be? This is the only circumstance that requires applying a brow color that matches the hair on your head. It will look the most natural. Use the wedge brush and powder to follow the bone above the eye, using whatever hair is there. Usually there's enough shape to create a natural, shaded impression of a brow. Use a light touch; use short, quick motions; and avoid the temptation to exaggerate the shape, arch it severely, or extend it into the temple. Downplay the fact that there is no hair, and don't overexaggerate the brows with a strong, eye-catching line. Also, don't place a highlighter or light-colored eyeshadow under the brow to further emphasize the brow. Putting something dark next to something light makes it look even more prominent. Use what you have as the basis for any makeup application; do not make any obvious, theatrical changes.

Powder eyebrow colors: Eyebrow color should be applied using a soft-textured powder (either an eyeshadow or a powder designed for the brow works great) that matches the brow color exactly, and a soft wedge brush or a tiny eyeliner brush (I prefer the control of a small eyeliner brush). Follow the basic shape of the brow, using the same guidelines as for tweezing. Fill in only at the front or underneath the brow, or through the brow itself. Avoid drawing on color above the brow.

I rarely recommend using eyebrow pencils. They can produce a greasy look and mat the eyebrow hair, and too often you end up looking like a leftover from another decade. If you are presently penciling your eyebrows, seriously consider changing to powder. If penciling doesn't look absolutely natural, don't do it. Better to go without any eyebrow makeup at all than to be adorned with a line of pencil above your eye.

Many makeup artists use both pencil and powder to create natural-looking brows for women with little to no eyebrow hair, and this can be a great alternative. This way you can get the control and delineation of a pencil, and then soften and shade the effect with a powder.

Application: To apply the powdered brow color, brush the brow up with an old toothbrush and then apply the color with an angled wedge brush, filling in the shape of the brow between the hairs where needed. If your eyebrows are set high, away from the eye area, and you want to reshape them, place the color directly under the eyebrow. The closer the brow is to the eye area (meaning the height from the brow to the lid or eyelashes is small), the more you should fill in the color in the existing brow itself rather than shading just below the brow. As much as possible, work only with the hair that is there. The idea is to shade rather than draw on eyebrows. Do not place your brow color, whether it is pencil or powder, more than one-quarter inch away from where the natural hair growth stops. It simply looks fake and accentuates the fact that there is no brow there in the first place. What you want is the suggestion, the shadow of a brow—not a line and not an obvious application of color (see the picture on page 274).

Colored eyebrow gels: These are a fairly recent development and a good option for making the most of sparse, light-colored eyebrows or for giving a thicker look to most other eyebrows. (My favorite brand is Borghese Brow Milano.) These products look like mascara, but they have a much lighter consistency.

Application: Apply the color through the brow in much the same fashion as you apply mascara to the eyelashes. Brush the wand through your brows, being careful not to get it on the forehead or other areas of the skin, or to have the brows standing straight up. It will probably take you a few times to get the hang of it. You also might have trouble at first controlling the amount of gel from the tube to the brow. But if you want your brows to look fuller, give this one a try—it really works.

Eyebrow Mistakes to Avoid

1. **Do not overtweeze, and never tweeze above the brow, only underneath.**
2. **Do not overstate the shape of the brow; minimal brow alteration is the best.**
3. **Do not pluck brows into a thin line thinking it will make your eyes look larger. It will only look strange, contrived, even sinister. It can also give the face a surprised look, and none of this is attractive or natural.**
4. **Do not use eyebrow pencil or eyeliner pencil to fill in your eyebrows unless you are adept at making it look very soft and shaded.**

5. **Do not apply eyebrow powders that are different from your own eyebrow color; it is best to always match your existing brow color.**
6. **Do not apply brow color that is noticeable or has a drawn-on look.**
7. **Do not forget that eyebrow color should look shaded and soft, not like a straight, hard line.**
8. **Be careful of brow colors that look red on the skin, which can make the eyebrow look fake and the skin irritated.**

Contouring

Contouring is the art of creating or increasing shadows in certain areas so the face appears to have more structure and definition. It involves using brown tones of blush to contour along the sides of the nose, at the sides of the forehead, under the cheekbones, and in the center of the chin to add color, definition, and shape to the face. Although contouring is an optional step for most daytime makeup applications, it is still rather intriguing and worthwhile for some women.

For the most part, using contouring to reshape the face has somewhat subsided. The likely reason for its demise is that believable-looking contouring is difficult to master (even more difficult than believable-looking blush). Contouring takes skill and patience, and very few women have the time to deal with it every morning. Women who do decide to take the time often end up with a brown stripe under their blush, and that is not the way contouring is supposed to look. Think twice before incorporating this step into your daily makeup routine until you've practiced and developed the skill to apply this look softly.

Contouring is always done as a separate step, using a completely different brush and shade of powder than for the blush application. Shades of pink, red, and orange are used as blushes; only shades of brown are used in contouring. The safest contour shade to use if you have fair to medium-dark skin tones is one that looks like your skin color when it is tanned. A soft or rich golden shade of brown is generally the perfect color to use when trying to produce realistic shadows on the face. Shades of gray-brown can look dirty, and shades of red-brown and mauve-brown can look like bruising on women with fair to medium-dark skin tones. For women of color, particularly African-American women, either an extremely dark shade of golden brown or a deep chocolate brown color work exceptionally well.

Types of Contour

Contour is essentially blush in a golden brown or reddish-brown color. For the varying types of contour, review the "Types of Blush" section later in this chapter.

Applying Contour

Instead of using a brush designed for contouring, use a brush designed for blush or rouge. Traditional blush brushes are too small for most cheeks, so they are a poor choice for blush application. Likewise, traditional contouring brushes are a poor choice for applying contour because they are usually too stiff and have a flat edge, and can leave visible edges when you apply your color. Use the full end of the blush brush when contouring. Knocking off the excess powder before applying and brushing in short, quick motions going back to the ear should net the best results. Here are some rules of placement to help you most effectively contour your face.

Contouring under or along the jawline: Avoid contouring or shading along any portion of the jawline. After you've gone through all the trouble to find a foundation that leaves no line of demarcation at the jaw, it makes no sense to add a brown stripe there and hope people will believe it is a natural shadow. However, shading the jawline or just under the chin can be passable for pictures or possibly for evening, but it must be applied very carefully. Shading under the jawline can also result in shading your collar at the same time. Be careful! Be sure to blend well and soften any noticeable edges or concentrations of color.

Contouring under the cheekbone: Place the center of your brush about one-quarter to one-half inch behind the laugh line, and stroke the color straight back, aiming toward the middle of the ear. The area of application should be approximately a half inch in width, with no definite edges visible. Use your sponge to soften hard edges. The starting point for under-cheekbone contouring is almost always the same regardless of the face shape, because the cheekbone corresponds nicely to the laugh line and middle ear area for most women. You can adjust the angle depending on your preferences. The steeper the angle going toward the top of the ear, the longer the face will appear. If you have a square or round face, you might want to try contouring at a steeper angle. The longer the face (as an oblong or triangular face might be), the more horizontal (straight back toward the middle of the ear) the line can be. This, in effect, deemphasizes the length of the face. All this takes experimentation, so be patient until you achieve the look you want. Be sure to blend well and soften any noticeable edges or concentrations of color.

Caution: When applying the under-cheekbone contour, be sure never to blend or place the contour color below the mouth area, below the middle of the ear, or onto the cheekbone itself. There is also no need to suck in your mouth to help find your cheekbones—that will help you find the sides of the mouth, not the cheekbone.

Contouring the sides of the nose: Although most women think that contouring the nose is done strictly to make it look smaller or narrower or longer, there is actually a more artistic reason for using this shading technique. If you're applying full makeup, particularly for evening, and you ignore the nose, you will have color everywhere on your face except for a blank spot in the center of the face. Contouring the nose helps to achieve color balance for the whole face when you choose to wear a formal, full makeup application. It isn't essential, but it's a great trick.

The goal is to make the contour color look absolutely as soft as possible. The challenge is that you have to restrict the color to the sides of the nose. You never want to accidentally blend the color of the nose contour onto the area under your eyes or onto your cheeks. Take extra care to blend only a small amount of contour color on such an obvious focal point.

The best technique for applying the nose contour is to place the brush itself between your fingers and thumb, so the brush tip becomes somewhat flattened. This way the brush tip can more easily follow along the sides of your nose. (You can use the brush you usually use for contouring or a very large, flat eyeshadow brush.) Now, take the index finger of your other hand, place it flat down the center of the nose, and apply the contour color along the side of your finger. Where the brush falls against your finger is the area to be contoured. Once you've done this, remove your finger and softly apply the contour fully around the tip of the nose and on the flare of the nostrils. Continue the contour in a narrow, soft line up under the eyebrow, avoiding the corner of the eye and the area between the eyebrows. Be sure to blend well and soften any noticeable edges or concentrations of color.

Contouring the temple area: Temple contour is a traditional step that is as basic as applying blush. The difference is that most women don't know about it. Take a look at the cover of any fashion magazine or ads for designer clothes, and you will notice this contouring on most of the models. When temple contour is neatly applied, the eyeshadows at the back of the eye can be blended into it so they don't end abruptly with a harsh edge of color. Without temple contour, the forehead becomes a great bare wall against the colored background of the cheeks and eyes.

The temple contour is placed next to the back third of the eye near the brow bone, directly out and up onto the forehead like a pie wedge, but without the edges. Temple contour can be applied either before or after the eye makeup design is in place. If you apply the contour after the eye makeup design, it is important to place the brush directly over the eyeshadows at the back third of the eye and then brush the contour all the way back to the hairline. If you do the contour first, apply it in the exact same place and in the same way, but when you apply the eyeshadows, blend them directly over and onto the temple contour. Either way, the contour softens the back edge of the eyeshadows.

When temple contour looks bad, it's usually for one of three reasons: (1) forgetting that this step begins at the back third of the under-eyebrow area, right on top of and over the back third of the entire eye area; (2) not brushing the contour directly over the eyebrow itself, which can make the application look choppy instead of smooth and even (you should apply the eyebrow color after the temple contour); and (3) applying the color in a straight one-inch strip next to the eye instead of in a softly blended two-inch pie wedge that is partially blended onto the forehead. Temple contour is a shaded area, like the blush area, and it should never look like a stripe. Be sure to blend well and soften any noticeable edges or concentrations of color.

Contour Mistakes to Avoid

1. **Do not use a blush color to contour any part of your face. Contour only with golden brown, chocolate brown, or dark brown shades.**
2. **Do not use contour under the jaw or chin area during the day; it will look too obvious and possibly get on clothing.**
3. **Do not apply contour until you get used to blending it on softly: it should never look like stripes or brown lines on the face.**
4. **Do not forget to blend hard edges; contour should always look soft and as natural as possible on the face.**

Blush

Blush is one part of makeup application many women take for granted. The comment I hear most often is "I've been doing that for years. I know how to put on blush." Yet it is so easy to make mistakes, and I see them all the time. Blush is one of the more prominent parts of any makeup routine, so if you do make a mistake—such as applying it too close to the lines around the eye, applying it like a stripe of color across the cheek, applying the wrong color, or applying it underneath the cheekbones as if it were contour—it is very noticeable. I urge you to take time to learn how to apply blush properly.

I can't say that everyone agrees exactly where you are supposed to place blush. There are many opinions on where it should start, where it should end, and how high or low to place it along the cheekbone. My strong preference—one I believe is shared by many—is to keep the blush on the cheekbones and away from the eye area, blending the color just on the cheekbones and starting it about a half inch behind the laugh lines. Some women start the blush no farther into the center of the face than the center of the eye. That can make the blush look very strange. The idea is to blush the entire cheekbone, and that means full across the cheek.

Types of Blush

Compact powder blushes: Powder blushes are an excellent choice for all skin types. They go on easily, blend beautifully, and come in great colors. A brush is essential for applying these smoothly, softly, and evenly.

Application: To find the area to be blushed, place the full end of your brush about one-quarter to one-half inch behind the laugh line. Starting here, brush downward and back toward the center of your ear, being careful not to place any color below the level of the mouth. Applying your blush by brushing down as opposed to back and forth eliminates a stripe effect. The blush area should be about two inches thick, with no hard edges. Always use your sponge to soften edges.

Pros: There are only pros to this type; it works for everyone!

Liquid, gel, and cream blushes: These are not my favorites and I strongly recommend staying away from them. Liquid, gel, and cream blushes sound good when the salesperson is explaining them, but they don't perform reliably for most skin types. (They can be very awkward to blend evenly; they tend to streak, whether you use your fingers or a sponge; they can stain the pores, making the face look dotted with color; and they don't work well over foundation—the foundation gets wiped off as you apply the blush.) If you have flawless, poreless, smooth skin (no dryness and not oily) and have a deft touch at blending, you are a candidate for liquid, gel, or cream blush. Just don't buy anything until you check it out in the daylight and see how it wears during the day.

Application: There isn't one best way to apply these types of blushes. A sponge is my first choice, but some women do fine using their fingers. Use whatever works best for you.

Ultra-matte cream blushes: Several companies, particularly Revlon and Almay, have added ultra-matte cream blushes to their line. These ultra-matte blushes come in a cream-to-powder form that you apply like any other cream blush, but the ultra-matte dries very quickly and has impressive staying power.

Application: As with any cream blush, it takes skill to blend it on smoothly and evenly, but with these, if you make a mistake, there is no fixing it once it dries. However, applied with a good-sized sponge applicator and a deft hand, it can look quite natural and soft, and it does stay put.

Applying Blush and Contouring

If you are applying both blush and under-cheekbone contour, apply the contour color first and then blend the blush on top of and gradually down into the contour color. Then, using your sponge, blend until you meld the colors together into an attractive design. The hallmark of an attractive design is not being able to see where one color stops and the other starts.

Choosing a Blush Color

How much color and which color should you use? That is not an easy question to answer. For the past several years, pale blushes have been in vogue, while mauve, peach, rose, pale red, and coral blushes have never gone out of style. Pale blush looks ghostly on most women; nothing brightens the face better than a little blush. Soft is better than vivid when it comes to cheek color, but some color is definitely desirable and ultimately more attractive.

I have never been one to recommend the no-blush look when a woman is wearing makeup. Leaving the cheeks pale or blank when the eyes and lips are done and foundation has been applied all over the face creates a gaunt, haggard look. That can make an interesting statement, but the statement doesn't say pretty or beautiful.

One option when choosing blush color is to go neutral; a soft golden brown, tannish-looking color is great for many skin tones. For darker skin colors, a deeper golden brown works perfectly. Whatever option you choose, be sure your blush matches the underlying tone of your lipstick (or the lipstick matches the underlying tone of your blush; either way, they need to be coordinated). If you are wearing red lipstick with a blue undertone, the blush should be in that same color family; rose lipstick means rose blush; coral lipstick coordinates with coral or coral/tan blush; and tan lipstick works with almost any color of blush. What you absolutely do not want to do is wear pink blush and coral lipstick or cranberry lipstick with mauve blush. The lipstick and blush must work together and not look like opposite, clashing ends of a rainbow.

Blush Mistakes to Avoid

1. **Blush and lipstick colors should never clash; they should either complement each other or be in a similar color family.**
2. **Never put blush close to the lines around the eye; it makes them look more evident, and if you are using a pink, peach, or coral shade of blush, the eye area can also look red and irritated.**
3. **Do not apply blush below the mouth or the laugh lines; blush is for the cheekbones only.**
4. **Do not blush your nose, forehead, hairline, or chin: it can make the face look overly pink or red or made up.**
5. **Do not forget to use your sponge to blend out hard edges or smudges of**

blush. Blush should always be well blended, with no visible edges where the blush starts and stops.

Lipstick and Lip Pencil

Most of you already know about lipstick, but I've talked to enough women to know that this next idea needs to be stated explicitly. Simply put, if you're wearing makeup, your lips need lipstick—not lip gloss, but lipstick. Lip gloss doesn't last, but lipstick does. Lip gloss provides a sheer, temporary look that can be great for teenagers. Lipstick (cream lipstick, not iridescent) provides a polished and put-together look that can last at least until your second cup of coffee. If your lips are naked while your eyes and cheeks are made up, you will look like you forgot you had a mouth when applying your makeup. For the sake of balance, remember lipstick.

Types of Lipstick

Is there a difference between lipsticks? Yes, there are vast differences between lipsticks. As you probably already know from experience, lipstick colors and textures can vary within the same cosmetics line. Some are creamy; others are dry, greasy, shiny, or flat. Some melt easily; others go on stickily, smearily, evenly, thickly, thinly, and combinations thereof. I recommend lipsticks that go on creamily, in an even layer that doesn't smear, look thick, or look greasy. The only way to find them is to be patient and try on the colors you like and see how they feel. But whatever you do, avoid wearing shiny lipsticks, particularly if you are an adult with a serious career. Iridescence is for evening, not for daytime.

Note: If your lipstick has a tendency to cake or get dry as the day goes by, avoid reapplying your lipstick over semi-worn-off lipstick. Wipe off all your lipstick first and then reapply it. You may also want to apply a bit of gloss under your lipstick if the problem of caking persists.

What about the ultra-matte lipsticks? The ultra-matte lipstick craze has been nothing less than amazing. Keeping up with the Joneses has taken over the industry. Ultra-matte lipsticks were first introduced by Ultima II as Lip Sexxxy, then reintroduced by Ultima II's drugstore sister, Revlon, as ColorStay Lipstick. Since then, knockoffs have been showing up in almost mind-boggling profusion. Maybelline Great Lip, L'Oreal Colour Endure, Lancome Rouge Idole, Cover Girl Marathon, Shiseido Staying Power Lipstick, Almay Lasting LipColor, and Estee Lauder Indelible Lipstick are the best of the bunch. Maybelline Great Lip is my favorite, but they are all virtually identical. They all go on moist and wet, then dry within a few seconds to form a dry, matte layer with no movement or creaminess. The dry texture does prevent transference to coffee cups, glasses, the food you eat, and the significant other you kiss. But it isn't indelible;

this stuff does eventually rub off. Actually, it tends to chip or peel off. These **ultra-matte lipsticks are not for everyone, particularly not for those with a tendency toward chapped lips, because it will make them even drier.** Ultra-matte lipsticks can feel very uncomfortable during cold, dry winters or in hot, arid climates. Also, while ultra-matte lipsticks tend not to bleed, if you have wrinkles on your lips, these lipsticks will accentuate them.

Choosing Lip Colors

When choosing lipstick colors, follow these basic rules: (1) Thinner or smaller lips look best with brighter, more vivid colors. (2) Avoid darker colors on thin lips; they make the mouth look severe and harsh. Brighter colors may take a bit of getting used to, but they truly make a smaller mouth more noticeable. Occasionally I read or hear that makeup advisors suggest applying a neutral color on small lips and playing up the eyes instead (as if the notion is ever to play down the eyes or ignore the mouth). Test this technique for yourself before you give in to this nonsense. (3) Larger lips can wear just about any color, but softer shades look better because darker or vivid colors can make large lips look too prominent.

Applying Lip Color

A lip brush or lip pencil is an optional accessory. You can use a lip pencil to draw a definitive edge around the mouth to follow when applying lipstick, and a lip brush to control your application. A tube of lipstick is too big for some lips and too small for others. If your lips are small, it is best to use a lip brush; if your lips are large, the only reason to use a lip brush is for improved accuracy.

If you do choose to work with a lip pencil, always place the color on the actual outline of your mouth. Do not use corrective techniques that make the mouth look larger or longer, especially for daytime makeup. **If you try to change the outline of your mouth with a lip pencil by drawing outside the lips, two hours later, when your lipstick wears off, the lip liner, which lasts longer than the lipstick, will still be in place and it will look like you missed your lips.** Always line the lips following their actual shape, then fill in with your lipstick, using either the tube or a lip brush (see the picture on page 275).

What about the center outline of the mouth? Do you round the point of the lips or make the point more obvious? As a rule, a softer appearance is better than a hard one. Leave the points neither rounded nor pyramidlike; someplace in between with a soft arch is best.

To prevent lipstick from gunking up in the corners of the mouth, don't place lip liner or pencil in that area. Stop before you get to the very corners of the mouth.

Lip pencils should never create an obvious dark, brown, or definite line around the mouth. This obvious delineation keeps showing up and women hold on to it for some unknown reason, but I've yet to see a professional makeup artist apply this look on anyone. **Your lip pencil should not make an obvious line that shows up as a colored border around the lipstick. The goal is to have the lipstick and lip pencil meld so that you can't see where one starts and the other stops.**

If you wear lip liner and you want to help your lipstick last longer, apply the lip pencil all over the lip area, including the outline of the lips, and then apply your lipstick over it. This places a more permanent color on the lips, so the lipstick won't wear off as quickly as it normally does. **As you already know, there is no such thing as all-day lipsticks. I wish there were, but they don't exist.** For years the cosmetics industry has been proclaiming new "all-day" or "long-wearing" lipsticks, yet women continue to reapply their lipstick. It is still impossible to go past lunch, or even past midmorning, with your lipstick looking the same as when you first applied it.

How can you stop lipstick from traveling into the lines around your mouth? The first step is to stop wearing greasy lipsticks and lip glosses. **The greasier the lipstick or lip pencil, the faster the color will slip into the lines around your mouth.** The drier-feeling lipsticks are best for conquering this problem. Powdering the mouth with loose powder before applying the lipstick also helps, but can be a bit messy. Lip pencil will not stop greasy lipsticks from traveling, but it can slow them down.

A few years ago, some cosmetics companies came out with new products that were supposed to prevent lipstick from bleeding. I tried a lot of them and many never worked, but I finally found three that changed the way I wear lipstick, because now I don't have to worry about my lipstick bleeding. Revlon ColorLock, Coty StopIt and HoldIt, and The Body Shop No Wander pencil really stay put—beautifully.

Does using a lipstick brush help keep lipstick on longer? Why a brush would serve this purpose has never been explained to me in a manner that makes any logical sense, and it simply doesn't work. Lipstick stays on longer when you put on a lot of lipstick; wear strong, vivid colors that are not greasy; and avoid wearing lip glosses.

Lipstick and Lip Pencil Mistakes to Avoid

1. **Do not use a lip pencil that contrasts with your lipstick; it is out of date and can look severe.**
2. **Do not wear lipstick that is a different color tone from the rest of your**

makeup. For example, if you are wearing blue-toned blush, wear a blue-toned lipstick.

3. **Do not use lip gloss in place of lipstick during the day; it can bleed and won't last as long as lipstick.**
4. **Do not wear iridescent lipstick; when it wears off, it can look dry, white, and caked; it also looks too distracting for daytime.**
5. **Do not exaggerate or change the shape of your mouth with your lip pencil or lipstick; it will look like you missed your mouth.**
6. **If you want your lipstick to last, wear more of it and don't blot; blotting takes off several layers before you've even left the house.**

Touching Up

As the day goes by, even the best-applied makeup can slip, fade, and get phone- or finger-printed. Lipstick can get thick and clumped. Long days require quick touch-ups to revive beautifully applied makeup. Following the steps below, in order, will revive the look you started with.

- If you have oily skin, you can blot away the excess oil by laying either a tissue or one of the face-blotting papers sold by some cosmetics companies over the face and blotting. Perm end papers also work well. Do this before you do anything else.
- Remove all of your lipstick so you can start over after you have touched up your face makeup.
- Once the excess oil on your skin has been absorbed, take a fresh sponge and smooth out the foundation, blush, and contour (women with dry and normal skin should also follow this step). Use a gentle buffing motion, being sure to smooth things as you go.
- Apply a little extra concealer under the eyes if that area is looking a bit dark.
- If you need a little more foundation over blemishes or discolorations, blend it on now, avoiding the blush and contour area.
- Dust a light layer of powder over the face.
- Apply more blush or contour if needed, but only if needed, and be careful: color grabs more over makeup that has been on the face awhile.
- If you want to touch up your eyeliner, particularly under the eyes, where it might have smeared, use a powder shadow instead of a pencil.
- If your eyeshadows have creased, blot gently with a tissue or blotting paper and then use a brush to smooth out the color. Apply a powder over the area

to even out the shadows and add whatever color is needed to make things look balanced.

- Finally, reapply your lipstick. (Lip liner is always optional.)

Please note: If you are wearing one of the new ultra-matte foundations, you may find touch-ups to be tricky, because stay-put makeup doesn't move and reblending is almost impossible. In that case, you may very well be stuck with starting over, but it's worth a shot to see if you can blend things smoothly and do a simple touch-up. For me, stay-put foundations stay so well that my makeup never slips in the least once it's on and in place.

Turning Daytime Makeup into Night

Now that you've touched up your makeup but you want to change it from your office or daytime look to a knockout evening visage, consider the following.

- Add a dark or black shade of eyeshadow to the back corner of the lid or in the crease.
- You can also use this same shade of dark or black eyeshadow to create a more dramatic liner around the eye.
- With a powder that has shine, add some shimmering highlights to the cheekbones, center of the forehead, chin, neck, shoulders, or décolletage.
- A vivid red lipstick always makes a dramatic evening look, especially if you are wearing black.
- Avoid using more blush. Making the cheeks more colorful doesn't improve an evening look.

Balance, Proportion, and Detail

Have you ever wondered exactly what it is you admire when you see a well-made-up woman? You may not know exactly what it is you like, but you probably envy her skill and wish you could figure out how she did it. At the airport the other day, I noticed such a woman and watched other women (and a few men) turn their heads and take notice. It wasn't just that she was attractive and her clothes were stylish, but her makeup in particular was impeccable. Her face looked smooth and was accented with rich though subtle blush and contour tones. All the colors, from her lipstick to the eyeshadows, softly mingled into a harmonious sweep of light to dark, with just the right amount of shading—not too much and not too little.

It occurred to me that anyone can spruce up her makeup by going over a list of everyday makeup mistakes that detract from rather than enhance her appearance. Knowing about the nuances of a well-done makeup application versus one that is poorly done can make all the difference in helping a woman look great all day long. With all the time most women spend putting on makeup, getting it on wrong is not acceptable.

Besides the essential rules regarding application and blending techniques, there are three basic concepts you need to keep in mind in order to achieve a flattering look: balance, proportion, and detail. **Balance** is about making sure the different elements of your makeup go together and that no one aspect is more prominent than any other. In other words, if you are wearing a dark, rich brownish red lipstick, you must choose blush in a harmonious color (shiny pink blush is not going to work with an orange-red lipstick) and make sure your eyeshadows accent the eyes so they don't get lost because of too much attention to the lips. When colors and tones are in balance and no one aspect of the makeup shouts over another, you don't notice the makeup as much as you notice the woman. Don't forget little things, like lining the upper lashes if you line the lower lashes (otherwise the line underneath will look too heavy and obvious all by itself). If you choose to wear blush, blend the color well so it doesn't stand out as a visible swipe of color across your cheek.

Proportion is about the total package of selecting what to wear. It's about paying attention to symmetry, to how your makeup colors, wardrobe, and hairstyle work together. If you are wearing a business suit and the eyeshadows you have on range from tan to black, with a wine-colored lipstick and blush, that may indeed be a stunning combination, but not with what you are wearing. The same is true for someone with very light hair and fair skin: the color combination may be dramatic and beautiful, but it will look out of place in sunlight or office light. Proportion is making sure that everything works together, with nothing looking out of place, so your makeup doesn't upstage you.

Detail is the most essential and perhaps the most difficult area, because it takes so much effort and concentration. Pay attention to every nuance of your makeup. If necessary, apply your makeup using a magnifying mirror so you don't leave the house with eyeshadow sprinkles on your cheek or mascara smudges at the back corner of your eyelid. Do not be satisfied with doing a ten-minute makeup application in only five minutes when you are in a hurry. If you don't have enough time to do your normal makeup routine, do only what you have time for.

I can't tell you how often women have asked me what they can do differently with their makeup, and I have said something about how they needed to blend the foundation better because it looked patchy and uneven or the eyeshadows were smeared and poorly blended. Often these women responded by saying, "Well, I didn't have much time, and this was the best I could do." I then say, "I notice you have your blouse buttoned and your skirt zipped up." Typically their answer to that is, "Of course!" I in turn comment, "Well, even though you didn't have much time, you didn't leave the house undressed. You should apply the same rule to your face." It doesn't mean being late because of your makeup; it means doing less so it goes faster. But whatever you do, take the time to do it right. Because when makeup is sloppy, it just looks wrong.

As I mentioned above, I use several levels of makeup application, depending on the time I have and what the makeup is for. For me, full makeup for a television appearance takes 20 to 25 minutes. Makeup for a business meeting or a formal event takes 15 minutes. Makeup for casual daily business or informal get-togethers takes 5 to 10 minutes. Makeup for running to the gym to work out takes a minute and a half (lipstick and mascara only).

Getting Your Makeup to Look the Way You Want

- Don't apply anything you don't have time to apply well. If you don't have time to make sure every part of the makeup you are applying is going on smoothly and evenly, don't apply it. Never leave the house with streaked, smeared, or blotched makeup. You wouldn't leave your house with your blouse undone, nylons hanging down, or a pant leg dragging behind you, so don't do the same with your makeup.
- Foundation should always match the skin exactly—no exceptions. Avoid lines of demarcation in any light, but most of all in daylight.
- Be sure your foundation is best for your skin type. If you have oily skin, do not use a foundation for dry skin, and if you have dry skin do not use a foundation for oily skin.
- Colors on the face should blend softly and without definite lines: no stripes of blush, no stripes of eyeshadow.
- Go light with the powder. After you find a foundation that matches your skin exactly and blend it on smoothly and sheerly, loading your face with powder negates all your previous efforts. As a rule of thumb, the more wrinkles you have on your face, the less powder you should wear.
- Powder should either match the color of the foundation or be translucent and have no color effect on the foundation at all.
- Powder without any added oil is best for oily skin; powder with some amount of oil is best for dry skin.
- You can never blend too much. Soften blush and contour colors several times.
- I know you have been staying away from shiny eyeshadows if you have wrinkles on your eyelids (right?), but some cosmetics lines are sneaking them back into their collections and calling them matte, even though they have some

amount of shine. Stay away from them. No matter how minimally shiny they may appear in the container, when they are applied to your eyelid, the shine will make the skin look wrinkly, plus they don't wear as well as matte eyeshadows during the day. Unless that's the look you want, and you can always check this out in daylight, don't wear them.

- Always check for eyeshadow that has flaked onto your cheek while you were applying it.
- If your eyebrow and eyeliner pencils smear during the day, try using powder instead; don't continue using products of any kind that don't hold up during the day.
- Thickly clumped-on mascara does not look like natural, long eyelashes. It looks like thickly clumped-on mascara.
- Greasy lipstick or gloss can look wet and sloppy as opposed to creamy and smooth. Be certain your lipstick looks soft, not damp. Also, the greasier the lipstick, the more quickly it will come off.
- Lip liner is a nice touch, and using a lip brush can provide a great professional flair, but if you don't have time, you can apply lipstick evenly from the tube and still look terrific.
- Dark lipsticks can be quite attractive, but if you look like Brad Pitt in *Interview with the Vampire,* rethink your makeup (unless you are going Gothic on purpose). Also, wearing dark lip liner with a lighter shade of lipstick inside hasn't been in fashion since 1980, and even then it looked bad. It is too obvious and makes your mouth look hard and angry.
- Don't ever do your makeup like Tammy Faye Bakker!
- When you apply makeup, take into consideration how it will look by midday and at the end of the day. Don't buy products that look great for an hour or two but by lunchtime make you look like you forgot to wash your face the night before. If you have a problem with eyeliner or mascara that smears, reconsider the products you are using or the look you are trying to achieve.
- If you buy a gray eyeshadow and it goes on blue, even though it looks gray in the container, it isn't gray, it is blue. If you buy a foundation that is the right color in the bottle but looks peach, ash, or rose when applied on your skin, it's the wrong color. Believe what you see on your face, not what you see in the container.

Choosing Color

Ah, now here's the most difficult subject of all to discuss, at least on paper. I would love to have the time to sit down and create a makeup look that works for everyone. That isn't humanly possible, but I do have some rules that can help you create the makeup look you want.

Color Choices

- Foundation matches the skin exactly so there are no lines of demarcation (I know this is getting repetitive, but I can't emphasize this point enough).
- Concealer is only a shade or two lighter than the foundation.
- Powder should match the foundation exactly or go on translucent so as not to affect the color of foundation in the least.
- Eyeshadow colors should be neutral shades ranging from pale beige to tan, brown, dark brown, and black, and thousands of shades in between.
- Eyebrow color should match the exact shade of the existing brow hair.
- Eyeliner on the upper lid should be a darker color (all the way to black, depending on the look you want) than the line along the lower lashes, which should be a softer shade of brown.
- Blush can be almost any color as long as it coordinates in some logical fashion with the lipstick color, but it must be blended on softly, without any noticeable edges whatsoever.
- Lipstick can be bold to neutral, but there is a wide range for it, with the only suggestion being that smaller lips should wear brighter shades than larger lips.
- Less is best.
- To create a tanned appearance, use golden brown and chestnut shades for your blush, eyeshadows, contour, and lipstick, but do not under any circumstances apply a foundation or bronzer all over the face if it leaves a line of demarcation at the jaw or hairline.
- If you are wearing clothes in a strong color such as red or pink, you may wish to match your lipstick with that color. However, it is best not to clash color tone. For example, if the outfit you are wearing is peach or coral, your blush and lipstick should have that same underlying color tone or be neutral enough not to clash.

Color Mistakes to Avoid

- Don't wear white or very pale lipstick with a white cast to it. This can look ghostly and ghastly.
- Don't wear blue, green, or violet anything, including eyeliner, eyeshadow, and mascara.

- Don't wear navy blue eyeshadow. (Stick with black; it looks smoky, while navy tends to look "dirty.")
- Don't wear dark brown or black lipstick. (On Dracula it's great; on women it looks like death.)
- Don't wear shiny eyeshadows (unless you like having your eyes look wrinkled).
- Don't wear rainbow-style eyeshadow designs.
- Don't wear eyeshadow applied as a smudge of black around the eye, unless your career objective is to be in a punk rock band.
- Don't wear clashing blush and lipstick; they should be in the same color family, not glaring opposites.

Correcting Some Popular Makeup Myths

- Some makeup artists declare that you shouldn't be afraid to touch your makeup. The truth is, you should be very afraid to touch your makeup. After you've taken time to apply your foundation smoothly with a sponge and your eyeshadows evenly with brushes, there's no reason to use your fingers unless absolutely necessary, and only lightly at that. Touching your face during the day will rub off all your nicely applied makeup.
- Don't spray water or toner on makeup to set it or freshen things up. It doesn't work. A mist of water can streak foundation, powder, and mascara. How this makeup mistake got circulated is anyone's guess.
- Don't change every part of your makeup with every season. If you want to go softer during the spring and summer, that's fine, but it isn't an absolute must.
- Don't use makeup to correct the shape of anything on your face, especially the lips. In person you can absolutely tell when lipstick has been applied beyond or inside the natural lip line. If you overcontour, you will look like you have brown stripes all over your face.
- Don't use foundation or color correctors to change the color of your skin. Foundation must match the underlying skin tone exactly. That will soften any skin discoloration or redness. If you have yellow or olive skin, there is nothing you can or should do to change that. Any correction will look strange next to your neck and along the hairline.
- To keep pencil eyeliner in place, many makeup artists recommend going over it with a matching powder eyeshadow. That works, but why do two steps when only one is needed? Forget the pencil and just use dark eyeshadow to begin with.

- Glowing skin does look nice, but mostly just in pictures. In real life, the skin looks like it is covered with glitter. That isn't bad, but it doesn't look the way it does in the pictures, and it just makes wrinkled skin look more wrinkled. It is an option for an evening out, but that's about it.
- There is no set of colors that is absolute for any skin color. The days of being typed into one color grouping are gone. Just because you have red hair doesn't mean you have to wear corals and avoid blue-red lipstick. It's all up to experimentation and finding what looks best.

Teenagers and Makeup

My experience with teenagers and their impressionable egos has been an eye-opener. Here's what I've learned over the past few months as I've talked to them about skin care, makeup, and the pursuit of looking beautiful.

In our society, one of the emotional mileposts for young girls on the perilous journey between preadolescence and adolescence is the social awareness and self-awareness that it's time to start wearing makeup. Putting on blush, lipstick, mascara, and eyeshadow has become one of the primary rites of passage when changing hormones begin to influence both mind and body. Just as this new style of expression is developing, teenage anxiety is beginning to take on a whole new depth (witness the explosive desperation at a single perceived insult or problem). What do you do when the little girl in your life (who is looking less and less like a little girl) wants to start wearing makeup? Particularly when her sensitivities are overflowing but her sophistication is lagging? And it isn't just that she wants to wear makeup—she *has* to.

Feeling attractive is overwhelmingly important for many teenage girls. It is often complicated by well-meaning adults who don't quite know what to do or say. "You look beautiful—you don't need to wear makeup" is just as irksome as "A little pink blush, rose lipstick, and brown mascara will make you look beautiful." One discounts what the teenager intuitively knows—that women can look more exciting with makeup on (or why else would Mom and the rest of the world be wearing it?)—while the other suggests that the girl is unattractive and would be better off hiding her face behind a layer of cosmetics (albeit a light one). Then there's the ever-popular "You can start wearing makeup when you're 16, and that's that." An arbitrary date ignores the specific needs and development of each teen.

What to do? I wouldn't recommend any of the above approaches, that's for sure. Instead, I suggest incorporating all three positions into a compassionate compromise. The goal is to acknowledge your teenager's needs, letting her know they are valid and important. Tell her, "I know wearing makeup is important to you and it could look lovely on you. But at the same time, I want you to know that I think you are beautiful just the way you are." Then the two of you can decide together what is appropriate, each giving in a little as you go. Gloss yes, lipstick no; blush yes, but only a little; mascara yes, but only brown; concealer yes, but foundation no; and so on. Remember, what you think is important may not be what your teen thinks is important. Mostly this process is about being gentle and respectful of (not controlling or contradicting) the teen's feelings as they come up.

Another option is going together to a professional makeup artist or makeup demonstration. It can be a positive experience as long as you are careful to ward off any attempt on the part of the salesperson to foster insecurity and vulnerability via sales techniques. Let the salesperson know ahead of time, in no uncertain terms, that you don't want him or her to use any language that suggests something is unattractive or wrong with any aspect of your teen's appearance. If the salesperson wants to introduce something different, he or she can easily say, "I think a softer blush can be an attractive look," instead of "The blush you have on is all wrong for you." Don't let salespeople get away with statements like "You have small lids, and a bright color will make them look larger," when a simple statement such as "A pale brown eyeshadow on the lid is a good color choice for you" can go a long way toward building self-esteem instead of makeup addiction and insecurity.

If you do decide the age of your teen is an important factor in determining when makeup is allowed, you can put off the inevitable by intervening with an emphasis on skin care (which is a good starting point in general). Encouraging the everyday use of sunscreens, cleansing with a water-soluble cleanser, exfoliating gently with baking soda or an AHA or BHA product, and using 3% hydrogen peroxide over blemishes is a great way for a teenager to pay attention to beauty issues without getting into makeup. (This is also a great skin-care routine for teenage boys, who are starting to have skin-care concerns of their own.) At the same time, it is essential that you take the time to share information about how the cosmetics industry can take advantage of women and why expensive products are a waste of money. That combination is an excellent and beautiful introduction to the world of cosmetics.

You and your teen can even read a copy of this book together, marking areas to discuss. If there are points you disagree on, both of you can write me a letter and let me try to mediate.

Most of us grown-ups started off on the wrong foot with makeup and skin care, thinking incorrectly from the outset that it would make us perfect and correct all our flaws (of which there were many: eyes too close together or too far apart, nose too broad or too narrow, face too square or too round, skin too yellow or too pink, and on and on). Or we were left on our own with little information about color choice and application technique. We are now in a good position to hand the next generation a measure of self-worth and tell them the truth about cosmetics and what they can and cannot do.

Is It Safe?

Mascara, eyeshadow, and eyeliner are intended to make women more attractive. One thing they shouldn't do is harm the eyes. Yet each year, many women suffer eye infections from cosmetics. At the time of purchase, most eye cosmetics are free from bacteria that could cause eye infections. The problem is that they may not be adequately preserved against microorganisms or they may be misused by the consumer after they are opened. Poor preservation or misuse of an eye cosmetic can cause dangerous bacteria to grow in the product. Then, when the cosmetic is applied to the area around the eye, it can cause an infection.

The Food and Drug Administration has taken numerous steps to make sure that eye cosmetics are free from contamination when they reach you, and that they contain preservatives to inhibit the growth of bacteria. The cosmetics industry generally makes products that will not harm you. Nevertheless, the FDA urges you to follow these 11 tips on the use of eye cosmetics.

1. **Discontinue immediately the use of any eye product that causes irritation. If irritation persists, see a doctor.**
2. **Recognize that bacteria on your hands could, if placed in the eye, cause infections. Wash your hands before applying cosmetics to your eyes.**
3. **Make sure that any instrument you place in the eye area is clean.**
4. **Do not allow cosmetics to become covered with dust or contaminated with dirt or soil. Wipe off the container with a damp cloth if visible dust or dirt is present.**
5. **Do not use old containers of eye cosmetics. If you haven't used the product for several months, it's better to discard it and purchase a new one.**
6. **Do not spit into eye cosmetics. The bacteria in your mouth may grow in the cosmetic, and subsequent application to the eye could cause infection.**
7. **Do not share your cosmetics. Another person's bacteria in your cosmetic can be hazardous to you.**
8. **Do not store cosmetics at temperatures above 85 degrees Fahrenheit. Cosmetics held for long periods in hot cars, for example, are more susceptible to deterioration of the preservative.**

9. Avoid using eye cosmetics if you have an eye infection or if the skin around the eye is inflamed. Wait until the area is healed.
10. Take particular care in using eye cosmetics if you have any allergies.
11. When applying or removing eye cosmetics, be careful not to scratch the eyeball or some other sensitive area.

Now This Is A **Great Brush Collection**

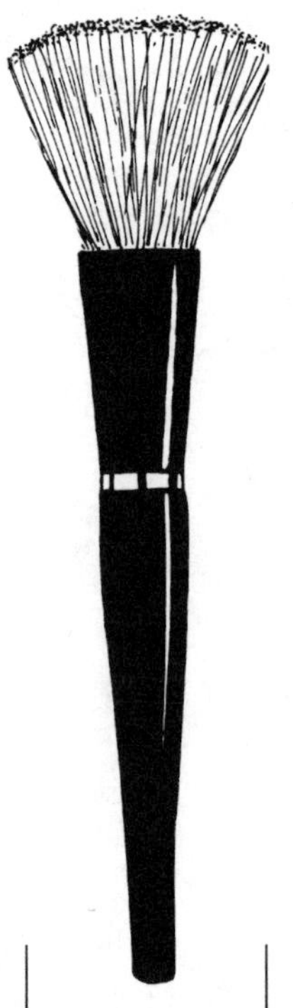

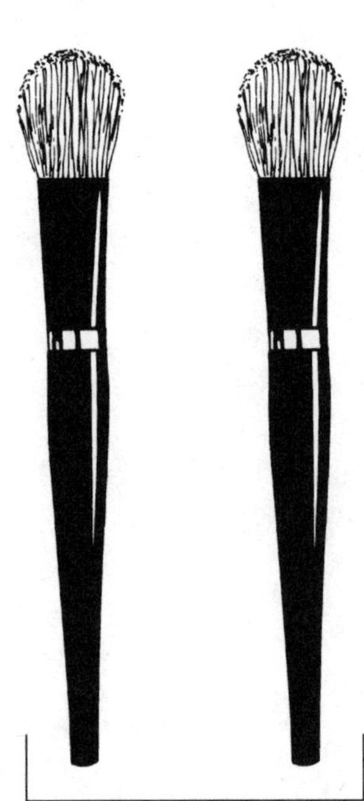

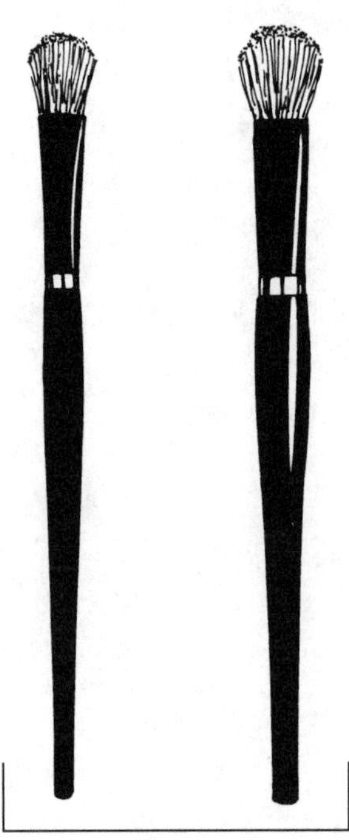

1 powder brush (don't get one that's too big or you will end up spreading too much powder over your face or powdering areas you don't want powdered)

2 blush brushes (one for blush and one for contouring)

2 eyeshadow brushes (one small rounded brush for the crease and back corner of the eye and one large rounded brush for the lid and under-brow area)

Now This Is A **Great Brush Collection**

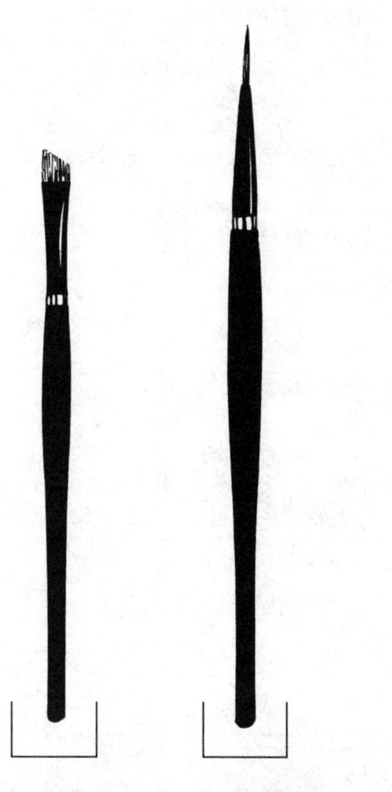

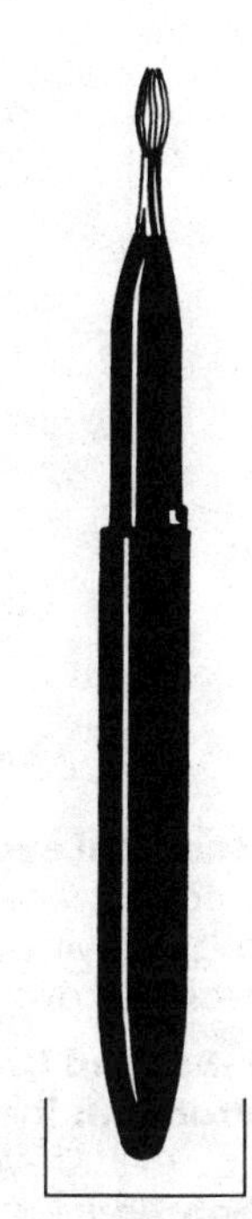

1 angle brush (for shaping eyebrows)

1 eyeliner brush (for lining eyes or for shaping eyebrows)

1 toothbrush (for combing through eyebrows and eyelashes)

1 mascara wand (for combing through eyebrows and eyelashes)

1 retractable lip brush

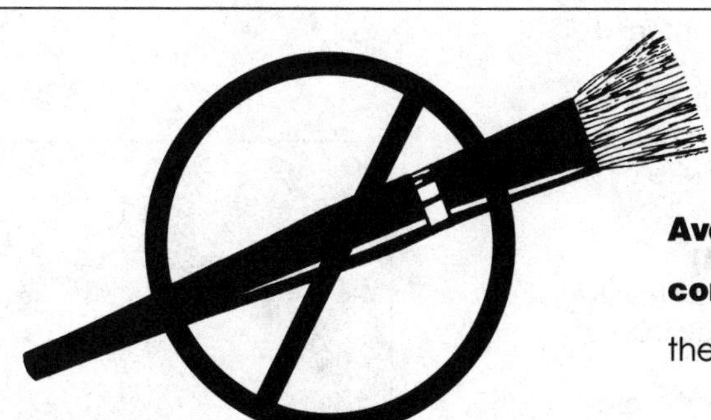

Avoid sharply angled contour brushes — they can leave streaks.

Beautiful
Eyebrow Solutions

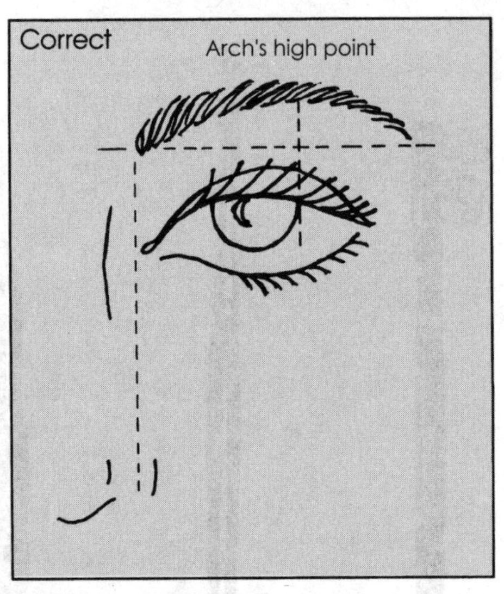

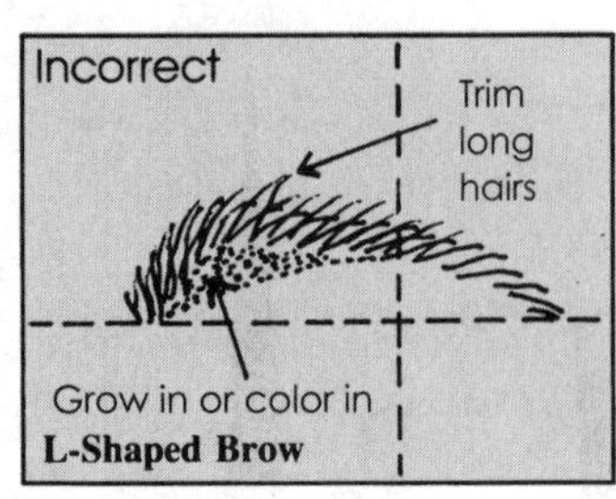

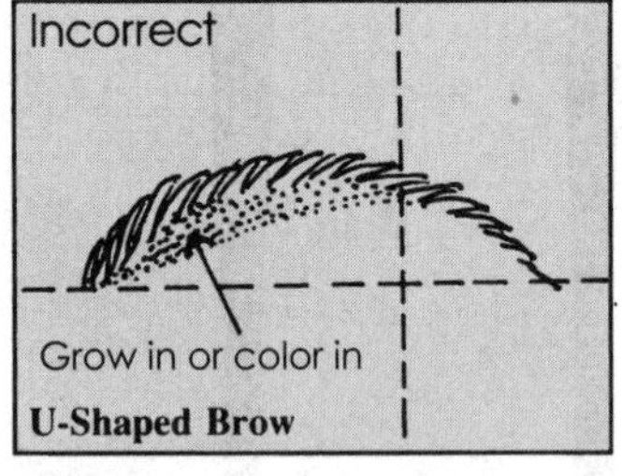

Beautiful eyebrows: The shape of the eyebrow is correct when the beginning of the brow is aligned with the center of the nostril and the arch falls over the back third of the eye.

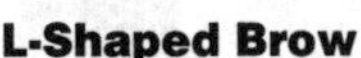

L-Shaped Brow
Problem: The arch is over the front third of the eye.
Solution: Grow in or color in the indicated area.

U-Shaped Brow
Problem: The eyebrow has no arch.
Solution: Grow in or color in the indicated area.

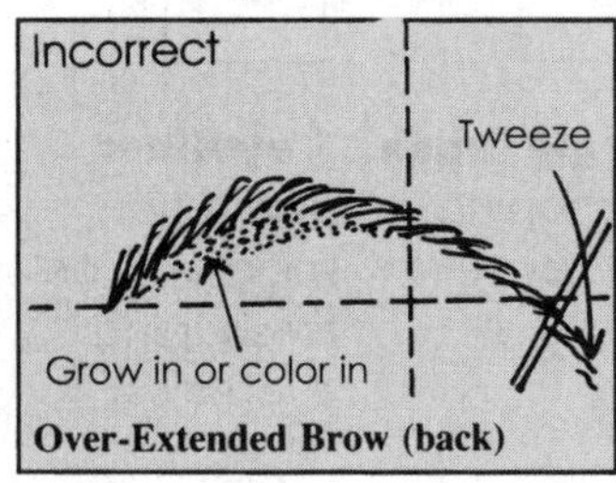

Over-Extended Brow (back)
Problem: The back third of the brow is lower than the front third of the brow.
Solution: Grow in or color in the indicated area and tweeze the end of the brow to align it with the front of the brow.

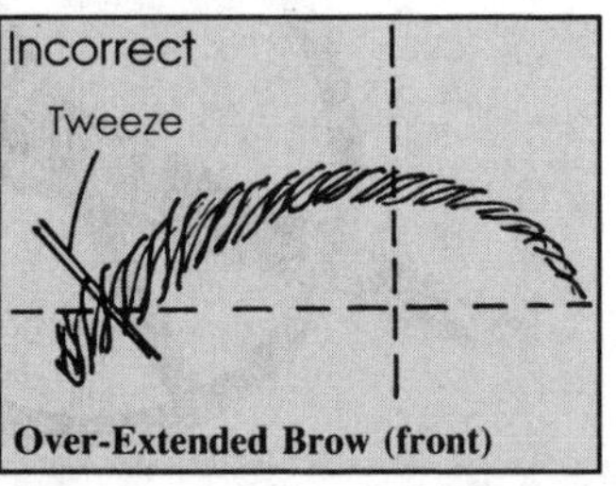

Over-Extended Brow (front)
Problem: The front third of the brow is lower than the back third of the brow.
Solution: Tweeze the front of the brow to align it with the back of the brow.

Creating **Shapely, Natural-Looking Brows!**

Tweezing a soft natural shape is the goal; eyebrows that are too thick or too thin can take attention away from the rest of your face. Follow these steps to create beautiful eyebrows.

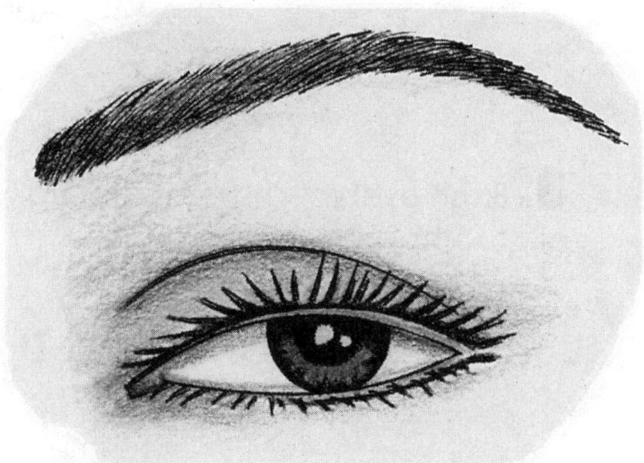

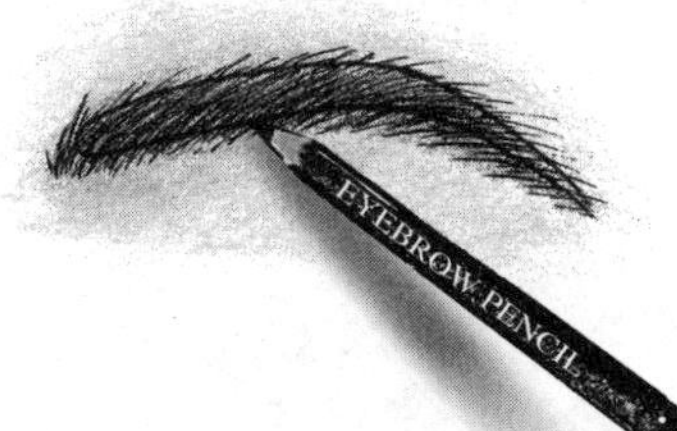

1. Draw on the shape you want with an eyebrow or lip pencil, following the natural growth as much as possible. Take your time with this step, repeating it until you get the look you want.

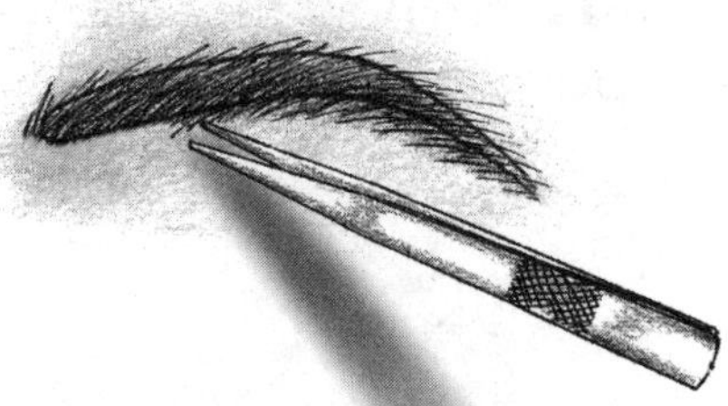

2. Tweeze hairs that fall outside the brow you penciled on. Use rounded or needle-nose tweezers for accurate removal.

Creating **Shapely, Natural-Looking Brows!**

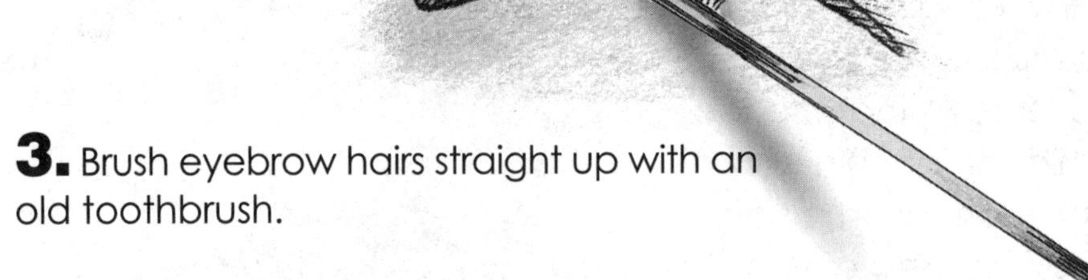

3. Brush eyebrow hairs straight up with an old toothbrush.

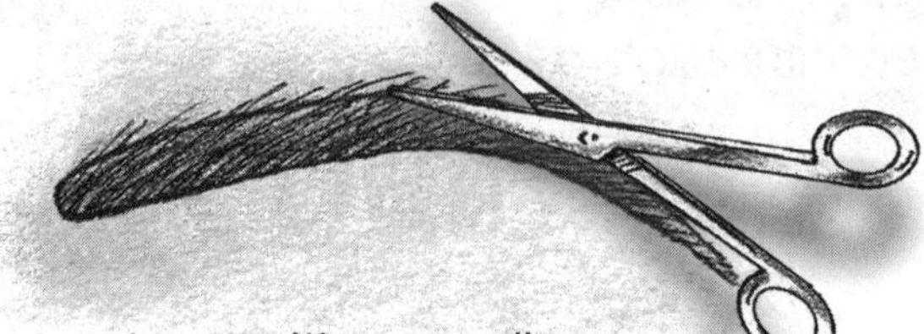

4. Trim hairs that are too long with a small pair of scissors.

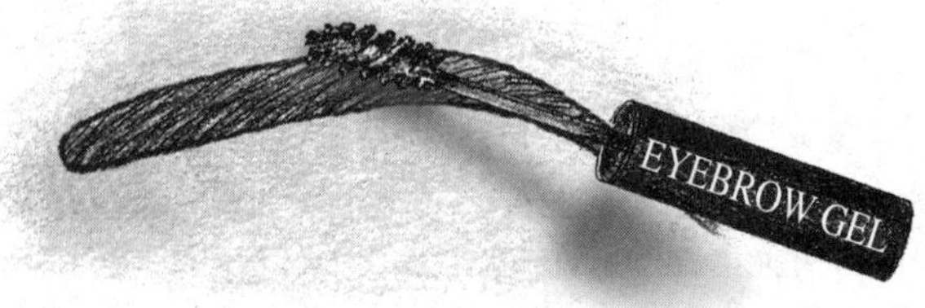

5. To keep brows in place, smooth the hairs with an old mascara wand and then apply brow gel or clear mascara, or spray the mascara wand with hair spray and then comb it through the brows.

CHAPTER NINE

Body Care

Body Neglect?

I receive over 10,000 questions from readers every year, and almost 85% of them concern the face. Does this emphasis on the face reflect a lack of care about the rest of the body? Hardly, but facial problems are more obvious and therefore much harder to ignore. The face prominently displays all kinds of flaws, it is more exposed to the elements, and it has more oil glands and nerve endings than the rest of the body. Problems from the neck down are less conspicuous, more spread out, and far less disconcerting. They are not only easy to cover up, but they also tend to be less severe.

From the neck down, women worry about their weight, not the condition of their skin: excess pounds can't always be hidden under clothing. From the neck up, women worry and obsess about every blemish and line, seeking remedies for a myriad of woes with endless anti-wrinkle concoctions, cosmetic surgery procedures from facelifts to eye tucks, and an arsenal of makeup products. These extreme approaches leave the face cared for too much and the rest of the body cared for too little, at least when it comes to good, effective skin-care choices.

Hundreds of women tell me they would never tan their face, even though they happily brown and bake the rest of their body. Many think their legs and arms aren't subject to the same ruination when it comes to sun damage, but nothing could be further from the truth. Lots of women also don't care if their skin from the neck down wrinkles, but that is a mistake. Bodies that aren't protected from sun damage run the risk of developing thickened, yellowed, brown-spotted, lined, and crepey-looking skin, along with skin cancer. Many women who fly into a tizzy at the appearance of one blemish will ignore breakouts on their chest and legs, never thinking of applying the fighting basics for blemishes to any other part of the body but their face. But this is also a misguided notion. **Scarring and worsening breakouts can result from ignoring blemishes anywhere on the body.**

The number of products dedicated to bathing and body care is growing, but they tend to be aimed at pampering and indulging ourselves rather than addressing concerns about blemishes, wrinkles, sun damage, and exfoliation. A veritable deluge of moisturizers, cleansers, bath salts, exfoliants, bubble baths, hand creams, massage oils, and aromatherapy products in every aromatic combination imaginable promises to soften, scent, stimulate, smooth, and soothe your body. Occasionally some company puts out a laughable cellulite cream that promises to undimple dimpled thighs or an even more laughable bust cream that claims it can raise sagging breast tissue, but these products are far outnumbered by the horde of preparations offering more sensual pleasures.

There isn't a square inch of the body that has been neglected by the cosmetics industry. Large cosmetics companies, small cosmetics companies, prestigious lines, simple lines, and even businesses to whom body care is just a sideline, such as Victoria's Secret and The Gap—all want us to soak, scrub, and moisturize everything from dry skin to stress and emotional woes out of our lives with bath oils, bath salts, loofahs, body masks, fragrant moisturizers, and perfumes. And we love buying the stuff: bath and body-care products and fragrances account for more than 33% of all cosmetics sold!

One interesting wrinkle (no pun intended) is the number of body-care lines that include the word "spa" as part of their name. **Marketing finesse has given spa lines the aura of being authoritative and healthful when it comes to skin care, particularly from the neck down. This misperception can waste money and also cause skin problems.** Spa products are not the result of any particular enlightenment, nor are they specially formulated in any way. In fact, spa products sold at cosmetics counters and specialty spas are notoriously similar to the ones sold in drugstores. I think most women would be in shock if they knew how close to identical the formulations for various body washes, bath salts, body moisturizers, and bath oils really are. Plus, spa lines, like most body-care products, are highly fragranced, and fragrance is no better for the body than it is for the face.

Far be it from me to deny anyone the pleasure that can be derived from pampering, soothing body care. Taking care of the body should include relaxing in deliciously warm, fragrant, oiled, and/or salted water, rather than concentrating only on skin-care issues. But skin-care problems can occur all over the body, and they require more than sweetly scented bath salts and oils. Problems such as dry skin, blemishes, irritation, rashes, surfaced veins, cellulite (the dimpled appearance of fat on the thighs), rough elbows and knees, badly needed manicures and pedicures, and sun damage can affect the way we see ourselves as well as relay information about the health of our skin and nails. Sun damage is as serious an issue for the body as it is for the face; irritation can cause breakouts or dry, flaky skin anywhere on the body; and overmoisturizing can clog pores and prevent skin from exfoliating naturally, causing skin to look and feel dry and scaly. Overly fragrant, overly emollient, pore-clogging body-care products will only make matters worse.

Skin-care products designed for the body tend to be rather ordinary, with no specific directions as to which ones should or should not be used by particular skin types and why. I am going to provide you with a realistic program for paying attention to the body's skin-care needs, because the current approach doesn't necessarily lead to good, healthy skin.

The Joy of Bathing

I think it is appropriate to start with the luxurious, sensual side of body care, and there is no denying the relaxation one can derive from a quiet interlude in a serene, carefully prepared bath. By adding just a few cosmetic preparations to the tub (and locking the bathroom door), you can create a tranquil refuge right in your own home. And none of these products have to be expensive. In fact, the less expensive ones (like pure almond or sunflower oil, Epsom salts, or body moisturizers like Lubriderm, Eucerin Light, and Cetaphil Moisturizer) are preferred because they contain no fragrance. Where the body is concerned, fragrance can be a serious skin irritant. If you use fragranced oils and salts in the bath, the perfume component can be especially sensitizing for the vaginal area and other parts of the body as well.

But back to the indulgent part. Simply feeling beautiful and tranquil is the main goal of a leisurely bath. Imagine steamy water, drizzled with oils or foaming with rich bubbles, a scented candle flickering in the mirror (that way you don't need to put fragrance in the bathwater), and at least a half hour to an hour of spare time. Even the thought is gratifying. Later, when you're done soaking, after gently exfoliating your skin, shaving unwanted hair from your legs and underarms, and applying a moisturizer over your slightly damp, plumped skin, your body will feel silky in a way it doesn't after your usual morning ritual of shower and moisturizer.

Without trying to burst anyone's bubble, because my job is to tell you what I know to be true from the research I've done, I should mention that, as blissful as all this can be, the only benefits are psychological. Regularly soaking for long periods, especially in hot water—and that includes Jacuzzis—is not best for the long-term health of the skin. As I mentioned in Chapter Two, "What Works and What Doesn't," **oversaturating the skin with water can break down its immune/healing response and can actually make it drier.** The best approach is to keep the temperature of your bath water warm but not hot, and, if you bathe regularly, soak for no more than five to ten minutes. Occasionally it is fine to soak for longer periods of time, but make that the exception instead of the rule. Whether it's for five or ten minutes, or the infrequent 20- to 30-minute soak, the repose and quiet serenity of a bath can give you the time to feel the texture changes in your skin and to calm stressed-out, responsibility-weary nerves.

In short, bathing can be a grand sensual experience. And it is so easy to do. Turn on the tap; pour in the bubble bath (preferably fragrance-free), oil (fragrant bath oil if you prefer, but fragrance-free is best), and/or bath salts (again, fragrance-free is best); then lie back on a bath pillow with a few strategically placed candles and let the world float into oblivion. OK, so long soaks can be a bit damaging (the skin does get pruny and thick from water overload), but the skin will get over it if you don't do it regularly, and how often do you have the time to do this anyway?

What is the best way to go about this indulgent ritual? It is definitely easier and far less expensive if you use something other than the products lined up at the cosmetics counters and specialty salons, that's for sure.

Start running the bath using **water that's slightly hotter than normal**, but only slightly; water that is too hot can be hard on the skin and may cause problems over the long haul.

If you have normal to dry skin, **drizzle in some almond or sunflower oil** (but use only a teaspoon or two or you'll feel like you're soaking in an oil spill). You can use fragrant oils, but only if you don't have sensitive skin and aren't predisposed to allergies. If you have oily, blemish-prone skin from the neck down, oils of any kind are not the best idea, fragrant or otherwise.

Add a teaspoon of bubble bath or bath salts. As I mentioned above, these should preferably be fragrance-free to avoid irritation and breakouts. **Epsom salts are a great, incredibly inexpensive addition to any bath.**

If you chose bath items that are fragrance-free but still want to add fragrance to the bathwater, you can **sprinkle in a few drops of your favorite fragrance** for an overall aromatic experience (but only if your skin doesn't mind this addition to the water). Boutiques such as The Body Shop and Garden Botanika, and many health food stores, carry an array of fragrant extracts and oils you can use separately or in combination to create your own personal blends.

Rather than pouring fragrance into the bath, which can be irritating for the skin, you can **light a scented candle or two** (more than that and it will feel like church, despite what it looks like in the movies) and place them in strategic locations so the light can flicker on the water and in the mirror. You can also buy tiny oil lamps that help radiate fragrance throughout the room.

If you plan on giving yourself a manicure or pedicure after your bath, take the time now to **file your nails into the shape you want.** Filing nails when they are wet can damage them and cause splitting. If you plan on cutting your nails, wait until after you are done soaking, when they are softer and less likely to be damaged.

Turn down the lights or turn them off altogether and **bathe by candlelight.**

Enter the bath slowly, even gracefully, trying hard not to disturb the water or bubbles.

Prop a towel or bath pillow behind your head, and stretch out.

While you're soaking, take the time to **gently, and I mean gently, buff a washcloth or loofah over your body.** (Be careful with loofahs—they can be hard on most skin types and overuse can encourage the growth of dry, callused skin.)

You can **use a body cleanser or wash** alone or with the loofah (again, be very gentle on the skin when using a loofah) or washcloth. Don't use soap: it leaves a film on the tub, discolors the water, dries skin, and clogs pores.

If you have dry skin, use a **body wash that contains moisturizing agents.**

For obvious reasons, **save shaving your legs till the end**, when the water is going down the drain. Use shaving cream or your hair conditioner for the smoothest results. (Shaving the legs is much easier and causes far less irritation and fewer bumps if the legs have been soaked for at least two or three minutes, and preferably more. Also, sitting in water filled with used shaving cream is hardly luxurious.)

You may want to **shower off as your final step.** If you don't like the feeling of bath oils left on your feet, underarms, or genitals, this is the time to wash those areas again to remove the oil or bath salts from your skin.

When you're done, **exit as slowly as you entered.** This is still part of the ceremony, so keep the candles lit.

Dry your skin with a fresh **towel, dabbing your skin lightly.**

If you haven't used a body exfoliant in the bath, you can **use your towel to give your legs and arms a good rubdown.** But take it easy; hard rubbing can irritate the skin.

Applying a moisturizer over slightly damp skin is a nice way to get more water in the skin if you have very dry skin. (Do not apply moisturizer to areas of the body that tend to break out.)

If you didn't use a loofah or washcloth in the tub, you may want to **use an AHA product in a moisturizing base over your legs and arms, especially on your knees, elbows, and heels.** (I don't recommend pumice stones for the feet: the pressure and roughness can actually encourage the formation of calluses. AHAs work far better, more consistently, and more evenly than scrubbing can.) AHAs also come in gel form if your skin needs the exfoliation but not the moisturizing.

If you bathe in the morning it is essential to apply an effective sunscreen over those parts of the body that will be exposed to daylight.

Finally, **slip on something very soft**, like cotton leggings and a cotton top, or a silky robe, and enter the world slowly, refreshed and renewed. **Don't forget to blow out the candles.**

If you have the extra time, this is the perfect opportunity to **give yourself a pedicure and manicure.**

Body Basics

Here is a game plan you can use to pick body-care products that will work wonders for every part of you from the neck down. It means paying attention to many of the issues I've been discussing throughout this book.

Body Washes

Body cleansers, body washes, and body shampoos are just what they sound like—they use the detergent cleansing agents typically found in hair shampoos to clean the body—and they are excellent for all skin types. They tend to be less drying than bar soaps and cleansers, they leave no "bar" residue on the skin, and the chance of irritation or dryness is greatly reduced. (A moisturizing body wash can leave a slight film due to oils being left behind on the skin, but that's how these cleansers moisturize.) **Bar soaps and bar cleansers can be problematic for the body, just as they are for the face.** Body washes are just as effective as soaps are, without any of the problems soap can stir up.

Many body washes designed for dry skin claim all kinds of moisturizing properties. What they contain is simply some kind of oil. Vitamins, proteins, amino acids, and other fancy water-binding agents may be in there too, and while these ingredients can be good moisturizing agents, in a body wash they are just rinsed down the drain. Oils tend to stick around a bit longer and are not easily washed away, so they do provide some emollient benefit for dry skin. Personally, I don't feel quite as clean after using a moisturizing body wash. I prefer the gentle cleaning effect of a regular body wash, followed by a moisturizer applied after I get out of the shower, but the choice is up to you.

Body Scrubs

There are lots of ways to help get dead skin cells off the body. You can use anything from a washcloth to a loofah to a body cleanser with almond pits or bits of silica. The skin on the body can handle mechanical scrubbing a bit better than the skin on the face can, but only a bit. You still need to be gentle with this kind of physical scouring. If you're careful, scrubbing can be a good way to immediately exfoliate the skin, principally on elbows, heels, and knees. Exfoliating skin from the neck down provides the same benefits as it does from the neck up: it helps the skin to absorb moisturizer better, unclogs pores, and allows healthier skin cells to surface.

Loofahs have two major drawbacks you need to be aware of. Because they hang around in the shower and are often not cleaned or rotated with a new one, they are an optimum breeding ground for bacteria such as staphylococcus. **Overscrubbing or scrubbing over blemishes and cuts with an old loofah that**

has not been properly cleaned is unwise. Also, zealously scouring the skin with a loofah can actually encourage the growth of dry, callused skin. The pressure and the scrubbing kill more skin cells and can stimulate the growth of thickened skin. By the way, washcloths work just as well as loofahs, if not better, for exfoliating. Washcloths are easy to throw in the wash and tend to be less rough and less irritating on the skin.

Unequivocally and without exception, no amount of scrubbing or beating at the skin will change or eliminate one dimple on your thighs. The only benefits from exfoliation are those discussed earlier in this book and above, and that's it. You might feel that your thighs look better after you have scrubbed them and applied various lotions ands gels, but all these products do is temporarily swell the skin on the thighs, making them look momentarily smoother.

When it comes to cosmetic cleansing scrubs (tiny particles suspended in some type of cream base), good old-fashioned baking soda is still one of the best options for this kind of mechanical (though gentle) scrubbing, whether it be for the face or the body. Baking soda is a "pure" ingredient that, much like other mineral salts, can work as an anti-inflammatory agent. It doesn't contain any of the "creamy" ingredients that cosmetic scrubs do, so there's no risk of pores getting clogged, and it is astonishingly inexpensive.

Please keep in mind that all of these scrubs can prove way too irritating for some skin types. Be very careful about getting carried away and overdoing it. Scrubbing can tear skin down, not build it up. The idea is to get dead skin cells off, not rip off layers of skin. Actually, in many ways chemical exfoliation with an AHA product, Retin-A, or Renova is preferable and provides more long-term benefits.

AHAs, BHA, Retin-A, and Renova for the Body

Treatments for dry or sun-damaged skin on the face can also be used on the body. AHAs, BHA, Differin, Retin-A, Renova, and Azelaic Acid are all excellent choices for taking care of sun-damaged skin, dry skin, and areas that break out. AHAs, Retin-A, and Renova are superior options for parts of the body, such as the neck, chest, and arms, that have been exposed to the sun and are showing signs of sun damage. AHAs can also be excellent for reducing or eliminating roughness on elbows, knees, and heels, and for minimizing dry skin. (It is completely unnecessary and useless to use AHAs, Retin-A, or Renova on areas of the body that have no sun damage and are not dry.) In regard to application, follow the same course of action for the body as for the face. During the day, after cleansing, apply an AHA product in a moisturizing or gel base over dry skin, or Retin-A or Renova over sun-damaged areas. (If you use a gel-based

AHA product, you can use a moisturizer over dry areas afterward.) You should then apply a sunscreen over areas of the body that will be exposed to daylight.

BHA, Differin, or Retin-A can be used for areas of the body that are prone to breakouts. In regard to application, follow the same course of action for the body as for the face. After cleansing, disinfect areas of the body that have breakouts with any of the topical disinfectants mentioned in Chapter Six, "Special Battle Plans for Blemishes." Then apply BHA, Differin, Retin-A, or Azelaic Acid. It is extremely helpful to apply a moisturizer to dry skin, but do not use a moisturizer over any areas where you have breakouts. During the day, you should then apply a sunscreen over areas of the body that will be exposed to daylight.

Just one more reminder: If you are going outside, it is absolutely essential to wear an SPF 15 sunscreen in a moisturizing base that contains the sunscreen agents avobenzone, titanium dioxide, or zinc oxide. Apply it to any area of the body that will be exposed to the sun for any length of time, no matter how brief. Sunscreen can and should be worn over AHA gels, lotions, or creams as well as over Retin-A or Renova.

Bath Oils

Bath oil is one bath preparation I don't care for in the least. (I dislike feeling like an oil slick, although lots of women say they feel silky and soft after using it.) It can be a good treatment for dry skin, but this step is not for someone who has problems with breakouts on any part of the body.

Bath oils are primarily just that: oils derived from all sorts of sources, including sunflower, almond, coconut, and jojoba—a virtual plethora of plants and flowers. Some bath oils contain volatile (fragrant) oils with potential for causing allergic reactions. Some bath oils are formulated with slip agents (ingredients that help the oils move over the skin) as well as mineral oil (mineral oil can be more soothing for the skin and it poses little to no risk of irritation). Some even contain water-binding agents, which are hardly necessary because the skin will be water-laden regardless of their presence and their effect is washed down the drain.

If there is any distinction between oils, it has more to do with how greasy they feel and how much irritation they can cause rather than any healing benefits. **Plain mineral oil can be an excellent bath oil because it is fragrance-free, gentle and emollient, and unlikely to cause irritation or breakouts. However, it is also not absorbed by the skin.** Plant oils tend to be a bit more problematic in terms of clogging pores, but they are absorbed far better than mineral oil. Safflower, sesame, almond, avocado, jojoba, and even olive oil can add the slip and emollience needed by dry skin.

Bath Salts

Bath salts can be beneficial for many skin types. **Salts and minerals, regardless of their source, can soften water and, depending on the specific salts used, reduce inflammation and swelling. Epsom salts are probably the best-known type; they work quite well and are shockingly inexpensive.** Most of the salts added to bath products are just fine, although ingredients such as borax, sodium sesquicarbonate, sodium carbonate, and phosphate can cause irritation and probably should be avoided. Table salt and sea salt can also be a problem, because if they don't get rinsed off well they can pull water from the skin and cause dryness and irritation.

Many cosmetics lines, particularly spa lines, brag about how their products contain minerals from all kinds of sources: mineral springs in France, volcanic waters in Italy, Dead Sea salts from Israel, and on and on. The question is whether minerals and salts from exotic sources have any special effect on skin. The answer is no (see Chapter Two, "What Works and What Doesn't"). In the long run, Epsom salts are preferred for their skin-softening and anti-inflammatory properties, and because they pose a minimal risk to sensitive skin.

Body Masks

I hate the sensation of clay drying on my body, and most body masks are clay. Clay masks don't hurt the skin as long as they contain no irritating ingredients, but they can be quite drying for someone with dry skin. The only benefits they offer are some amount of exfoliation and oil absorption (particularly for areas that are oily). They don't detoxify the body and they definitely don't affect cellulite or improve circulation (only exercise can do that). Some women love masks and feel utterly pampered and silky smooth afterward. Me, I just feel icky and itchy all over. Besides, unless you have a helpful roommate or significant other, and a place to lie down that is OK to get messy (because this is one messy process), it is hard to use these products on your own with any finesse or comfort. Body masks are the centerpiece of most spa treatments, and while they won't make one bit of difference in the health of your skin, they can feel great when they are applied and washed off by someone else.

If you do tend to break out on your back and chest or if those areas are extremely oily, it is completely acceptable to use the same milk of magnesia mask recommended in Chapter Six for those areas too. Again, the back is a hard area to work with unless you have help, but this step can make a big difference in reducing breakouts and absorbing excess oil.

Plants in Your Bath

All those herbs, flowers, vegetables, fruits, and other botanical marvels found in bath products are essentially a waste, just as they are in products for the face. They won't hurt the skin, at least the ones that aren't irritating won't, but there isn't any evidence to support their claims about healing or firming or anything else. Essential plant oils (I'm still trying to find out what a nonessential oil is) are popular because they smell great and make any product sound more exotic, and, as I mentioned above, some plant oils can be excellent for dry skin, but aside from the emollient and moisturizing effect, they don't heal or reverse damage or render any other skin-care miracle, particularly in bathwater.

Aromatherapy?

Fragrance is one of the most important aspects of body care, at least to many consumers. Ironically, it is one of the least important for the health of the skin. For some people, fragrance can be as much a problem from the neck down as from the neck up. Although the body is generally less susceptible to allergic reactions than the face, that varies from person to person, and there can be a problem even if you don't feel a reaction. Yet, with the advent of aromatherapy, scent has taken on new prominence in the world of body care, and it can be difficult to avoid. Despite the risk to the skin, most body and bath products are highly fragranced, and things are getting worse, not better. While women are becoming more and more aware that fragranced skin-care products can cause problems for the face, they are nevertheless likely to purchase bath and body-care products because of their scent.

Can a particular scent or blend of scents provide special benefits for your skin or your emotions? When it comes to skin, fragrant oils are not helpful for any part of the face or body because they can cause irritation, skin sensitivities, rashes, inflammation, and allergic reactions. Fragrance is especially problematic for the genital area. As far as your emotions are concerned, only you can know for sure. **Make aromatherapy decisions based on fact rather than on what your nose is telling you. Don't be swayed by the inflated claims being made about aromatherapy, which range from renewed energy to euphoria.** Lots of women indeed feel less stressed out after indulging their senses with interesting fragrant blends, but they are also taking time out from their busy day while doing it. Does the fragrance or the time out cause the effect? That's hard to say. What is easy to say is that scent is better for the nose than it is for the skin.

Most people are greatly influenced by pleasing aromas, and almost everyone feels invigorated or supremely relaxed after a good long soak. (I know I do.) Because fragrance can play such a significant role in this experience, there is no reason not to partake. **I would encourage you to find other ways to please your olfactory sense than putting fragrant products in the bathwater or all over your skin.** Scented candles, plain candles drizzled with fragrant oils, and oil lamps (you can purchase the latter at most health food stores or specialty body-care shops) are a great way to fill the air with sublime scents and leave your skin unaffected.

By the way, many cosmetics boutiques are dedicated to helping you find just the right personalized scent. Everything in these stunning little shops is immaculate, with the accent on fragrance and aromatherapy. You may find a tiered bar with more than 50 extremely pretty bottles filled with exotic and standard fragrances, allowing the salesperson to custom-design an eau de toilette, lotion, or bath oil just for you. Scents such as Egyptian musk, mango, freesia, and gardenia mingle, filling these stores with an intoxicating aroma. Once inside, you may find it hard to leave without your own little mixture. But beware: the experience is more about seduction and olfactory enticement than it is about the health of your skin.

Perfume

Women the world over use perfume and have been doing so for eons. Smelling nice seems to be as much a human need as breathing, eating, and sleeping. When it comes to buying perfume or cosmetics, one of the first things a consumer does is smell the product. Why? Because a pleasing scent can make a woman feel confident, sensual, and happy. With all that, who cares if it helps the skin?

Buying perfume is an entirely sensory experience. Minute drops applied to the "warm" spots on the body—behind the ears; along the cleavage; inside the thigh; and on the pulse points on the wrist and neck, inside the elbow, and behind the knee—can provide all the radiating scent you need to attract someone's attention. Perfume is almost exclusively about love and sex, and not necessarily in that order.

Unless you've been visiting another planet for the last 30 years, you won't be surprised when I say that sex is used as a sales tool for almost every product from shoes to deodorant (if advertisers could figure a way to make the Pillsbury Doughboy into a sex symbol, they would do it to sell more biscuits), but only young sex. Images of older people (meaning over 30) being sexy aren't used to sell anything in this country. Perfume ads feature young, sultry, long-legged, breathless women; half-clothed, hard-bodied men; or both, in couples who can barely keep their hands, lips, or gaping eyes off each other.

Most of us throw logic out the door when confronted with the hope of increased desirability, and that's what sells perfume, because there is nothing utilitarian or professional about it. In short, perfume is a difficult subject for a consumer reporter because it defies logic, and it should. But let me throw in just a little information to help you in making a selection. Other than allergic reactions, there are no risks when it comes to wearing perfume. How much you like a scent and how it affects the people around you, specifically the people who get close to you, are all that count.

Speaking of the people around you, it is a complete mystery to me why some women feel a need to saturate themselves with a conspicuous amount of fragrance. The air around women who have generously anointed themselves with their favorite perfume or eau de toilette is so thick and pungent that their presence is announced by an overpowering hit of fragrance. This is definitely one of those beauty steps that can be overdone and lose its original purpose, which in this case is to exude a subtle scent for those you want to be close to. Perfume should not be so pungent an emission that it overwhelms strangers in an elevator or business associates around a conference table. In addition, an overpowering scent can trigger allergic reactions in others. I suspect many women put on extra fragrance in the morning to make it last longer. Yet it is simple enough to touch up fragrance as the day goes by, just as you would makeup. Most women who overdo their perfume would never apply 20 layers of makeup to make sure it stayed all day.

While we're on the subject, the endurance of a fragrance has nothing to do with natural ingredients versus synthetic ones or with how many products you apply. If anything, synthetic ingredients take the unreliability of plant extracts and oils out of the equation to create more stable products. Yet there is no way to know which ingredients are used in any perfume or eau de toilette because this is the sole area where the cosmetics industry doesn't have to reveal formulas. Consequently, fragrance recipes truly are secrets. I have been told by several master perfumers that most fragrances are created from a vast combination of fragrance components that are both natural and synthetic. The art of creating a nuanced, resplendent bouquet involves bringing together varying aromas in a cohesive, unified scent that pleases the olfactory sense. **The secrecy and complexity is why fragrance knock-offs, inexpensive imitations, just don't work.** Some perfumers have blended hundreds of flower oils, plant extracts, and synthetic scents to create one perfume. How can a formula that complex be duplicated? It can't, which is why a cheap version of the perfume you like won't make your nose happy.

Without ingredient lists to turn to, there are only two ways to determine how long a fragrance will last on your body: product type and testing. In terms of product type, you can count on cologne (which is about 1% to 3% fragrance) and eau de cologne (about 3% to 5% fragrance) lasting two to three hours; eau de toilette (about 5% to 7% fragrance) lasting two to four hours; eau de parfum (about 12% to 18% fragrance) lasting four to six hours; and perfume (about 15% to 30% fragrance) lasting six to eight hours or more. Consider purchasing perfume (which is oil-based) instead of cologne or eau de toilette (water- and alcohol-based) if longevity is an issue for you. Perfume is more expensive, but it does have a better potential for lasting the whole day because the oil and the fragrance concentration cling better to skin, so it tends not to wear off as easily as alcohol- and water-based fragrances.

Testing is the next step. Body chemistry can greatly affect any fragrance a person applies; how long any fragrance, regardless of type, will last or how well it will retain its scent during the day is anyone's guess. A fragrance can smell different at the beginning of the day than it does by the end. Trying on a fragrance (only one at time) is the best way to determine how well it endures and which one you prefer. Do not choose a fragrance based on the way it smells in the bottle or on a card, because that is not usually representative of what it will be like on your skin.

Should you buy body products that all have the same fragrance? As you already know by now, I would rather you *not* apply scented skin-care products of any kind all over the body. It is best if your fragrance comes from a perfume or cologne applied to the inside part of your elbow, knee, neck, and cleavage. That's plenty. You do *not* need an additional bath product, powder, body cream, perfume, or cologne to make a fragrance stick around longer; that's fragrance overkill. But to answer the question, clashing fragrances can end up smelling unpleasant, or at least not the way you want.

One more point of interest: the most expensive part of any fragrance is the bottle (about 40% of the cost), the advertising (another 30% of the cost), and the celebrity endorsement or designer insignia (another 10% to 15% of the cost). That leaves about 15% to 20% actual fragrance cost. Now that stinks.

The Smoothest Legs in the World

One of the best-kept beauty secrets women have is what they hide under pants and dark nylons: namely, unshaven legs. If you're running late in the morning during the winter, it doesn't matter in the least because if you don't get a chance to shave no one knows except you and possibly your significant other.

Shaving legs isn't a lot of fun and it's time consuming. Most women barely get out the door on time with their teeth brushed, their kids off to school, and their makeup on straight before they commute to the office, so shaving is a luxury that gets put on the bottom of the to-do list. But when the long, cold days of winter are a memory and the shorts and no-nylons time of year begins, there is no more hiding. Women, bring out your razors.

Several lines of cosmetic products are dedicated to the art of shaving. A brochure for one of these lines says a perfect shave requires an understanding of the fundamental principles of wet shaving and the use of five easy products (theirs, of course). But what's easy about applying five of anything to the skin? Shaving should take no more than four steps (getting the legs wet, applying shaving cream, shaving, and rinsing) and two shaving products (the razor and a shaving cream or gel), followed by moisturizer.

There is no real trick to shaving. We all know how to do it, but not everyone knows how to get the best results and the softest legs. The following tips are the basics of a great, smooth shave.

It is essential for your legs to be wet for at least two or three minutes, or longer, before starting. Nothing is as irritating or chafing as shaving dry, unsoaked legs.

Finding a razor that works well for your skin, given the pressure you use while shaving, the texture of your skin, and the density of hair growth, takes some experimentation. No one type of shaver works well for everyone. Personally, I have a tendency to nick and slice myself when shaving, and finding a razor that doesn't let this happen every time I shave my legs took a while. I found disposable razors to be excellent for me, and foolproof, but many women prefer standard razors with replaceable blades.

When it comes to shaving creams, for both men and women, those that contain emollients (usually those identified as being good for sensitive, dry skin) work perfectly on the legs! There is absolutely no reason to buy shaving gels or creams in pretty pink containers when in truth they are virtually identical to those in more masculine or unadorned packages.

Avoid shaving products that contain irritants. Used over newly shaved skin, irritating ingredients can cause red bumps and ingrown hairs. When I find myself without shaving cream in the shower, I use hair conditioner or a body wash instead, which is far easier on the legs than bar soap or bar cleanser.

For best results, shave against the growth of hair and be careful.

After you are done, do not use a loofah or washcloth. They can cause irritation and create problems.

Once you are out of the shower or bath, dab your legs dry gently.

Apply a moisturizer over slightly damp skin. Do not use an AHA product over newly shaven skin; it can be unnecessarily irritating.

During the day, if you are going out bare-legged, use an SPF 15 sunscreen with avobenzone, titanium dioxide, and/or zinc oxide.

Preventing Red Bumps

As many women know, in addition to the occasional nicks and cuts incurred during shaving, it isn't unusual to also have an aftermath of uncomfortable and unattractive razor bumps (red, inflamed blemishes), particularly along the bikini line. Hair follicles are attached to oil glands, and both are attached to nerve endings. Shaving can easily irritate the skin, the hair follicle, and the oil gland, causing a rashlike breakout of annoying bumps. Ingrown hairs can also be a dilemma. Ingrown hairs are curly, wiry hairs that curl and dig into the adjacent skin as they grow out or hairs that grow back in the wrong direction, causing a bump that can become infected.

As widespread a beauty problem as this can be, for women and men alike, the lack of products addressing the issue is surprising. The only product I know of that is specifically aimed at reducing or preventing these red bumps is called **Tend Skin** *($50 for 16 ounces).* It contains isopropyl alcohol (70%), propylene glycol, acetylsalicylate, and glycerin. This is a very interesting formulation that is ridiculously overpriced, and the alcohol part of it is self-defeating! Alcohol causes irritation and redness, the very problems this product is supposed to address. How absurd! As it turns out, Tend Skin is nothing more than aspirin (that's what acetylsalicylate is) suspended in alcohol with a slip agent (glycerin). Aspirin is an anti-inflammatory, and a very effective one at that. The notion that you can put it on your skin to reduce irritation is intriguing and completely worth trying. However, the $50 is best kept in your pocket because there is no reason why you can't put this concoction together yourself with a small bottle, one or two aspirins, a quarter cup of tap or distilled water, and perhaps a touch of glycerin (which can be purchased at a drugstore; just ask your pharmacist). The drawback to creating this yourself is guessing at the proportions, but with a little experimenting you should be able to produce an interesting toner for ingrown hairs and for areas that get inflamed after shaving, including the face (for men), bikini line, legs, and underarms. You can apply your moisturizer after the aspirin solution is absorbed into the skin.

If you find the bumps do not respond well to the aspirin, try an over-the-counter cortisone cream to reduce the redness and irritation. However, if the bumps get infected you will need to disinfect them with an over-the-counter antibiotic like Neosporin, Polysporin, or Bacitracin. All three are excellent for quick relief from a small topical infection.

What Are All Those Bumps on My Arms and Legs?

Some people have a troublesome inherited skin problem called keratosis pilaris. This is the technical name for a condition in which hundreds of hard, clogged pores cover a person's shoulders, upper arms, buttocks, and upper thighs. It can seem to be a persistent case of acne, but these lesions never become inflamed and never come to a head. They only become inflamed if you pick at them. On darker skin the plugs can look like a sea of blackheads. What to do?

Just like acne, this problem can be cured only with Accutane (see Chapter Six for more information about Accutane and its risks), but there are ways to minimize it. Gentle cleansing, exfoliating, and disinfecting can make a huge reduction in the number of bumps. First, wash and exfoliate the area with a soft loofah (you must keep it scrupulously clean and use it gently), a washcloth, or baking soda. If you are using a washcloth or loofah, use a body wash that does not contain moisturizing ingredients or irritants. It is best to avoid bar soap or bar cleansers of any kind because the ingredients that maintain the bar shape can clog pores. Do not overscrub. You can't rip these bumps off, and inflaming the area will only make matters worse.

After bathing, dry the area gently. Using a cotton ball, apply a topical disinfectant such as 3% hydrogen peroxide, 2.5% benzoyl peroxide, 5% benzoyl peroxide, or one prescribed by a physician over the problem area. When that has dried, you can apply an AHA gel or BHA gel or lotion to the area (a properly formulated BHA product—see Chapter Two, "What Works and What Doesn't"—is probably the best one to start with because of BHA's ability to get through the sebum causing these bumps). Do not apply moisturizer to these areas; it can make clogging worse. It is essential to use sunscreen over these areas if they will be exposed to sun during the day, but be aware that sunscreen ingredients can also make matters worse.

Seriously Dry Hands

Struggling with dry hands can be painful. Even if you are diligent about keeping them protected when doing housework or gardening, and unfailingly apply moisturizer whenever the opportunity arises, you can still suffer from bone-dry, cracked, parched hands. Clearly, it is essential to protect your hands from dish detergent, laundry detergent, excessive washing (medical professionals have a rough time with this one), and irritating ingredients, and also when doing potentially irritating manual work. Wearing gloves to prevent contact with these types of products and ingredients is of the utmost importance. However, a significant number of women may be allergic to latex gloves. About 10% of the population has negative reactions ranging from mild to severe if they come in contact with latex. If this turns out to be a problem, ask your physician or pharmacist where you can find nonlatex gloves.

The more emollient the moisturizer, the faster you get it on your hands after washing, and the longer you can keep it on, the better. It helps to keep small tubes or bottles of emollient moisturizer all over the house, including near the kitchen sink, in the bathroom, at the bedside, and in the garage. Keep more in your car, purse, briefcase, and desk drawer. That way it is never out of reach for a quick application. The best moisturizers for daytime are any moisturizing sunscreen whose active sun-blocking ingredient is titanium dioxide or zinc oxide. Titanium dioxide and zinc oxide provide an occlusive barrier that can act as a protective layer to retain moisture in the skin while keeping the sun's rays off the skin. (Bear in mind that brown sun spots on the back of hands and arms are a direct result of relentless, daily, unprotected sun exposure.)

Moisturizers such as Palmer's Cocoa Butter Formula, Eucerin Light, Jergens Advanced Therapy Lotion, and countless others are all excellent for use at night. The notion is to apply moisturizer every chance you get. It is also incredibly helpful to purchase an over-the-counter cortisone cream such as Lanacort or Cortaid to help treat cracks and fissures that may occur.

Body Itches

If you find that every time you shower, your entire body begins to itch and the problem lasts for a brief span of time or longer, you may have an allergy to the bath or hair-care products you are using. It will take experimentation to find out exactly what the culprit is, but the best strategy is switching to products that have no fragrance whatsoever. However, you may also want to check out the possibility that the laundry detergent or fabric softener you use for your clothes or linens may be the real offender. Fabric softener sheets pose an interesting chemical problem. These sheets are heat activated in the dryer. When you shower and towel dry, a little of the fabric softener residue comes off on your skin. Then, the next time you take a hot shower, the residue is heat activated on your skin, causing the itching. The itching stops after about 20 or 30 minutes, as your body cools down again. Laundry detergent can also be a problem. Using laundry detergents that have less potential for causing skin irritation, such as Cheer Free, All Free & Clear, Arm & Hammer Free, or Tide Free, can make a huge difference. Sleeping on pillowcases and sheets that have detergent or fabric softener residue can be a serious problem when you have dry, sensitive, or acne-prone skin.

Hot water and showering can also cause problems for sensitive skin and can stimulate itching. I have advocated the use of tepid water for some time, particularly for the face, and it can make a difference for the neck down if itching and rashes are an issue.

Another source of body itches can be the extremely irritating and drying salts that get deposited on the skin when you sweat. Instead of washing with bar cleansers or soaps, consider using a fragrance-free body wash. You will also want to avoid scrubs, loofahs, washcloths, bubble baths, and bath salts, all of which can trigger itchy skin.

Tight clothing such as jeans, nylons, tights, and leggings can also stimulate itching. The only way to prevent that situation is to loosen things up or do without. Nylons may be hard to give up, but for those with itchy thighs, wearing pants and cotton socks may be the only way to solve the problem.

Hard as Nails

While some women have naturally great nails, others search endlessly for anything that will help make their nails strong, thick (but not too thick), and long (sometimes too long). Sadly, you can't fool Mother Nature. What is genetically predetermined cannot be permanently transformed. If you are lucky enough to have strong, fast-growing, perfectly shaped nails with smooth, even cuticles, only trauma and damage to the nail bed will change the health and appearance of your nails. If you have naturally brittle, soft nails and thick cuticles, there is no way to alter what you've inherited. There is a lot you can do to make your nails look and feel better, and there is a lot you can do to make matters worse, but changing the way your nails naturally grow is as impossible as changing the way your hair grows.

I know there are dozens of nail products made by everyone from Revlon and Sally Hansen to Barielle, Orly, and Cutex, plus new ones being introduced monthly, all claiming they can repair the irreparable. Don't any of them work? If they did, we'd all have long, beautiful nails. Yet millions of women have struggled with weak, brittle, soft nails, trying an endless assortment of strengthening, lengthening, and body-building nail products, only to give up in frustration. It is almost impossible for a woman who wants to improve the appearance of her short, fragile nails not to wonder about all of the products that claim to feed the nails, engorge them with vitamins, or build them up from the outside in. **I would love to say those claims are legitimate and tell you which ones perform the best, but all the claims are bogus; changing the growth of the nail can't be done cosmetically, and there is no research anywhere proving that vitamin supplements can change the way the nails grow either.**

Physiologically speaking, the nail is simply a protective covering composed of dead cells filled with a thick protein called keratin, quite similar in essence to the hair. While the part of the nail you can see is dead, the matrix (the part of the nail under the skin) is very much alive. The white crescent area of the nail is called the lunula and is part of the matrix. The nail grows out from the matrix. As the growth of new cells builds up and dies it is pushed forward and out toward the surface. The cuticle is the protective layer of skin between the outside environment and the matrix. Keeping the cuticle intact is perhaps the single most important element in preserving the health of the nail.

Despite the nail's basic attributes. several long-standing myths about getting the talons of your dreams make the coffee-klatch rounds every now and then. Perhaps you've heard some of these nail delusions before, such as the idea that tapping your nails on a hard surface will help them grow and make them stronger. That isn't true in the least. You can't strengthen the nail by exercising it, assuming the nail needs the same training as a muscle. If anything, tapping will do just the opposite of what you want. Repetitive pressure or strain on the nail will lead to breakage and splitting. Another inane nail fiction is the notion that eating gelatin makes nails healthier. Gelatin probably got its reputation as a nail builder because of its relationship to protein. Like your nails and your hair, gelatin contains protein, but no form of food goes directly to the nail or hair to help it grow. There are no studies or data demonstrating that eating gelatin will improve the condition of anything. Eating a balanced, low-fat, nutritious (meaning lots of fresh fruits, vegetables, and whole grains) diet is certainly an important factor in overall good health, but feeding the nail directly isn't feasible. Perhaps the last piece of nail improbability is the belief that applying calcium to your nails will make them strong. Calcium, along with lots of other vitamins and minerals, shows up in many nail-care products because of an assumption that you can feed the nail from the outside in. **You can't feed the nail directly, though even if you could, calcium and other minerals are unlikely ingredients for this purpose. Calcium and minerals may help build strong bones (bones are primarily calcium), but they cannot build strong nails. There is virtually no calcium in nails; they're made of keratin and that's about it.**

Cuticle Care

While trying to affect the matrix and change the inherent growth of the nail with nail-care products is a waste of time and money, there are many things you can do to improve your nails. Without question the most important element to pay attention to is the skin around the nail, namely the cuticle. **The best way to keep your nails healthy, whole, and as free from problems as possible is to keep your cuticles intact.** Aside from inherited problems and physical trauma (getting smashed by a hammer or door can permanently alter the physical attributes of the nail), damage from manipulating or cutting the cuticle is the number-one cause of nail problems. I know this may seem shocking and contrary to much of what you've heard, but pushing back the cuticle and cutting it off is a huge no-no. Simply put, there is no way to remove a cuticle without hurting the nail. **Any kind of cuticle prodding may impart a shapely appearance, but it destroys the integrity of the matrix, which is the source of healthy nail growth. There is no way around this one. The cuticle is the body's form of protection for the area between the exposed, dead part of the nail and the living matrix the nail grows from. Anything that tampers with this seal puts the nail at risk.**

Pushing on the cuticle can result in weak, brittle, ridged, dented, peeling, or unevenly growing nails (where one part of the same nail grows at a different rate); once these problems occur, they won't go away until the nail grows out, and that can take anywhere from three months to a year. Orange sticks and metal cuticle tools, even when padded with cotton on the tip, even when you think you are using them gently, can cause damage to the nail. Almost every dermatologist I interviewed agreed that cuticle damage negatively affects nail growth. You can test this for yourself. Stop manipulating, pushing, or cutting your cuticles. Then, for the next six months, simply take care of your nail shape (I'll explain more about that later in this section) and only minimally trim hangnails or excess skin around the nail. Do not move or force the cuticle in any manner whatsoever. Within a relatively short period of time you are likely to see a radical change in the growth of the nail. I know this is a hard one to get used to. It was for me. Even, well-trimmed cuticles that don't grow up on the nail are definitely more attractive, but the improvement in the strength of the nail is worth the trade-off.

Another thing you can do for the cuticle is to moisturize it as often as possible, and during the day be sure you use a moisturizing sunscreen with avobenzone, titanium dioxide, or zinc oxide. It doesn't have to be a special nail or hand moisturizer with sunscreen; as long as the SPF is 15 and the active ingredients are the ones I've been mentioning, it will do just fine. If the cuticle becomes dry and flaky, or sun damaged, the protective barrier for the matrix will break down, which can absolutely and quickly hurt nail growth. In some ways it is almost impossible to keep the cuticle moist and healthy. Think about how often you wash your hands and use them every day for everything from office work to housework to sports. Also, the hands are incessantly exposed to the sun and it is difficult to keep them constantly protected with sunscreen. Yet doing so is essential. **In short, don't push back your cuticles, keep them protected from the sun, and use a moisturizer to prevent dryness.**

Manicures—Keep It Simple

While leaving the cuticle alone is the best thing you can do for the growth of the nail, leaving the length of the nail alone is also a wise part of nail care. The part of the nail that extends past the quick is long dead and vulnerable to damage. Overfiling can tear at the nail's structure, and that can never be replaced. Once filing tears or starts lifting the fibrous nail material, it can begin a cycle that is hard to stop. Nails are softened by water, and soft nails are more susceptible to damage and tears. Shape the nails only when they are completely dry. It is also essential to avoid metal or extremely coarse nail files. Use the gentlest file with extremely gentle pressure to achieve the shape you want. You'll use up more nail files than before, but the result will be stronger nails. You've probably heard the one about filing in one direction only. That is completely unnecessary. Regardless of the direction you file, if you don't do it gently you will damage the nail.

When you do take the time to indulge in a full manicure, it is essential to **keep it simple.**

First, remove any previously applied nail polish. **It doesn't matter whether you use a nail polish remover that contains acetone. It also doesn't matter whether the nail polish remover contains moisturizing ingredients. If a nail polish remover can remove nail polish it is going to be harsh stuff, but that is the price of nicely painted nails.** Use as little nail polish remover as necessary to remove the polish. Never soak the nail in nail polish remover. Minimal contact with nail polish remover is crucial for the well-being of the nail and cuticle. Nail polish remover is extremely drying and damaging to the entire nail, especially the cuticle.

Gently file the nails into the shape you want, using the least abrasive emery board you can find. **Don't create long talons or severe squares; these draw too much attention to the nails.**

Softening the cuticle around the nail is needed only if you plan to remove excess skin and cut the nail. Soak the nails in plain warm water for no more than three minutes. **Oversoaking hurts the nail and the cuticle. Avoid soapy or detergent-filled water, which only dries out the skin and damages the cuticle.** If the hands or feet are dirty, wash them first and that's it. Minimal contact with cleansers is best for every part of your body, including the nails!

Trim the cuticle and avoid pushing it back as much as possible, being exceedingly careful not to pull, lift, tear, rip, force, or cut into the cuticle in any way.

Trim nails carefully, using sharp manicure scissors or nail clippers. Nails are definitely easier to trim after bathing or soaking. Fingernails should be given a slightly rounded edge to protect the nail growth; toenails should be trimmed straight across, slightly above the quick. Avoid cutting nails too short to reduce the chance of developing ingrown toenails.

Moisturize the cuticle with an emollient moisturizer. Almost any moisturizer for dry skin will do. It is unnecessary to purchase special cuticle creams: they contain absolutely nothing special for the nail or cuticle.

Before you polish your nails it is essential to remove the moisturizer from them. **Moisturizing ingredients prevent nail polish from adhering to the nail.** Use nail polish remover just over the nail's surface to take off any moisturizer. Avoid getting nail polish remover on the cuticle; that's the area you want to keep the moisturizer on.

Polish your nails in layers, allowing them to dry between coats. A minimum of three coats is standard. **If you have weak or brittle nails, place one or two coats of ridge-filling nail polish on the nail as the base coat.** This is the best way to shore up the nail. Two coats of a colored nail polish are next, followed by a top coat to add shine and luster.

Allow plenty of time for the polish to dry. Quick-dry polishes and some quick-dry top coats of polish often contain alcohol, which can cause the polish to peel and chip more easily, so you will want to avoid those. Using a quick-dry oil or spray after you're done polishing is a great way to ward off smudges, but they won't prevent nicks or dents in the polish, so be careful.

Do not dry your nails with a blow dryer or any other heat source. Heat causes the polish to expand and lift away from the nail.

Touching up polish every other day with a layer of top coat can help make a manicure last longer. Carry a bottle of top coat in your purse, and when you have a moment or a break in your day, quickly do a once-over. A single layer dries quickly and makes all the difference in keeping up appearances.

Nail Polish That Lasts

After spending way too much money on nail-care products and nail polishes, many women complain that for this kind of money their nails should be ten times stronger and the polish should last ten times longer, but that isn't the case. Price has no relation to how long a nail polish will last. Nail polishes are produced by only a handful of manufacturers, so there are no secrets, and the formulations vary only slightly because only a handful of ingredients can stay on the nail.

Lots of women complain that if they want their nails to look good it takes practically a full-time effort, and they can't live life like a normal person. I myself have gone around walking like a surgeon to be sure my nails didn't come in contact with any surface anywhere. Though it doesn't take money to improve the appearance of your nails, it does take diligence and care. Those two things can't be avoided. Unfortunately, some polishes do tend to chip more than others (this is determined by formulation, not cost). I wish I could offer some insight into which formulations work best, but no matter how many surveys I do or how many cosmetic chemists I interview, there is no consensus as to which products stay better. More often than not, polish longevity has to do with the process of applying the layers in the right order, including base coat (preferably a ridge-filler-type product), color, and top coat; applying layers that are thick enough but not too thick; leaving plenty of time for drying; and then treating your nails carefully (wearing gloves, avoiding water, having minimal contact with soaps or cleansers, and not using the nails as tools).

Polishes are often given names like SuperWeave Base Coat, Color Lock No-Chip Sealer, Strong Wear Nail Strengthener Polish, Extra Life Top Coat, Nail Building Base Coat, Color Shield, Fortifier Hydrating Base, and Nail Protector. They are all great names that promise great things they can't even begin to deliver. Take **Markron's Five Minute Nail Miracle**, for example. This product isn't even a minor miracle. It contains standard nail polish ingredients and tiny amounts of protein and amino acids, as well as formaldehyde. Nails are dead, and all the protein and amino acids in the world won't help. Formaldehyde can toughen nails, but it can also seriously dry them out and damage the cuticle. What kind of miracle is that?

I wish I could find a line of nail polishes that last, but it doesn't exist. So many factors affect how well your nail polish holds up: Do you wear gloves when you clean? What kind of daily work do you do with your hands? Are your nails oil- and cream-free before you start polishing? I also get frustrated trying to separate one nail product from another because they have so much in common. The resins, lacquers, and basic products are all essentially the same. Most women experience about the same amount of wear from product to product: about one to three days. All nail polishes begin to chip on the third to fourth day after application, regardless of the claim on the label (but you already knew that, didn't you?). Reapplying your top coat daily and avoiding fast-drying nail polishes will increase the chances of getting your polish to last. Finding the discipline to do that isn't easy, but it is the cheapest and most reliable way to make a manicure stick around until the end of the week.

By the way, it is completely unnecessary and actually a bad idea to store nail polish in the refrigerator. Condensation and cold negatively affect nail polish, making it too thick to use reliably.

Fake Nails

Fake nails of any kind, whether they are painted on with a paste that is left to dry or glued on, are another problem for nails. Acrylic nails contain chemicals that can cause allergic reactions, damage the nails, and encourage fungal infections that can turn the bed of the nail green. Acrylic nails prevent proper ventilation of the nail, allowing fungi and bacteria to grow. Because fungi and bacteria are already present on the skin naturally, and because no matter how well you clean the nail, they can reappear in seconds, picked up from the rest of the body or from the air, very little can be done to prevent contamination. Acrylic nails provide a hothouse for microbial growth; once these nasty bugs are trapped underneath the dried cast, they continue growing. There is also some evidence that the ingredients in acrylic nails can penetrate the nail's matrix. The side effects of that are not known, but penetration into the living part of the nail is probably not a good thing.

Those are a lot of strikes against this time-consuming, expensive, and, I hope, passé fashion trend. My strong suggestion is to give up on fake nails. Shorter nails are not only in, but more practical and, in my opinion, more attractive. Fake nails, no matter how well done, always look fake, and when you lose or break one, and you usually do, you have to wait until you can get an appointment with the manicurist to get it fixed. Let me emphasize the foolishness of this process in regard to the outrageous monthly expense (and don't forget the amount of time it takes). Even if you can get your nails done at a bargain rate (say, $25 a visit), when you include the occasional broken nail repair, we are talking well over $500 a year! I know acrylic nails keep the polish in place longer, but there are other options for a long-lasting manicure without any of the potential risks or expense.

While I know lots of manicurists will bristle at my comments about fake nails, let me mention that my comments are supported by countless dermatologists and cosmetic chemists in various articles and research papers. My critique of these products is hardly the first one of its kind, just the first one many of you may have read. A manicurist can mix the ingredients in acrylic nails in any proportion she likes, and the risk to the nail stays the same. Acrylic ingredients by their very nature are potential allergens. Not only are the fake nail formulations a problem, but the process the nail has to go through to get the acrylic to stick to the nail—the sanding, buffing, and drilling—is extremely damaging to the cuticle and nail.

Yes, there are indeed fake nails that don't look all that fake, but come on—for the most part, you can always tell when someone has fake nails. Many women and the manicurists who serve them may consider fake nails a continuing fashion trend, but this is one of those rare areas where the fashion magazines and I agree. Long fake nails have been out for a long time, and I have heard that from several nail artists who specialize in fashion photography for magazines. (One appeared with me on *The Oprah Winfrey Show* and told everyone the same thing on national television.)

While acrylic nails are one issue, glue-on nails are another kettle of fish altogether. These preposterous little imposters look entirely fake, they have incredibly poor staying power, and the glue is damaging to the nail and cuticle. Thankfully, most women don't use glue-on nails.

Nail Strengtheners

If only nail-strengthening products really existed. What I wouldn't give to find one, and I've tried them all! As it turns out, many of the products that claim to strengthen nails contain extremely drying ingredients such as formaldehyde or toluene, which toughen the nail temporarily but also make it more brittle. Formaldehyde goes by other names on ingredient lists, so watch out for names like toluene, toluene sulfonamide, and toluene sulfonic acid. Toluene and toluenelike ingredients are illegal in the state of California because of serious health risks, including cancer and respiratory problems.

Some formaldehyde-free nail strengtheners just coat the nail, like the ridge-filling products. So-called strengthening creams contain thick waxy ingredients, like lanolin, that smooth over the nail and are hard to wash off. If you are good about reapplying these several times a day (sans polish, of course, because they can't penetrate polish), you might just see a change in your nails because they help to protect the cuticle and prevent the nail from drying out, but it takes discipline. Keep in mind that you can't wear polish over any kind of moisturizing product because polish won't adhere to a moist, lubricated surface. You can apply these products over polish; they won't help the nail, although they can moisturize the cuticle.

Nail Do's and Don'ts

Surprisingly, there are more don'ts than do's when it comes to taking care of your nails. Most dermatologists will tell you that what you don't do to your nails is far more important than what you do to them when healthy, strong nails are what you want. This list summarizes some of the things I've mentioned above, but they bear repeating given the amount of deceptive nail information and nail products being sold and advertised all over the cosmetics world.

Do coat the outside of the nails with nail polish or ridge fillers, which can help protect the nail and prevent breaking and splitting, at least while the manicure lasts.

Do moisturize the cuticle area to prevent cracking and peeling, which can hurt the matrix.

Do wear gloves to protect nails and cuticles from housework, gardening, and doing dishes.

Do be cautious when doing office work. Nails and cuticles can take a beating from filing, opening letters (use a letter opener), typing (use the flat of your finger pads on the keyboard instead of the tips of your nails), and handling papers.

Do apply a hand cream frequently *before* and immediately after you're done washing your hands, and pay attention to the cuticle area.

Do wear a sunscreen during the day on the hands and cuticles to prevent sun damage, which can hurt the nail.

Do meticulously clean all nail implements and change nail files often. Bacteria and other microbes can get transferred by the nail tools you use, causing infection or harm to the matrix.

Do use quick-dry oils or sprays to help nail polish set faster. These products are all just forms of silicone, mineral, or plant oil. You can treat your nails with hair serum that contains pure silicone oil for a fraction of the price.

Do disinfect any tears or cuts to the cuticle, and treat ingrown nails as soon as possible. Nail infections not only are unsightly but can cause long-lasting damage to the nail. Any drugstore antibacterial ointment, such as Polysporin, Neosporin, or Bacitracin, will do.

Don't use nail products that contain formaldehyde or toluene. They pose health risks for the nail and for your entire body as well.

Don't use fingernails as tools to pry things open.

Don't use your fingers as letter openers; that destroys the cuticles, which in turn destroys the nail matrix and and affects nail growth and strength.

Don't soak nails for long periods, and never use any kind of soap or detergent when soaking. Nails and cuticles that become engorged with water weaken, and the longer soap or detergent is in contact with skin and nails (despite the advertisements for Palmolive dish detergent), the greater the potential for damaging the nail and cuticle structure.

Don't overuse any kind of nail polish remover. Use a minimal amount on the nail and avoid getting too much on the cuticle and skin.

Don't push back the cuticle. Leave the cuticle alone as much as possible. Trim only the part of the cuticle that has started to lift away from the nail.

Don't allow any manicurist to touch your hands with utensils that have not been properly sterilized. The importance of this cannot be stressed enough. Risking your health and well-being for a manicure is just not worth it, and that is a definite possibility with bacteria-laden nail instruments!

Don't use nail treatment oils or creams. These are nothing more than moisturizers; they are fine, but nothing unique or of special benefit to the nails or cuticles. Any oil or moisturizer will help your nails and cuticles.

Don't pull or tear at hangnails. Always gently cut them away, leaving the cuticle as intact and untampered with as possible.

Don't ignore nail or cuticle inflammation. Disinfect the skin as soon as you can with an antibacterial or antifungal agent. Any change to the nails' appearance (see the next section) needs to be checked out by a dermatologist.

When the Nail Gets Sick

There are times when nail care requires a dermatologist. Fingernails and toenails are extremely vulnerable to infection and damage. If you have been diligent about leaving your cuticles alone and avoiding all the don'ts and performing most of the do's in the list above and you are still having nail problems, making an appointment with your dermatologist is the next step. Nails that are brittle, discolored, dull, abnormally thick, distorted, crumbling, loose, or subject to unusual debris under the nail are a medical problem as opposed to a cosmetic one.

It is quite normal for the skin to host a variety of microorganisms, including bacteria and fungi. Some are useful to the body. Others can multiply rapidly and lead to infections. Fungal infections are caused by microscopic plants (fungi) that thrive on the dead tissue of the nails and outer skin layers, particularly the cuticle.

Fungal nail infections are most often seen in adults, can be difficult to treat, and often recur. Toenails are affected more often than fingernails. People who frequent public swimming pools, gyms, or shower rooms; people who perspire a great deal; and people who wear tight, occlusive shoes are most likely to develop toenail infections because the fungi flourish in warm, moist areas. Prolonged exposure to moistness on the skin, minor nail injuries, and damage to the cuticle area can also increase susceptibility to fungal infection. Please be aware that fungal and bacterial infections are extremely contagious and can be spread through direct contact with another person who has the problem or through contact with contaminated towels, shower and pool surfaces, and nail implements such as cuticle clippers, nail clippers, orange sticks, and cuticle pushers.

Nail infections can be cleared with the persistent use of a prescription antifungal or antibacterial cream or lotion. Because nails grow slowly, treatment must be continued for 3 to 6 months for fingernails and 6 to 12 months for toenails (the time it takes to grow a new nail). There are oral medications for these problems, but they are best discussed with your doctor.

In terms of preventing problems for the feet, it is essential to keep them clean and dry. Change shoes and socks frequently. Dry the feet and hands thoroughly after bathing. Powders such as baby powder or talcum may help to keep the feet dry. Of course, avoiding damage to toenails and fingernails is of utmost importance.

To minimize the risk of damage to the nails, keep them smooth and properly trimmed. Trim the fingernails weekly. The toenails grow more slowly and may be trimmed as needed, about once a month. Nail polish remover of any kind can weaken and dry the nails. Nail polish may coat and protect the nails slightly, but if you choose to use it remember that all polishes are basically identical, despite advertising claims to the contrary. Nail strengtheners can discolor or break the nails and damage the nail. Artificial nails may produce allergic reactions under the nail and can create a perfect environment for bacterial or fungal growth.

Ingrown Nails

Ingrown nails are another inelegant but typical nail problem. Often they are the result of cutting the nail too deeply or filing the nail too much, forcing abnormal growth. Pain, swelling, infection, and discharge can result when the nail edge then grows into the surrounding skin. Many women love wearing shoes that crunch their toes into unnatural positions, and this too can interfere with nail growth and impede a normal healing process.

How can you prevent ingrown nails? Give your toenails plenty of room. That means changing to shoe styles that do not force the foot into an unnatural shape. Also, when you trim your fingernails and toenails, it is essential to avoid radically changing the natural shape of the nail by overfiling or cutting the nail below the tip of the finger or toe. Also, do not cut or push the cuticles; this can significantly affect the nail's growth.

If an ingrown nail does become infected, thoroughly clean the area and try to minimally trim away the portion of the nail that is digging into the skin. Overcutting can simply re-create the problem, so be cautious. Disinfect the area with an over-the-counter antibacterial ointment like Polysporin, Neosporin, or Bacitracin. If the problem does not improve, it may require medical care.

CHAPTER TEN

Problems? Solutions!

Dark Circles

Problem: I have dark circles that seem to get worse as the day goes by! What can I do to make my concealer last?

Solution: Be sure you are using a lightweight moisturizer (gel moisturizers are best for this) under the eye area that isn't making your concealer slide off. Matte-style (rather than creamy or greasy) concealers are best, particularly the new ones such as Almay Amazing Lasting Concealer, Maybelline Great Wear Concealer, and one made by Zhen (a department-store line). The color of the concealer must be light enough to cover the dark circles, but not so light as to give the appearance of a white mask around the eyes. Don't use greasy pencils along the lower lashes and don't use mascara that smears; these can slide during the day, making matters worse. Use only a powder to line the lower lashes, and then the tiniest line possible, or wear no lower liner at all. If you have allergies that get worse as the day goes by, you may want to consider an antihistamine. City pollution can get to your eyes by day's end, so you also may want to consider using an air filter in your home or office (talk to management).

Lashes Falling Out

Problem: My lashes are falling out! Is there anything I can do to stop this from happening?

Solution: It is natural for lashes to shed and then regrow, but if you are noticing bald spots along your lash line, you may need to change some habits that are making the condition worse. Do not wipe off eye makeup (or any makeup, for that matter). Wiping and pulling at the eyes can pull out lashes. Do not rub your eyes, even if they itch, especially when you are wearing mascara. Do not overuse mascara. I know it is tempting to have long, fat lashes, but the weight and subsequent removal can be too much for delicate lashes. Waterproof mascaras are the most difficult to remove and often take too many lashes with them. You might also want to change mascaras. It is unlikely that you are allergic to the mascara you are using, but on the remote possibility that it may be the cause of the new fall-out, switch brands and see how that works.

By the way, you aren't using an eyelash curler, are you? Over time, that consistent tugging can certainly pull out lashes. One more possibility: noncosmetic allergies may also be playing a part in your eyelash dilemma. Your only recourse, if that turns out to be the cause, is using antihistamines or eliminating from your environment the allergens causing the problem. For example, if you are allergic to the down in your pillows, change to a synthetic fill. Hay fever can be causing the eyes to severely swell, damaging eyelashes, which could be alleviated by using antihistamines.

Self-Tanners

Problem: I tried an expensive new self-tanner from a line called DeCleor at Neiman Marcus. It just smelled so much better than the one I was using from Coppertone. Now my palms are striped, one leg is darker than the other, and my knees and elbows look mottled!

Solution: Believe it or not, the DeCleor product, though absurdly expensive, is not at fault for your chameleon dilemma. First, all self-tanners, regardless of price, use the same ingredient, namely dihydroxyacetone, to create the color change in your skin. The fragrance that attracted you to the DeCleor product (some women tell me the Clarins and Bain de Soleil self-tanners smell great too) helps mask the chemical smell of this ingredient. But the smell is temporary and fades in a brief period of time. Nonetheless, once the color is in place, it will take time to get your skin back to normal. Because self-tanners affect skin cells, it is virtually the cell itself that changes color. Sloughing removes the altered skin cells, but you can't all at once slough off all the layers of skin that have been affected. That takes time. Loofahs, baking soda mixed with Cetaphil Cleanser, sea salt scrubs, and even a washcloth massaged over the problem areas twice a day will help a lot, but time is the real cure.

Once your skin is back to normal, you can try again. Remember, when it comes to self-tanners, application is everything. Be patient. Apply the self-tanner only over a clean, dry, exfoliated body, with special attention to the knees, elbows, and heels. Do not apply self-tanner in a steamy, hot room where perspiration or condensation may make it run. Do one area of your body at a time. Watch what you are doing, and apply the self-tanner thoroughly and evenly. If you miss an area, you will look noticeably streaked or blotchy. Wash the palms of your hands as soon as you are done applying the self-tanner, then stand still until it is completely absorbed, with no after-feel. Some women think that using a fast-darkening self-tanner is best because it changes the skin's color immediately and you can more easily see your mistakes and correct them. Others feel a self-tanner that changes color slowly is best so you can build a tan slowly and evenly. The choice is yours.

Seriously Oily Skin

Problem: I have seriously oily skin in the T-zone, and it is driving me crazy. I've tried matte foundations, even Lancome MaquiControle, all kinds of oil-control gels and powders, and my face still feels like an oil slick by midday.

Surely there must be something I can do?

Solution: In addition to doing the right things, it is essential to be sure you aren't doing anything to your face to make matters worse. For example, if you are using a moisturizer, even an oil-free moisturizer, stop immediately. Your oil glands are working overtime as a result of hormonal activity, but this oil is also your own built-in moisturizer. There is no reason to add more. If your oily skin is still driving you nuts, my favorite trick is to take Phillips' Milk of Magnesia (the one I recommend as a facial mask for oily skin) and apply an extremely thin layer of it over the most oily areas. Let it dry, then apply your foundation over that. It works great! When it comes to powdering, try loose powder instead of compact. Even when a pressed powder is oil-free, the waxlike ingredients that keep it in a pressed form can add to a slick feeling on the face.

Small Lips

Problem: I have small lips. Any lipstick color I put on seems to make this more noticeable. What should I do?

Solution: To deal with small lips, do not overline your lips to make them look larger. That technique of creating a new lip line works great in photographs, but in real life it looks like you missed your mouth. Also, to keep up the alteration you have to diligently touch up your lipstick and pencil the second any wears off. What works best is lining just to the outside or edge of your true lip line with a natural-colored lip liner. Do not wear dark lipstick. When dark colors are applied to any surface, they make things look smaller. A true red or any vivid color will make your lips look bigger, while a more neutral shade of lipstick with just a hint of color can also help. Of course you can always consider cosmetic surgical procedures that enlarge lips, but that would be a last resort after experimenting with lipstick options.

Flaking Eyeshadow

Problem: Whenever I apply eyeshadow, I always find eyeshadow sprinkles on my cheeks and under-eye area. What am I doing wrong?

Solution: Be sure you are knocking the excess powder off the brush before you apply your eye makeup; that will help a lot. Some eyeshadows are more "powdery" than others and cause more sprinkles. Eyeshadows made by M.A.C., Physicians Formula, Prescriptives, Ultima II, and Iman are more reliable in this respect. Another option that some makeup artists use is to apply foundation and concealer to the eye area first; then add the eye shadow, liner, and mascara; and then apply foundation to the rest of the face, touching up the concealer if "drippies" have made a mess of things. Although I find that approach time-consuming, it does help eliminate any trace of stray eyeshadow.

Bleeding Lipstick

Problem: I like a sheer lipstick look, but every one I've tried (and I've tried them all) just feathers into the lines around my mouth and looks like a mess! I've tried several of the stay-put lipsticks, but they look so hard and dry, and pencils are useless. I'm too young to have this problem. Is there something out there I've missed?

Solution: No, you haven't missed anything; sheer lipsticks (which are just glosses in a stick form), both expensive and inexpensive, are slippery by nature and don't stay put. Pencils are helpful, but they can't block a creamy, glossy lipstick all day. If you have any lines around your mouth—which are not necessarily related to age—sheer, creamy lipsticks and lip glosses in general will follow those pathways. Your only option is to give up the notion of a completely sheer look. Try a semi-matte lipstick such as Coty "24," Clinique Long Lasting, Zhen Matte Lipstick, or Revlon Velvet Lipstick. Once you apply it, blot with a tissue until it looks more or less sheer. I know it won't have the sheen you're looking for, but it also won't travel into the lines around your mouth. Don't try to put a gloss over that; it will only encourage the lipstick to bleed. The matte lipstick is not a shield impervious to the effect of the gloss. Gloss creates movement no matter what it goes over.

Bloodshot Eyes

Problem: I have red, bloodshot eyes that just look awful. It seems to have nothing to do with sleep and I don't drink alcohol, so what am I doing wrong, or, better yet, what should I be doing right?

Solution: Lots of things can cause the blood vessels in the eye to swell and look more obvious. Lack of sleep and alcohol consumption are only two possible causes; there are lots more. Contact lenses, exposure to smoke, rubbing the eyes, allergies, dry air (from heat or air-conditioning), makeup particles getting in the eye and causing irritation, bad pollution days, staring at a project all day without giving your eyes a break, and overusing eyedrops can all make the tiny blood vessels in the eye look like road maps.

A humidifier in your home or office can help, and regularly blinking during the day, not wearing contact lenses all day, using antihistamine for allergies, keeping your hands away from your eyes, and zealously keeping makeup out of your eyes are all exceptionally helpful. To reduce dryness, the natural tear products and eyewashes found at the drugstore are a great option (but use only disposable cups; repeatedly using the same cup can cause or aggravate problems such as eye infection or irritation). Eyedrops such as Visine used repeatedly can aggravate the problem and cause a rebound effect, making the blood vessels swell even more.

Puffy Eyes

Problem: I have puffy eyes every morning that sometimes don't go away until midday. They look awful and I've tried lots of eye products that don't change a thing.

Solution: There are no cosmetics or miracle eye moisturizers that can alter puffy eyes, but lots of things can cause the skin around the eye area to swell. Lack of sleep is probably not as big a factor for puffy eyes as it is for bloodshot eyes. If anything, sitting up instead of lying down prevents fluids from collecting in the tissues around the eye. Of course, no one should sit up day and night. Sleeping with your head slightly elevated, being sure to give your neck the support it needs, can prevent fluid retention. Alcohol consumption and a diet high in salt can cause water retention and increase puffiness around the eyes. Contact lenses can cause irritation and swelling of the eye, so be sure you are wearing the most comfortable type for your vision correction. Exposure to smoke, rubbing the eyes, allergies, dry air (from heat or air-conditioning), makeup particles getting in the eyes, allergic reactions to skin-care or makeup products, bad pollution days, and leaving makeup on overnight (which cause inflammation) can all make the eye area swollen.

Be sure to take your makeup off meticulously at night, do not rub your eyes during the day, and take an antihistamine if you have allergies. If you are allergic or sensitive to skin-care or makeup products, avoid them. Preventing dryness around the eyes can also be very helpful in reducing irritation and swelling that can cause a puffy appearance. If that is your problem, a lightweight moisturizer will help a lot. Be certain the moisturizer does not contain any irritating ingredients that could make matters worse, such as witch hazel, volatile plant oils, and sensitizing plant extracts like lemon oil or menthol. If you have time in the morning, place cool compresses on the eyes (low temperatures can make the skin contract); if you don't have time, leave your moisturizer in the refrigerator to apply when you wake up.

If none of these things help alleviate the problem, the natural appearance of your eyes may just be puffy, especially the under-eye area. If that is the case, the only way to get rid of the problem is with cosmetic surgery.

Chapped Lips

Problem: What should I do about my eternally chapped lips? No matter what I use, they never go away.

Solution: Whether they are from cold weather, from an arid climate, or just naturally dry lips, chapped lips are a pain. Cracking, flaking, and chapping is not only uncomfortable but unsightly, and lipstick only seems to make the situation worse. You can solve those dry lips blues with consistency and patience. Chapped lips are not going to disappear in a day, and missing even one day of treatment can drive lips to dryness.

Lips are more vulnerable to the environment than any other part of the face. This means that keeping your lips moist and sealed against the weather is essential. There are lots of emollient lip products that do just that, and the more emollient the better. Ingredients like lanolin; oils of any kinds, including castor oil, lanolin oil, safflower oil, almond oil, and vegetable oil; and shea and cocoa butter are all excellent, especially if they are listed at the beginning of the ingredient list. However, many lip products are little more than waxy coatings that make lips feel thick and protected when they are on (Chapstick is a great example), but they don't really moisturize or provide adequate protection from the weather outside or dry heat and air-conditioning inside.

Lots of lip products claim to be medicated. "Medicated" is a dubious term at best, with no regulated meaning. These products usually contain camphor, peppermint oil, eucalyptus, or menthol, but these are not medicines for dry lips. They mostly irritate and can actually make lips burn, which is neither disinfecting nor helpful for already dry, chapped lips. Products like Blistex, which includes 0.5% phenol, are the exception, because they truly are medicated; phenol kills anything that gets in its way. However, phenol is strong stuff and actually can trigger some serious problems, the least of which are drying and irritation. It is not something I would recommend for anything but extremely limited use.

You may have heard a rumor that lips can adapt to or get used to lip balm. It isn't possible. But if the lip balm you are using contains irritating ingredients (and lots of them do), your lips will stay dried up. When a lip product contains irritating, drying ingredients, there is no way the other, more emollient ingredients can help. Likewise, if you are using a lip product that is just waxy, with no emollients or oils, it only plasters down dry skin; it doesn't reduce the dryness.

I am quite fond of BeautiControl's LipApeel. This two-step product exfoliates the chapped skin with a waxy cream you rub over the lips; then, after that's rubbed off, you apply a very emollient balm. It is the only really gentle and effective exfoliating product I've ever seen for lips. It's a bit pricey, but it can last for years. BeautiControl's ordering number is (800) BEAUTI-1.

At night you can apply almost any lip balm that contains some of the emollients I mentioned above, but no irritants. **For daytime care, it is best to use an SPF 15 lip balm that contains avobenzone, titanium dioxide, or zinc oxide.** However, if you wear an opaque lipstick, it may not be essential to have that kind of SPF protection. Research has shown that women are at a much lower risk of getting lip cancer then men. The theory of why this might be true is based on the fact that most women wear opaque lipsticks during the day, which can block most, if not all, of the sun's skin cancer–causing rays.

Dry Skin Around the Lips

Problem: For some time now I have had a strange red, dry irritation, just along the skin around my mouth. Moisturizers don't seem to help.

Solutions: One of the first things you can do is determine whether you've developed an allergic reaction to fluoride toothpaste. Fluoride can cause irritation around the mouth. Try a fluoride-free toothpaste for a while and see what happens. If fluoride-free toothpaste is the solution, check with your dentist to see how this will affect your dental health.

The dryness and irritation around your mouth could also be caused by a significant other who happens to have a rough beard. There isn't much you can do about that, but occasionally using a little cortisone cream around the area can help keep irritation from almost any source to a minimum. Another possibility is frequent, unconscious licking of the lips. Saliva can be an irritant for the lips, causing flaking and dryness. Lip balm won't be able to keep up with this bad habit.

If the area around the mouth is dry and irritated, that can also affect the lips. It is important to treat the root of the problem, which in this situation may require an emollient moisturizer used around the edge of the mouth as well as a lip exfoliant and lip balm for the lip area.

Expensive vs. Inexpensive

Problem: I'm not one to fall for a company's enthusiasm for its product, but surely some companies can have secret or special ingredients and formulas, or use more expensive, superior ingredients. A friend mentioned that her chocolate chip cookies contain flour, sugar, shortening, eggs, vanilla, chocolate chips, and nuts, but they still don't taste like Mrs. Fields'. I have used your inexpensive recommendations and they have worked great, but I am so tempted by the more expensive stuff!

Solution: I understand the concept your friend is suggesting when it comes to her cookies. However, some people may prefer Mrs. Fields' cookies while others would prefer your friend's. If she does have a secret ingredient, that may taste great to you but not to someone else. When it comes to shopping for makeup and skin-care products, there are unquestionably great formulas out there that work better for different skin types and different needs, in all price ranges, but the notion that expensive is better isn't supported by any of the research I've seen or done. We know this is true, because we've all bought expensive products we didn't like. After interviewing dozens of cosmetic chemists and cosmetic ingredient manufacturers, I have yet to find any that agree with this notion of secret ingredients providing superior benefits for the skin. There are ingredients that can make a difference but almost without exception, they are accessible to everyone. I rate lots of expensive and inexpensive products as excellent and lots as poor, but judging by price alone can hurt your skin and waste your money.

Using Different Products from Different Lines

Problem: I've been following your advice and using products from several different lines. My skin is doing great, but all the cosmetics salespeople say it is a mistake to mix and match. They say products are designed to work together, and that is what helps the skin best.

Solution: Stop listening to the cosmetics salespeople; they are wrong. If every line had SPF 15 sunscreens with the new FDA-approved ingredients, gentle cleansers with nonirritating ingredients, foundations that aren't peach-colored, and on and on, I would agree that you don't need to mix and match. But I have found good and bad products in every line (and I've reviewed more than 250 lines and thousands of products). Most lines don't have adequate sunscreens, and they have products that contain irritating ingredients, shiny eyeshadows, and rose, peach, and ashen foundation colors. Staying with the same line for all your skin-care or makeup needs assures that you will end up with some bad products. Mixing and matching is the only way to go. You don't wear clothes from one designer, buy furniture from one manufacturer, take medicine from one pharmaceutical company, or eat food from one company. The only way to develop a successful skin-care or makeup routine is to select what works best for your skin type, not what one line happens to be selling.

Hair Removal

Problem: I'd give anything not to struggle with shaving every day. Plus, I have a slight facial mustache that my doctor says is a result of starting menopause! Please tell me there is something I can do about all this. I'm tempted to try a hair-removal product called Sweet Simplicity that I saw advertised in an infomercial. They made it look so easy and wonderful.

Solution: All infomercials make everything they sell seem easy and wonderful, providing just the results we've always longed for. I have reviewed Sweet Simplicity and I found it to be neither sweet nor simple, but instead rather messy and difficult to use. Believe me, I would love to find an easy way to achieve a smooth bikini line or a hairless upper lip without trouble or bother, but hair removal just isn't that simple. Here are your options, depending on your budget, available time, and the area you want to have hair-free.

Waxing is an excellent and inexpensive way to deal with most hair removal on the body or face. Waxing leaves the area smoother than shaving does because it pulls the hair out below the top layer of skin, which makes grow-back slower and less uniform. Waxing can be done at home by yourself, and beauty supply stores sell all the equipment you will need, from the wax to spatulas, strips of cotton, and anti-inflammatory lotions. There are even hair remover kits with strips of wax or waxlike ingredients that you just peel off, place on the skin, and rip off. No heating or mixing. This is by far the most convenient and easiest way to go about peeling off hair from large areas such as the legs, bikini line, and arms. For smaller areas such as the upper lip, a wax that is melted in the microwave (instead of on the stove) and applied with a small spatula offers the most control.

In hot waxing, a thin layer of heated wax is applied to the skin in the direction of the hair growth. The hair becomes embedded in the wax as it cools and hardens. The wax is then pulled off quickly in the opposite direction of the hair growth, taking the uprooted hair with it. Cold waxes work similarly. Strips precoated with wax or a cool sugar-based substance are pressed on the skin in the direction of the hair growth and pulled off in the opposite direction.

Before you consider doing this yourself, visit an aesthetician with experience in this method of hair removal. It's tricky to get the technique right, and getting it wrong can mean a sticky mess on your body, in your kitchen, and around your bathroom. It also smarts a bit when the hair is ripped off. You can't wax again until the hair grows out to a noticeable length.

Tweezing is not only a painful option, but also extremely time-consuming. It is OK for occasional stray hairs, but not the best for large areas or areas with dense hair growth. Tweezing works virtually the same way as waxing—pulling the hair out from the root—which means it lasts far longer than shaving. Some women worry that tweezing will increase the growth or texture of the hair, but it won't. If plucking (or waxing and shaving) altered hair growth, we would all have bushy eyebrows. Actually, pulling out hair can shut down the hair follicle by causing repeated shock and injury. If there is any texture change, it is just during the initial grow-back phase, when the hair reemerges from the pore.

Bleaching is a great, inexpensive option if the issue is not the density of the hair but the darkness. This method is particularly effective for the upper lip or other parts of the face, neck, and arms. To this day I still use my mother's hair-lightening formula: 2 teaspoons of **Clairoxide 20 Volume Peroxide** *($1.95 for 4 ounces)* to 1 teaspoon of **Lady Clairol Instant Whip** *($3.95 for 2 ounces)*. (Both can be found at beauty-supply houses.) I mix the two together and apply the solution to my upper lip with a cotton swab. I leave it on for no more than 10 minutes maximum. The result is bleached white hair along my upper lip. A friend uses this same recipe, doubled, for her arms, which have sparse but dark hair growth. I prefer this to the facial hair–bleaching products you find at the drugstore. They tend to turn the hair yellow-blonde, while this recipe strips color from the hair and turns it white and relatively invisible.

Electrolysis is the only permanent form of hair removal, at least so far, but it takes repeated treatments that aren't inexpensive and a skilled technician for satisfactory results. Before you see someone, check out clients of theirs who have had permanent success with this tricky but effective method of hair removal.

Two types of devices use electric current to remove hair: the needle epilator and the tweezers epilator. Needle epilators introduce a very fine wire under the skin and into the hair follicle. An electric current travels down the wire and destroys the hair root at the bottom of the follicle. The loosened hair is then removed with tweezers. Every hair is treated individually. Needle epilators are used in electrolysis. Because this technique destroys the hair follicle, it is considered a permanent hair-removal method. The hair root may persist, however, if the needle misses the mark or if insufficient electricity is delivered to destroy it. However, the stimulus for hair growth in an area is never permanently removed. For instance, you can't control hormonal changes that cause new growth.

The major risks of using electrolysis include electrical shock, which can occur if the needle is not properly insulated; infection from an unsterile needle; and scarring resulting from improper technique. In addition, there are no uniform licensing standards regulating the practice of electrology. Only 31 states require electrologists to be licensed, and among those the license requirements vary from as few as 120 hours to 1,100 hours, which means all that most electrologists need to set up shop is a machine and very little else.

The American Electrology Association and the Society of Clinical and Medical Electrologists have certification programs, based on a written exam. A list of licensed and certified electrologists is available from the International Guild of Professional Electrologists, 202 Boulevard Street, Suite B, High Point, NC 27262; (800) 830-3247.

Home electrolysis devices technically work the same way as those for professional use and carry the same health risks. However, the risks for the home-use machines are not very great because the voltage and current output are not very high, which also means they aren't as effective. I know we've all seen those little machines you can buy via mail order (for about $100) that claim to remove hair painlessly and permanently. They've been advertised for years and years. I remember them from when I was a kid. The chances of operating these successfully yourself are at best slim. You probably would end up just tweezing instead of zapping the hair because getting the device to work right is extremely tricky and incredibly time-consuming. Given the time it takes for a hair to grow back, it could take months before you knew if it was really working.

The Soft Light Hair Removal System is a laser treatment for hair removal, developed by the Thermolase Corporation. It is still not certified by the FDA as being permanent, but a few plastic surgeons I've spoken to say they find its effectiveness compelling. The Soft Light laser is basically the same as other dermatologic lasers, but this one is used with a heat-conducting topical ointment that sends the laser beam down the hair shaft to zap the follicle, which slows hair growth. At least, that's the theory. If you're thinking this sounds pricey, you're right. It can cost $1,000 for a one-time complete leg and bikini-line hair removal or, to repeat the treatment as many as times as you need (and, depending on your hair growth, it can be four to eight times per year), $5,250! That's a hefty price tag without any guarantee the hair won't grow back. For more information, call (800) 76-THIRA to find out if and where this option may be available near you.

Shaving is fine, but we all know the problems associated with it. Shaving is the method most of us go back to for our legs and bikini line, but the hair grows back way too fast and the stubble or redness it can cause on the thigh and crotch is obnoxious. There are ways around the redness, such as shaving with a good topical lotion like a hair conditioner or Cetaphil Cleanser and applying a moisturizer afterward. On the legs, an AHA product can help keep flaky skin at a minimum, which means you can get a closer shave. **Alpha Hydrox Lotion for Dry Skin 8% AHA** does a great job. Skin should never be shaved while dry; wet hair is soft, pliable, and easier to cut. Contrary to what many believe, shaving does not change the texture, color, or rate of hair growth. Hair density is genetically and hormonally determined; it has nothing to do with what you do topically to the skin (unless you damage the hair follicle via trauma or burns).

Depilatories literally melt and dissolve hair with ingredients like calcium hydroxide and sodium or calcium thioglycolate. There are many reasons why this group of products is not great for everyone: the most compelling is the risk of burns to the skin and eyes. It is essential to test the depilatory on your arm first as a precaution against allergic reactions or skin sensitivities. Hair and skin are similar in composition, so chemicals that destroy the hair can also destroy the skin.

Depilatories, like shaving, remove only the hair on the surface, which means the hair comes back in just a few days. To get the best results from your depilatory, first apply warm to hot compresses, which help soften the hair and open the pores (where the hair is growing), allowing the depilatory to be absorbed better. Then apply an extremely thick, generous layer of the depilatory completely over the entire hair shaft and let it stay on the full recommended time, but no longer than between four and 15 minutes, depending on how fine or coarse the hair is. Because depilatories dissolve the hair, applying pressure can help remove more of the shaft. Instead of simply washing the depilatory away, use a washcloth and wipe the cream off, using a firm back-and-forth motion.

Depilatories should never be used for the eyebrows or other areas around the eyes, or on inflamed or broken skin.

Note: The above treatments for hair removal are all contraindicated after any facial peel. It can take six to eight weeks for the skin to completely heal after a peel. Any trauma to the skin can cause discoloration or even scarring.

Feeling Beautiful During the Trauma of Cancer

Problem: I have a dear friend who has just been diagnosed with breast cancer. I want to be a support for her. I know how important feeling beautiful is for her. Any suggestions from you would be truly appreciated.

Solution: I've spoken with many women who have lived through the ordeal of radiation and chemotherapy, and they all agreed that paying attention to how they looked helped a lot during the trauma of diagnosis and treatment. Having gone through this life-threatening event with my older sister, who was diagnosed four years ago with breast cancer, I appreciated the opportunity to look further into the issues and share some solutions and possibilities with you and your friend. Given the number of women who have breast cancer or other cancers, surely almost all of us know someone who can benefit from this information. One thing my sister found immensely helpful was when we talked openly about her cancer experience without embarrassment or reservation. Perhaps someone in your life would appreciate that kind of support and openness.

Body care: Because chemotherapy and radiation make the skin ultra-sensitive and even sunburned, as a general rule it is best not to use any types of adhesives, tints, bleach, wax, harsh or irritating chemicals, or hot baths or showers. Even deodorants and shaving can be a problem. Irritation can also be exacerbated by saunas, Jacuzzis, loofahs, strong soaps, and washcloths. Anything you can do to reduce the hypersensitivity will go a long way toward making the skin feel soothed and less irritated.

Instead of bar soap, which can be extremely drying and harsh on sensitive skin, try a gentle liquid body cleanser such as Nivea Moisturizing Shower Gel, Capri French Formula Foam Bath, or Oil of Olay Moisturizing Body Wash. Keep the skin moist with lightweight gels that don't trap heat, such as pure aloe vera (found at most health-food stores). If the skin becomes dry, use a nonfragranced, nonirritating moisturizer (the fewer plants the better) such as

Lubriderm Seriously Sensitive Lotion for Extra Sensitive Dry Skin. Take tepid or slightly warm showers and baths, and try to enjoy cool baths whenever possible with a little bit of light oil, such as safflower or sunflower oil, in the water. Avoid heavy oils such as vitamin E. In spite of the fact that vitamin E has a reputation for healing the skin and can help the skin after the radiation and chemotherapy are over (as can other antioxidants), in the midst of treatment keep in mind that vitamin E is a potential allergen, and its occlusive attributes can trap heat in the skin that needs to dissipate.

To keep her skin feeling soft and light, one of the first things my sister and I did before she went in for her radiation was to buy silk underwear, including T-shirts, underpants, teddies, and pajamas. She had to give up wearing a bra because the irritation from the straps and the tightness around the breast were just too uncomfortable. The silk not only was soothing but also helped her feel more feminine and attractive.

Hair care: Some women feel compelled to shave their head in anticipation of losing their hair. According to one woman, that is the worst possible solution for dealing with the inevitable. Shaving your head may look exotic, but unless you plan on shaving every day, it can itch like crazy when your hair starts to grow back between treatments. It is best to cut your hair very short and consider the option of wearing designer caps or wigs. Scarves always look like something is wrong, while caps and wigs can look quite normal.

By the way, the American Cancer Society can provide you with a free wig; call (800) 227-2345. These wigs have been donated and are clean, but use them as a springboard for finding one that is perfect for you. You can buy a wig at a specialty salon or wig shop; the trick is finding a good one and going to someone who knows how to style it. Wigs almost always need to be cut and styled to match your face. If you live in or near a large metropolitan area, your absolute best option is to find out who styles wigs for the women in the Orthodox Jewish community. For religious reasons, many Orthodox Jewish women cover their own hair with a wig. The shatel-macher (the wig maker) is a mainstay of the Orthodox community and knows better than anyone how to make a wig look natural and attractive. Just call the Orthodox synagogue in your area and ask for the number of the woman who styles wigs for the community. The larger the metropolitan area, the more choices there will be.

One woman told me that after she purchased her first quality wig (around $100 to $500), she was a changed woman. "Not only did it fit great, but it looked so real that no one could believe it was a wig. I still wear it now and then, and get the biggest kick out of telling people it's a wig."

When your hair starts growing back, you may find that it is rather thick and straighter or curlier than it was. As tempting as it will be to dye your hair or perm it, be patient. Wait for the hair to have a few normal cycles of growth before using chemicals on it. The skin and hair may still be sensitive or altered by the radiation and chemotherapy, and could react in a way that can cause problems.

Skin care: All of my recommendations for gentle skin care are doubly appropriate during radiation and chemotherapy. And it is even more imperative than usual to avoid the sun, because the skin can become photosensitive. Sunscreen is essential, and the less the body and face are exposed to the sun, the better. That means wearing hats, light cotton pants, and light long-sleeved blouses whenever possible. Because the skin can become dry, it is important to follow my recommendations for dry skin care, which include a gentle cleanser, a skin-softening toner, an emollient moisturizer, and the use of plant oils such as safflower or sunflower oil over dry patches.

Eyebrows and eyelashes: Accompanying the loss of hair on your head is the probable loss of eyebrows and eyelashes. Avoid the natural tendency to pencil in new brows, which will look fake and dated. Instead, try powder shadows to draw on a soft arch of a brow. If you have any eyebrow hair left, consider using the colored brow gels from Borghese, Ultima II, Lancome, or Chanel; these can add definition and shape to whatever hair you may have left. Another option is to use a waterproof mascara or a waterproof eye pencil that matches your brow color. Although waterproof mascara and waterproof eye pencils can look slightly more artificial, they are worth trying because chemotherapy or other drugs can bring on menopause or menopausal symptoms, and the accompanying hot flashes will wash the others away. This one takes some experimenting, so be patient until you find what works for you.

If you do lose your eyelashes, it is best to not use any mascara, even if you have a few lashes left. It is quite noticeable when there are gaps in your application, and mascara can shorten the life of the lashes you still have. Instead, consider lining the eyes with a dark brown shade of powder that you draw on more as shading than as a line. Lining with a pencil or liquid liner and no mascara can look odd, but shading the eye with a dark powder can look smoky and defining without making the lack of lashes more obvious.

Remember that brows and lashes grow back quickly, so that part is the most temporary!

Makeup: When it comes to foundation, concealer, blush, lipstick, and the rest, do whatever you are used to doing. Not only will it make you feel good, it will also normalize much of the process.

One woman who sent me a wonderful e-mail about this issue wrote, "I cannot stress enough the concept that *look good and feel better* really works. I thought I was doing OK and I was, until I found out what it felt like to go out in public with hair and makeup (eyebrows) that looked real. I never lost my sense of humor or my positive outlook; but when I got a great wig and wore makeup (and eyebrows), I felt fantastic."

One of the most powerful things you can do for yourself is to pay attention to your physical beauty and experiment to find what works. Don't try to pretend that feeling and looking beautiful doesn't matter during this time or that it is a waste of your energy. It may provide some of your most pleasant and uplifting moments until you are on the other side of your diagnosis.

Foundation Settling into Pores and Lines

Problem: What causes foundation to just sort of settle into the pores and leave tiny little spots or settle into laugh lines? I do not know whether my moisturizer is too heavy or not heavy enough, whether the foundation is too heavy or too light, or whether I have not waited long enough for the moisturizer to be absorbed.

Solution: Most foundations contain ingredients that provide some amount of movement. If they didn't, they wouldn't blend easily and would feel dry and matte on the skin, making wrinkles look worse. But that also means those foundations can easily slip into the pores, making the skin look mottled. Moisturizing when you don't need to would create even more slippage. Unless you have dry skin, there is no reason to wear a moisturizer under foundation. Most foundations for normal to dry skin have enough emollient ingredients, making an extra moisturizer unnecessary. Too much moisturizer (not too little) can absolutely cause slippage into lines and pores. Too much foundation can cause slippage into lines. Once you've blended on a foundation, apply a light dusting of powder to set your makeup. Also try blending on your foundation with a sponge and not your fingers. A flat sponge picks up excess foundation and blends it on in an even layer. Most importantly, you may want to consider changing to a more matte foundation (but not one of the new stay-put foundations; even though they don't slip into lines, they can make lines more noticeable because they go on so dry and matte).

Eyelash Dyes

Problem: A friend of mine gets her eyelashes and eyebrows dyed at the hair salon she goes to. The effect is really rather impressive and I'm tempted to try this myself. Her blonde lashes look dark and long, even without mascara. What do you think?

Solution: Unfortunately, my solution isn't much of a solution, because all I can do is strongly say, "Don't do it!" The only solution for making lashes and brows more visible is to use mascara on the eyelashes and shade your eyebrows with an eyeshadow that matches your hair color, an eyebrow pencil, or a brow mascara like Borghese's Brow Milano. Let me give you a little history first on why my answer to your question is such an emphatic "no." Back in 1933 a congressional controversy was brewing over the need for new and stronger food, cosmetic, and drug laws. At the time, the FDA had no authority to move against a cosmetic product called Lash Lure that was causing allergic reactions in many women. Two women, in fact, suffered severe reactions to the product; one woman became blind and the second woman died. When the new Food, Drug and Cosmetic Act was passed in 1938, Lash Lure was the first product seized under its authority. Although hair dyes have changed a great deal since then, they are still formulated with peroxide and ammonia or ammonialike ingredients. If a hair dye doesn't contain those ingredients, it can't affect hair color.

No one should ever dye her eyelashes or eyebrows. An allergic reaction to the dye could prompt swelling, inflammation, and susceptibility to infection in the eye area. These reactions can severely harm the eye and even cause blindness. The FDA absolutely prohibits the use of hair dyes for eyebrow and eyelash tinting or dyeing, even in beauty salons and other establishments. The FDA has continuously warned the public about the use of coal-tar dyes on the eyebrows and eyelashes, stating that such use could cause permanent injury to the eyes, including blindness. (Using eyelash and eyebrow dyes or hair dyes for the eyes or brows should not be confused with using mascaras, eyeshadows, eyebrow pencils, and eyeliners, which contain colors that have been approved by the FDA for use in the eye area.)

Be aware that there are no natural or synthetic color additives approved by the FDA for dyeing or tinting eyelashes and eyebrows—either in beauty salons or in the home. In fact, the law requires all hair dye products to include instructions for performing patch tests before use, to identify possible allergic reactions, and to carry warnings about the dangers of applying these products to eyebrows and eyelashes. The health hazards of permanent eyelash and eyebrow dyes have been known for more than 60 years. These dyes have repeatedly been cited in scientific literature as capable of causing serious reactions when placed in direct contact with the eye.

Seasonal Changes

Problem: During the winter I use an emollient moisturizer you recommend and it works great, but during the summer it seems a bit much. Should I change what I do with the seasons?

Solution: Summer can absolutely require a change in skin-care products, particularly moisturizers. Instead of the more emollient or rich moisturizers you were wearing at night to combat the dry heat indoors and the dry cold outdoors, consider lighter moisturizers that come in gel or gel/lotion consistencies. Keep in mind that the major notion is to cut back on the amount of moisturizer you are using. Moisturizer is for dry skin, so if you don't have dry skin, you really don't need moisturizer. Also remember that no matter how much moisturizer you wear, no matter how many antioxidants it contains, it won't change or stop one wrinkle on your face. What a lightweight moisturizer can do is soothe spot dryness and make fine lines less noticeable. Nothing is erased or changed, but things do look better, and that's great. And this is at night, right? Because during the day you should be using a sunscreen for your face and exposed parts of your body.

Please ignore the fact that many of the products recommended below are labeled as oil-free. This is meaningless. What makes these products good for those with minimally dry skin is that they contain fewer thickening agents and emollients. Also ignore words and phrases such as "oil-control," "lift," and "firming." None of these products can control oil, lift the skin anywhere, or firm it even a little. These are all good, very lightweight moisturizers, and that's enough.

Here's a list of some of the better lightweight gel moisturizers, regardless of price (price is not indicative of quality): Borghese Cura Notte Night Therapy for Normal to Oily Skin; Chanel Lift Serum; Clinique Moisture Surge Treatment Formula; Estee Lauder Future Perfect Skin Gel and Clear Difference Oil-Control Hydrator; Lancome Oligo Major Mineral Serum and Hydra Controle Oil-Free Fresh Gel; L'Oreal Revitalift Night; Prescriptives Line Preventor; and Revlon Results Line Diminishing Serum.

Makeup Color Selections for Redheads

Problem: I am a natural redhead and have problems finding makeup professionals who are trained to advise someone with my coloring (I have bright red hair, pale skin, and freckles). I've had lots of makeovers at department-store makeup counters and always walk out looking either overly made up or wearing colors that clash with my hair! What colors do you suggest?

Solution: The answer to your question seems rather simple to me, so I'm not sure what's going wrong when you get your makeup done professionally. For you, the sheerest foundation is best. If a makeup artist is trying to cover up your freckles, he or she should be shot. Neutral golden tan as well as shades of camel and chestnut brown for eyeshadows, blush, and lipsticks are made for your coloring. You can try a golden coral-brown for lipstick or blush if you want a dash more color. Although those colors are considered tried and true for redheads, there really is no color barrier these days when choosing colors. A vibrant red with a soft reddish brown blush can look wonderful and quite dramatic on someone with your coloring. In the long run, experimenting until you find colors you're comfortable with is the best way to go.

When it comes to mascara, stay with brown and avoid black, which can be too hard a look on fair freckled skin. Also keep in mind that makeup is not supposed to match hair color. A woman with gray hair doesn't wear gray colors.

Whiter Teeth

Problem: I would so love to have a perfect white smile. I hate my yellowing, stained teeth. What should I do?

Solution: Taking antibiotics for acne could have permanently yellowed or dulled your teeth; silver fillings might have grayed the surrounding tooth enamel; you might just have naturally off-white or yellow enamel; and lots of foods such as coffee, tea, and berries can cause yellow stains. You can cut back on the foods causing the problem, but whose going to give up their coffee in the morning or fresh berries? Serious staining and discoloration can not be corrected with toothpaste, even a so-called whitening toothpaste. Whitening toothpastes make the teeth maybe a shade lighter, but that's about it. These whitening toothpastes, regardless of the brand, all tend to work equally well, which isn't nearly as well as they claim. Abrasive toothpastes are a problem because over time they help erode the surface of the tooth, which further complicates yellowing. The external part of the tooth is white, but underneath the white is a yellow core. As the white part erodes, in part because of age, it is made worse by overbrushing with abrasive toothpastes and hard toothbrushes.

One remarkable solution is to ask your dentist to bleach your teeth for startling results. Teeth-bleaching treatments used by dentists come in two forms—one is done at the dentist's office and the other you purchase from the dentist and use at home. The dentist's whitening process done at the office can take several weeks, about a half hour per visit, for a cost of $300 to $800. The kit you buy from the dentist uses a similar carbamide peroxide-based bleaching gel. Your dentist will fit a mouth guard to your mouth that must be left on for several hours over several nights. These at-home kits can cost between $100 and $200. The teeth-whitening kits you buy at the drugstore ($15 to $25) use a substantially weaker peroxide-based bleach and the mouth guard is not specially fitted to your mouth. If your teeth are even that is fine, but if they aren't the mouth guard will not fit evenly and you can get uneven results. The mouth guard the dentist has made for your mouth has individual spaces for each tooth. If the teeth do not lighten evenly, you can do extra treatments for only the teeth that didn't become light enough. None of these treatments is very effective if your teeth are grayed instead or completely yellowed. Teeth-bleaching systems work best for partially yellow or food-stained teeth.

Other then bleaching, if the yellow or dull color of your teeth is from tartar buildup, get your teeth cleaned and have them cleaned regularly. If you can, avoid foods that can grab onto teeth and make them look darker, such as chocolate, dark-colored berries, red wine, and coffee. Milk can also grab onto front teeth and cause yellow tartar buildup. Clearly, it would be best to brush immediately after eating these foods, but if that isn't possible, rinse your mouth well with water and then chew sugarless gum. Many dentists recommend using the Sonicare automatic toothbrush as a way to prevent tartar or plaque buildup. You definitely cannot manually brush your teeth as well as the Sonicare can.

CHAPTER ELEVEN

Animal Rights

Beauty vs. Animal Testing

Politically, I'm a moderate. I haven't always been. I grew up in the 1960s, and my politics have ranged from idealistic liberal to confused bipartisan. Now, as I stand loosely planted in the '90s, leaning into the millennium, I can earnestly say I am convinced that few, if any, issues in life are black and white, or all or nothing. I find more and more often that there is truth on both sides of the issues and the middle ground is often the only reasonable position. At least the middle ground is the only position that acknowledges the whole picture and not just one side. I vote both Republican and Democrat, depending on the individual and his or her voting record.

This middle position also represents my perspective on animal testing as it pertains to cosmetics products and the health-care industry. While I unquestionably advocate the humane and ethical treatment of all life, especially unprotected and dependent life, I am not in favor of eliminating all forms of animal testing when it comes to health-care issues or human safety issues.

I feel terrible pain and anguish when I think of animals suffering in any way so I can put on mascara or clean my face. Many animal tests that are used to ascertain whether a cosmetic will hurt people are cruel and gratuitous. No one is ever going to eat 50 pounds of mascara. Forcing animals to do so in order to demonstrate how much mascara people can eat before they die makes me want to resign from the human race. How can anyone put an animal through such torture?

On the other hand, my older sister who had breast cancer, my father who had prostate cancer, my dearest friend's mother who has Alzheimer's, and my husband who has high blood pressure all take medication and have undergone medical procedures that have prolonged and improved their quality of life—and all of these medications and procedures have been proven effective and safe as a result of animal testing. I absolutely do not want to see even one animal die by being force-fed foundation or eyeshadow to prove a favorable formulation. Yet, if sacrificing an animal's life can help find the cure for Alzheimer's, prevent more cancers, or reduce the risks of high blood pressure and a host of other illnesses, I would and do support that research.

Most of us are aware of the dramatic pictures distributed by animal-rights groups showing the terrible torment of animals in research laboratories. This is indeed a grotesque and painful situation that all of us should be sickened by and do our best to change. But this narrow, shocking display does not address the results of animal research (the creation of safe products and medical treatments), nor does it represent the labs that treat animals humanely by caring for them and anesthetizing them.

Children who survive leukemia owe their lives to animal testing. Arthritis patients who can walk again owe their agility to animal testing. Successful excisions of brain tumors are due to animal testing, and on and on. Human health-care advancement and the use of animals to test various protocols and risks are inextricably linked and cannot be separated. This is the dilemma of animal testing.

There are many arguments surrounding this issue from both points of view. On one side are the animal-rights activists, who claim there is no need or reason to ever use animal testing (or eat meat, use leather goods, or employ animals for any purpose other than as pets). When it comes to animal testing, they point to alternative methods of research assessment that can be used. Spokespeople for People for the Ethical Treatment of Animals (PETA) and the National Anti-Vivisection Society (NAVS) claim that a preponderance of research proves that all animal testing is inconclusive and has no relation to what takes place in humans. Animal activists insist that all animal testing is motivated by financial profit and stubborn old-fashioned doctors or "good old boys" who refuse to change. Their reasoning is that animal testing is big business, and no one wants to alter what they are doing if it means they could potentially lose money.

On the other side are the vast majority of physicians, medical research groups from most major universities, national medical organizations representing everything from cancer to heart disease, and pharmaceutical companies, all of which believe the use of animal models for research is essential to evaluating new and old medical treatments and procedures. These physicians and organizations often agree that in vitro (test tube–oriented) tests and computer model studies can replace some animal testing.

However, no one among these countless medical professionals would concede that all or even most animal testing is futile and immaterial. They can point to thousands of chemical substances and operations that were first determined to be safe and effective or dangerous and deleterious because of animal testing. Stopping such testing would halt most medical research, from AIDS to Alzheimer's, and the development of all new drugs. Even physicians deeply involved in finding alternative research methods to replace animal testing would not agree that we should stop all animal testing now.

The truth probably exists somewhere in the middle. Medical, pharmaceutical, and cosmetics industry experts freely admit that in the past they conducted far more animal experiments than needed to prove safety. Animal-rights activist campaigns inspired a vocal consumer base to force a major change in the number and type of animal tests being done. Many companies responded by reducing animal testing, changing to alternative methods whenever possible, and instituting humane treatment of their animals. Yet all or nothing is the goal of animal-rights activists, and that may not be the goal of all consumers buying makeup, taking medicines, or considering medical procedures. Consumers should look at the whole issue and not just shocking pictures.

For example, according to an article in the January 1997 issue of *Drug and Cosmetic Industry* magazine, Gillette has been a boycott target of PETA since 1986. What PETA does not acknowledge is that since its boycott, Gillette has reduced tests on animals by over 90%, has contributed millions of dollars to alternative research, and has donated over $100,000 to the Humane Society. You would think PETA would ease up on Gillette, but that isn't the case. It still lists Gillette among its companies to boycott. As long as a company does any animal testing, humane or otherwise, it is a target for PETA's condemnation. That is regrettable, because as a consumer you get only a limited perspective.

As a result of PETA's and NAVS's black-or-white position, you may be led to believe that The Body Shop is the greatest ally of animal rights since the inception of the concept. Yet, when faced with the publication of an article exposing The Body Shop's ambiguous animal-testing policy, owner Anita Roddick had her cabal of attorneys prevent the story from running in *Vanity Fair.* That only fueled the ire of reporter Jon Entine, who was then able to get his story published in *Business Ethics* and *Drug and Cosmetic Industry* magazines. It seems The Body Shop didn't want people to know its product development included use of ingredients that had been tested on animals; in fact, The Body Shop was banned from using the term "not tested on animals" on their products by West German courts in 1989. (The company subsequently began using the term "against animal testing.") According to a January 1997 article in *Drug and Cosmetic Industry* magazine, a research executive at The Body Shop in 1993 was quoted as saying that "the technology of alternative testing for raw materials has not yet sufficiently advanced to guarantee product safety." This story about The Body Shop was overlooked or completely ignored by both PETA and NAVS.

Most of us are against animal testing, but we also have the right to safe products and straight information about how that can best be accomplished. It would be wonderful if alternative, computer-based, and test-tube models were sufficient for establishing a cosmetic, drug, or medical procedure's safety, but that doesn't seem to be true, at least not now or in the near future. If alternatives become common practice, it will probably happen in the world of cosmetics first, mainly because cosmetics are not ingested and alternative research methods for irritation studies are showing promise.

Frank Fairweather, head of clinical and pathological programs at the British Industrial Biological Research Association, is a frequent spokesperson in Europe on alternatives to animal testing of cosmetics. In a presentation Fairweather made in 1996 at the Second World Congress on Alternatives to Animal Use in the Life Sciences, he said that "none of the alternative techniques could yet be reliably substantiated." He hopes that research protocols can be quantified and then mimicked via in vitro methodology, but at this point they don't exist. He does feel optimistic, however, that in the next several years tests will be developed that finally do away with the need for testing cosmetics on animals. I hope so too.

I will continue to earnestly support the humane and ethical treatment of animals, but I do not at this time support a complete ban on animal testing. I personally do not use animal testing for any of my Paula's Choice skin-care products, either directly or indirectly (meaning I don't hire third-party testing facilities to do my testing for me). I use only proven, long-established formulations and ingredients, as do many other companies that make claims about "no animal testing." But because all of the cosmetic ingredients currently in use have at some point been tested on animals, no one can claim that the ingredients in their products involved no animal testing.

By creating products that are not tested on animals and by my support through financial contributions of such organizations as animal welfare groups and legal groups that fight for animal causes, I feel I am doing my part to help create a world where fewer and fewer animals will be used for testing, and those that are will be treated humanely and ethically every step of the way.

I want my readers to know that I believe their decisions and consumer activism in this area has been and continues to be vital. Cosmetics companies started changing and looking for alternative methods only because you, the consumer, brought pressure to bear and forced them to change. It is important to keep up this pressure. However, I feel it would be foolish to follow organizations like PETA and NAVS blindly unless you truly agree completely with their goal of abolishing all animal testing and creating a completely vegetarian society. **Instead, I encourage you to support organizations fighting for the welfare and safety of all animals, limited and humane animal testing, and continued research to find alternatives to animal testing in hopes that someday no animal will have to be used in any research experiments.** This is completely in your power, because you, the consumer, have everything to say about what you buy and whom you buy it from, and that speaks loudly and clearly to all kinds of corporations and enterprises the world over.

APPENDIX

Ingredient Dictionary

Understanding the Ingredients

Fortunately, in many countries (not Canada, but this could be changing soon!) cosmetics companies provide all of us with the very tool we need to implement our own objective evaluations—the ingredient list. These companies did not do this on their own. Rather, they went down kicking and screaming all the way, trying to keep this basic information hidden from the consumer. The FDA has made ingredient lists mandatory in the United States since 1978. For a long time, this information was left off the same products when they were sold in every other country in the world. Australia came on board in 1995, and the European Union countries followed suit in 1997. In all those countries, every skin-care and makeup item must list the exact contents on the box, container, or leaflet. One way or another, the information has to be available to the consumer, and if it isn't, the company is in violation of cosmetic regulatory law.

In cosmetics labeling, ingredients are listed in descending order of amount, so that the ingredient present in the largest amount is at the top of the list, and the ingredient present in the least amount is at the end. All of the information in that one small spot (often covered up by the price tag, unfortunately) has to be accurate, by law.

Ingredient lists can be your best friend, because they can't mislead you. They can be hard to understand, but once you get acquainted with the technical terms, you can at least start recognizing similarities between products.

Below is a list of some typical cosmetic ingredients. I briefly describe what each ingredient is and what it can or cannot do for the skin. This information is truly the nuts and bolts of the cosmetics industry. Understanding the ingredient list may not change the way you buy skin-care products, but I hope it will make you more aware of what you're buying. My major sources for this list were *A Consumer's Dictionary of Cosmetics Ingredients* by Ruth Winter (Crown Trade Paperbacks); the *International Cosmetic Ingredient Handbook* and the *International Cosmetic Ingredient Dictionary* (Cosmetic, Toiletry, and Fragrance Association); *Drug and Cosmetic Industry* magazine; and *Cosmetics & Toiletries* magazine. Keep in mind that this list is not complete; there are potentially thousands more cosmetic ingredients.

Acetone: Used in some astringents and toners for its ability to remove oil from the surface of the skin. Extremely drying; can cause severe irritation.

Acetylated lanolin: *See* lanolin.

Alcohol, SD alcohol 10-40: Alcohol is found in many types of skin-care products, but most frequently in astringents, toners, and fresheners. It can severely dry out the skin, and the resulting dryness can irritate the skin. Cetyl and stearyl alcohols, however, are merely thickening agents and should not pose an irritation problem.

Algae extract: Derived from seaweed. It is considered a good protective and emollient agent for the skin. All the miraculous claims about it healing the skin or getting rid of wrinkles are unsubstantiated.

Allantoin: Considered a good soothing agent.

Allspice: Whether as an oil or an extract, can be a skin irritant.

Almond: Whether as an oil or an extract, can be a skin irritant.

Aloe vera: Well known, legitimately, for its ability to soothe the skin.

Alpha hydroxy acids (AHAs): Please refer to Chapter Two, "What Works and What Doesn't," for specifics about AHAs.

Amino acids: Constitute the protein in human skin. Twenty-two of these extremely complex substances are used in cosmetics. Proteins provide a smooth covering on the skin and are considered beneficial in helping the skin absorb water. They provide no other benefit, such as building or supplementing the protein in your own skin. *See* protein.

Ammonium glycerhizinate: A very good anti-inflammatory agent. Helps soothe skin and reduce irritation.

Ammonium lauryl sulfate: *See* sodium laureth sulfate.

Amniotic fluid: Derived from the liquid surrounding an animal embryo. Some cosmetics companies claim this fluid can rejuvenate the skin. There are no independent studies that support this claim.

Angelica: Whether as an oil or an extract, can be a skin irritant.

Animal extracts: Animal extracts include the following: spleen, matrix, neural lipid, epidermal lipid, thymus, and animal tissue. These are dead fat or skin tissues from the thymus, testes, ovaries, udder, placenta, or other parts of a cow, pig, or sheep. The cosmetics industry would like you to believe that they have some rejuvenating effect on the skin. There is no evidence that these extracts can do anything for the skin, especially make it look younger. There is some evidence that these ingredients may be water-binding agents, however, which is good for the skin but hardly unique or unusual.

Animal thymus extract: *See* animal extracts.

Animal tissue extract: *See* animal extracts.

Arnica: Whether as an oil or an extract, can be a skin irritant. However, some studies indicate that arnica in small concentrations can be a healing agent.

Ascorbic acid: Considered a good antioxidant, which means it helps keep the air off the face, which helps prevent dehydration and possible free-radical damage.

Avocado oil: A plant oil that is a good emollient and water-binding agent.

Balm mint: Whether as an oil or an extract, can be a skin irritant.

Balsam: Whether as an oil or an extract, can be a skin irritant.

Bentonite: A clay that can help to absorb oil but can also be a skin irritant.

Benzalkonium chloride: Used as a disinfectant in cosmetics, but can be a potent skin sensitizer if it is found near the beginning of an ingredient list.

Benzoyl peroxide: A disinfectant. There has been some controversial evidence that benzoyl peroxide may have a negative impact on the skin. That research is not widely supported, and other research has disputed it. In my opinion, benzoyl peroxide is an effective option for someone with acne.

Bergamot: Whether as an oil or an extract, can be a skin irritant.

Beta hydroxy acid: *See* salicylic acid.

Bioflavonoids: Considered a good and effective antioxidant.

Bisabol: Considered a good and effective anti-irritant.

Butylene glycol: *See* glycerin.

Camphor: Found in many products intended to treat acne and chapped lips, but can cause contact dermatitis and be a potent skin irritant.

Caprylic/capric/lauric triglycerides: An oily substance derived from coconut oil; helps keep water in the skin.

Carrot oil: A plant oil that is a good emollient and water-binding agent.

Castor oil: A plant oil that is a good emollient and water-binding agent.

Ceramide: A component of skin. When used in cosmetics, can be a good water-binding agent.

Chamomile: Whether as an oil or an extract, can be a skin irritant if a lot is present in a product.

Cholesterol: Found in most living tissue, both plant and animal. An antioxidant, it is also considered a good emollient.

Cinnamon: Whether as an oil or an extract, can be a skin irritant.

Citrus: Whether as an oil or an extract, can be a skin irritant.

Clove: Whether as an oil or an extract, can be a skin irritant.

Clover blossom: Whether as an oil or an extract, can be a skin irritant.

Cocoa butter: A thickening agent and emollient. Considered very effective for dry skin but may cause skin irritation.

Coconut oil: A plant oil that is a good emollient and water-binding agent.

Collagen: A component of skin, and a well-known ingredient that helps keep water in the skin. The belief that rubbing collagen and elastin on the skin will somehow help rebuild the collagen and elastin in your own skin is, I hope, a thing of the past. The collagen and elastin found in cosmetics, because of their structure, cannot even penetrate the skin.

Coriander: Whether as an oil or an extract, can be a skin irritant.

Corn oil: Can be a skin irritant.

Cornstarch: Used as a thickening agent in cosmetics; can be a skin irritant.

Cottonseed oil: Can be a skin irritant.

Cyclomethicone: One of the many silicone oils used in cosmetics because of the incredibly soft, silky feel they leave on the skin and because of their versatility. They also are good water-binding agents. Cyclomethicone evaporates quickly, so it leaves little residue on the skin.

Dimethicone: *See* cyclomethicone.

Dmdm hydantoin: A common preservative in cosmetics that is also considered one of the more potentially irritating preservatives for the skin.

Elastin: A component of skin; when used in cosmetics, can be a good water-binding ingredient. *See also* collagen.

Epidermal lipid extract: *See* animal extracts.

Eucalyptus oil: Found in many products meant to treat acne and chapped lips, but can cause contact dermatitis and be a potent skin irritant.

Fatty acids: Stearic acid, the most popular fatty acid used in cosmetics, is a substance found in skin tissue. Used in a cosmetic, it helps keep water in the skin.

Fennel: Whether as an oil or an extract, can be a skin irritant.

Fir needle: Whether as an oil or an extract, can be a skin irritant.

Geranium: Whether as an oil or an extract, can be a skin irritant.

Glutathione: Considered a good antioxidant.

Glycerhizinate: Considered a good anti-irritant.

Glycerin: A fairly standard skin-care ingredient that helps attract water to the skin (an ingredient that can do this is called a humectant) and also helps deliver other ingredients into the skin. In large amounts, can be a skin sensitizer. Butylene, hexylene, and propylene glycol have similar properties.

Glycolic acid: An alpha hydroxy acid. Please refer to Chapter Two, "What Works and What Doesn't," for more information about AHAs.

Glycoprotein: *See* protein.

Glycosaminoglycans: A basic element found in skin tissue. When used in creams and lotions, helps water penetrate the skin. There is no evidence that glycosaminoglycans can aid the skin in any way besides keeping the surface soft and helping bind water to the skin.

Glycosphingolipids: A component of skin. When used in cosmetics, can be a good water-binding ingredient.

Grapefruit: Whether as an oil or an extract, can be a skin irritant.

Green tea: Considered a good and effective anti-irritant for the skin.

Hexylene glycol: *See* glycerin.

Horsetail: Whether as an oil or an extract, can be a skin irritant.

Hyaluronic acid: A component of skin; when used in cosmetics, can be a good water-binding ingredient.

Hydrolyzed animal protein: A component of skin; when used in cosmetics, can be a good water-binding ingredient. *See also* protein.

Hydroquinone: A skin-lightening agent considered most effective when combined with alpha hydroxy acids. Can be a skin sensitizer; many consider its skin-lightening effects to be minimal.

Imidazolidinyl urea: A common preservative that is also considered to have more potential for irritating the skin than other preservatives.

Isopropyl lanolate: A thickening agent and emollient. Studies show that it can cause breakouts or acne; however, it should not cause any problems if it is found at the end of an ingredient list.

Isopropyl myristate: A thickening agent and emollient. Studies show that it can cause breakouts or acne; however, it should not cause any problems if it is found at the end of an ingredient list.

Jojoba oil: A plant oil that is a good emollient and water-binding agent but can be a skin irritant or sensitizer.

Kaolin: A clay that can help absorb oil but can also be a skin irritant.

Kojic acid: Some studies indicate this is a reliable skin-lightening agent. Considered most effective when used with alpha hydroxy acids and other skin-lightening ingredients such as hydroquinone or song-yi acid.

Kola extract: Considered a good and effective anti-irritant.

Lactic acid: An alpha hydroxy acid. Please refer to Chapter Two, "What Works and What Doesn't," for more information about AHAs.

Lanolin: A superior emollient and lubricant for dry skin. There is evidence that it can be a skin sensitizer or can aggravate breakouts. Other than that, it is very effective at keeping the skin moist and supple. Several forms of lanolin show up on skin-care ingredient lists: lanolin oil, hydroxylated lanolin, lanolin alcohols, lanolin oil, and acetylated lanolin. All of these work as well as or better than pure lanolin to keep moisture in the skin.

Lanolin alcohol: *See* lanolin.

Lanolin oil: *See* lanolin.

Lavender: Whether as an oil or an extract, can be a skin irritant and a photosensitizer.

Lecithin: Found in most living tissue, both plant and animal. An antioxidant, it is also considered a good emollient.

Lemon: Whether as an oil or an extract, can be a skin irritant.

Lemongrass: Whether as an oil or an extract, can be a skin irritant.

Licorice root: Considered a good and effective anti-irritant.

Lime: Whether as an oil or an extract, can be a skin irritant.

Linoleic acid: A component of skin and plants known as a fatty acid. Considered excellent for keeping water in the skin.

Liposomes: Not a specific ingredient you would see on an ingredient list; rather, it is a unique delivery system that allows the penetration and slow release of water and lipids (oils and fats that act as water-binding agents) into the layers of skin.

Macadamia oil: A plant oil that is a good emollient and water-binding agent.

Magnesium laureth sulfate: *See* sodium laureth sulfate.

Marine extracts: Seaweed, algae, and other marine plants are used in cosmetics to justify claims of wrinkle prevention. None are substantiated and they are definitely not a unique or preferred source for antioxidants or water-binding agents. *See also* algae extract.

Marjoram: Whether as an oil or an extract, can be a skin irritant.

Melissa: Whether as an oil or an extract, can be a skin irritant.

Menthol: Although found in many products meant to treat acne and chapped lips, can cause contact dermatitis and be a potent skin irritant.

Methylacrylate: Forms a film or coating over the skin, similar to ingredients found in hairsprays that hold hair in place. It can temporarily make skin look smooth and hold it in place. Can be a potent skin irritant.

Methylparaben: *See* propylparaben.

Mineral oil: This widely used cosmetic ingredient has had a bad reputation in the past. In spite of the occasional bad press, mineral oil is considered one of the most nonirritating cosmetic ingredients available and is superior at keeping water in the skin.

Minerals: Minerals such as salt (sodium chloride), iodine, magnesium, chloride, and potassium are potential skin irritants when found in the first part of a cosmetic's ingredient list. However, minerals such as zinc, selenium, and choline are considered good antioxidants.

Mucopolysaccharides: A component of skin; when used in cosmetics, can be a good water-binding ingredient.

NaPCA: A component of skin; when used in cosmetics, can be a good water-binding ingredient.

Neural lipid extract: *See* animal extracts.

Oak bark: Whether as an oil or an extract, can be a skin irritant.

Oil: In general, oils of all kinds, whether plant, animal, or mineral, help keep water in the skin. A wide variety of oils are used in skin-care products, including plant oil, lanolin oil, castor oil, mineral oil, and silicone oil. If you have dry skin, buy a moisturizer that contains one or more oils as the primary ingredients. But be cautious of exotic plant oils such as ylang ylang, cardamom, lemon, and lavender oils that can be potential skin irritants, sensitizers, or allergens.

Palm oil: A plant oil that is a good emollient and water-binding agent.

Panthenol: Well known, legitimately, for its ability to soothe the skin.

Papaya: Used in skin-care products as an exfoliant; can be a skin irritant.

Peppermint: Although found in many natural products, can cause contact dermatitis and be a potent skin sensitizer.

Petrolatum: One of the more effective moisturizing ingredients around. Study after study indicates it performs as well as or better than any other skin-care ingredient for keeping water in the skin, and it does not clog pores. Mineral oil is derived from petrolatum. *See also* mineral oil.

Phospholipids: Found in human and plant tissue. In cosmetics, helps bind water to the skin and keep it there, and is considered a good emollient.

Placenta extract: *See* animal extracts.

Plant extracts: An endless array of plant ingredients that range from algae to chamomile. By far the most overhyped of all cosmetic ingredients. Some do benefit the skin, but no more or less than many other ingredients. More often than not, these ingredients offer little benefit other than boosting the appeal (and price) of a product. Many plant extracts can be skin sensitizers, particularly for people with plant allergies.

Plant oils: For the most part, these have a positive effect on the skin, helping to keep water in and lubricating and smoothing the surface. However, many plant oils can be skin irritants.

Polyacrylamide: *See* methylacrylate.

Polyethylene glycol (PEG): At least one member of this vast group of skin-care ingredients is present in practically every cleanser, toner, lotion, cream, and specialty product you will ever buy. These ingredients help attract moisture to the skin, help the product spread evenly, keep the other ingredients mixed together, and are good water-binding agents.

Propylene glycol: *See* glycerin.

Propylparaben: A standard preservative. All parabens are considered to be the least irritating of the preservatives used in cosmetics.

Protein: A component of skin. When used in cosmetics, can be a good water-binding ingredient, but won't add to the protein content of your skin.

PVP: *See* methylacrylate.

Quaternium-15: A common preservative that is also potentially irritating for the skin.

Retinol: A derivative of vitamin A. Vitamin A is also the source of the prescription drug Retin-A. This association with Retin-A misleads many consumers into believing that products containing retinol can provide benefits similar to those of Retin-A. At this time, there is no conclusive evidence to support this idea, although studies are being conducted. For the most part, vitamin A, retinyl palmitate, and retinol are simple but good antioxidants and help prevent free-radical damage. They may also have some benefits in terms of allowing moisture to penetrate the skin, but that's about it.

Retinyl palmitate: *See* retinol.

Rice bran oil: A plant oil that is a good emollient and water-binding agent.

Sage: Whether as an oil or an extract, can be a skin irritant.

Salicylic acid: A beta hydroxy acid (BHA) that is an effective exfoliant, but doesn't have a drop-off rate (meaning it doesn't stop exfoliating the skin) as AHAs do. Salicylic acid just keeps exfoliating, which can be too irritating for skin on a regular basis. Also, salicylic acid doesn't have the additional benefit of water-binding properties as AHAs do.

Sandalwood oil: A plant oil that can be a skin sensitizer.

SD alcohol: *See* alcohol.

Seaweed: *See* marine extracts.

Selenium: Considered a very effective antioxidant.

Serum protein: Derived from the blood of cows or pigs and used as a moisturizing ingredient. It may be a water-binding agent, but it isn't some miracle for the skin, despite its exotic sound.

Shea butter: A thickening agent and emollient derived from a plant. Considered nonirritating and very effective for dry skin.

Sodium C14-16 olefin sulfate: *See* sodium lauryl sulfate.

Sodium laureth sulfate: Along with a dozen or so similar-sounding ingredients, sodium laureth sulfate is considered a very gentle detergent cleansing agent. It is found most often in shampoos and water-soluble skin cleansers. It can be gentle, but it can also be somewhat drying.

Sodium lauryl sarcosinate: *See* sodium laureth sulfate.

Sodium lauryl sulfate: A cleansing agent found mostly in shampoos and skin cleansers. It is considered quite drying and potentially irritating when used as the primary ingredient in a skin cleanser.

Sodium PCA: *See* NaPCA.

Soybean oil: A plant oil that is a good emollient and water-binding agent.

Spleen extract: *See* animal extracts.

Squalane: A plant oil that is a good emollient and water-binding agent.

Squalene: *See* squalane.

Sunflower seed oil: A plant oil that is a good emollient and water-binding agent.

Superoxide dismutase: Considered a very effective antioxidant.

Sweet almond oil: A plant oil that is a good emollient and water-binding agent, but can be a skin sensitizer.

TEA-lauryl sulfate: *See* sodium lauryl sulfate.

Tea tree oil: Also known as melaleuca; almost identical to menthol. *See also* menthol.

Thyme: Whether as an oil or an extract, can be a skin irritant.

Tissue matrix extract: *See* animal extracts.

Tocopherol: The chemical name for vitamin E. Used in cosmetics as an antioxidant, which means it helps keep the air off the face, which helps prevent dehydration and possible free-radical damage. Vitamins do not feed the skin in any way from the outside in. The amount used is rarely enough to provide much benefit.

Triclosan: A disinfectant.

Triethanolamine: Typically used as a pH adjuster in cosmetics as well as, in combination with other ingredients, a detergent cleansing agent. Because triethanolamine is such a strong alkaline ingredient, it is also considered quite irritating.

Triglycerides: Found in human and plant tissue. In cosmetics, helps bind water to the skin and keep it there.

2-bromo-2-nitropane-1,3-diol: A less-than-common preservative that is considered potentially irritating.

Vitamin A: *See* retinol.

Vitamin C: *See* ascorbic acid.

Vitamin E: *See* tocopherol.

Water: Water is water—whether it is fancy water from the Swiss Alps, natural spring water, demineralized water, or water extracted from plants or flowers—and it must be present in your skin cells, or in your skin-care product, if you want to see positive effects on your face. Dry skin and mature skin contain an increased number of dried-out skin cells. Water rehydrates these cells.

Wheat germ oil: A plant oil that is a good emollient and water-binding agent.

Wintergreen: Whether as an oil or an extract, can be a skin irritant.

Witch hazel: A compound that is about 15% to 20% alcohol. Considered a mild skin irritant. Many products that claim to be alcohol-free contain witch hazel.

Ylang ylang: Whether as an oil or an extract, can be a skin irritant.

Zinc: Considered an effective antioxidant.

REFERENCES

Most of the information in this book was gleaned in large part from the following sources.

Industry Experts

Dr. Ronald Chez, professor of obstetrics and gynecology at the University of South Florida

Dr. Zoe Draelos, clinical associate professor of dermatology at Bowman Gray School of Medicine

Food and Drug Administration (FDA)

Dr. Ray Geronimus, director of the Laser and Skin Surgery Center of New York and clinical associate professor of dermatology at New York University Medical Center

Dr. Claude Hughes, research professor and attending physician in obstetrics and gynecology at Duke University

Dr. Cathy Kapica, Ph.D., professor of nutrition and clinical dietetics at Chicago Medical School

Dr. Richard Maloney, from The Aesthetic Surgery Center in Naples, Florida

Dr. Nia Terezakis, clinical professor of dermatology at Tulane University

Dr. Paul Weiss, clinical professor of plastic and reconstructive surgery at Albert Einstein College of Medicine

Books and Periodicals, by title

Chemical and Physical Behavior of Human Hair, 3d ed. Clarence R. Robbins. New York: Springer-Verlag, 1994.

A Consumer's Dictionary of Cosmetics Ingredients. Ruth Winter. New York: Crown Trade Paperbacks, 1994.

Cosmetics & Toiletries magazine. Published by Cosmetic Technology.

Drug and Cosmetics Industry magazine

Encyclopedia of Common Natural Ingredients, 2d ed. Albert Y. Leung and Steven Foster. New York: John Wiley & Sons, Inc., 1996.

International Cosmetic Ingredient Dictionary. The Cosmetic, Toiletry, and Fragrance Association. Washington D.C.: 1997.

International Cosmetic Ingredient Handbook. The Cosmetic, Toiletry, and Fragrance Association. Washington D.C.: Cosmetic, Toiletry, and Fragrance Association, 1995.

Journal of Cosmetic Dermatology

Medline Abstracts. Published by Health ResponseAbility Systems.

Personal Care for People Who Care, 8th ed. National Anti-Vivisection Society. Chicago: NAVS, 1997.

"Phytoestrogens: Friends or Foes?" *Environmental Health Perspectives,* May 1996.

Web Sites

ACS Polymer Web Site

http:/www.chem.umr.edu/~poly

American Academy of Dermatology

http://www.aad.org

American Chemical Society

http://www.acs.org

American Medical Association

http://www.ama-assn.org

ChemCenter

http://www.chemcenter.org

Chemistry Newspaper, e-mail

http://ci.mond.org

Contact Dermatitis

http://www.mc.vanderbilt.edu/vumcdept/derm/contact

Cosmetic, Toiletry, and Fragrance Association

http://www.ctfa.org

Environmental Protection Agency (EPA)

http://www.epa.gov

Federal Trade Commission (FTC)

http://www.ftc.gov

Food and Drug Administration (FDA)

http://www.fda.gov

Internet Dermatology Society
http://www.telemedicine.org/ids.htm

Occupational Safety and Health Administration (OSHA)
http://www.osha.gov

Medline
http://www.invivo.net/bg/medline.html

Medscape
http://www.medscape.com

National Institute of Health Sciences/Japan
http://www.nihs.go.jp

National Library of Medicine
http://www.nlm.nih.gov

National Science Foundation
http://www.nsf.gov

Patent Searching
http://www.spo.eds.com/patent.html

Pharmacy Web Site
http://www.mcc.ac.uk/pharmacy

Poly-Links
http://www.polymers.com

Science Sources
http://www.edoc.com/sources

U.S. Pharmacopeia
http://www.usp.org

Virginia Tech Chemistry Department
http://www.chem.VT.edu

Virtual Chemistry Library–UCLA
http://www.chem.ucla.edu/chempointers.html

World Health Organization (WHO)
http://www.who.ch

World Wide Chemnet Incorporated
http://www.chemnet.com